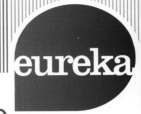

# Cardiovascular Medicine

**Paul Morris** MBChB MRCP BMedSci
Specialist Registrar in Cardiology
Sheffield Teaching Hospitals NHS
Foundation Trust
Clinical Research Fellow
University of Sheffield
Sheffield, UK

**Allison Morton** BMedSci MBChB
PhD FRCP
Consultant Cardiologist
Heartcare Western Australia
Bunbury, WA
Honorary Senior Lecturer
University of Sheffield, UK

**David Warriner** BSc MBChB MRCP
DipSEM
Specialist Registrar in Cardiology
Sheffield Teaching Hospitals NHS
Foundation Trust
Sheffield, UK

## Series Editors

**Janine Henderson** MRCPsych
MClinEd
MB BS Programme Director
Hull York Medical School
York, UK

**David Oliveira** PhD FRCP
Professor of Renal Medicine
St George's, University of London
London, UK

**Stephen Parker** BSc MS DipMedEd
FRCS
Consultant Breast and General
Paediatric Surgeon
St Mary's Hospital
Newport, UK

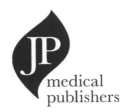

JP
medical
publishers

London • Philadelphia • New Delhi • Panama City

**ISBN: 978-1-907816-82-6**

British Library Cataloguing in Publication Data
A catalogue record for this book is available from the British Library

Library of Congress Cataloging in Publication Data
A catalog record for this book is available from the Library of Congress

| | |
|---|---|
| Publisher: | Richard Furn |
| Development Editors: | Thomas Fletcher, Paul Mayhew, Alison Whitehouse |
| Editorial Assistants: | Sophie Woolven, Katie Pattullo |
| Copy Editor: | Kim Howell |
| Graphic narratives: | James Pollitt |
| Cover design: | Forbes Design |
| Page design: | Designers Collective |

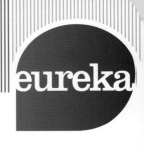

# Series Editors' Foreword

Today's medical students need to know a great deal to be effective as tomorrow's doctors. This knowledge includes core science and clinical skills, from understanding biochemical pathways to communicating with patients. Modern medical school curricula integrate this teaching, thereby emphasising how learning in one area can support and reinforce another. At the same time students must acquire sound clinical reasoning skills, working with complex information to understand each individual's unique medical problems.

The *Eureka* series is designed to cover all aspects of today's medical curricula and reinforce this integrated approach. Each book can be used from first year through to qualification. Core biomedical principles are introduced but given relevant clinical context: the authors have always asked themselves, 'why does the aspiring clinician need to know this?'

Each clinical title in the series is grounded in the relevant core science, which is introduced at the start of each book. Each core science title integrates and emphasises clinical relevance throughout. Medical and surgical approaches are included to provide a complete and integrated view of the patient management options available to the clinician. Clinical insights highlight key facts and principles drawn from medical practice. Cases featuring unique graphic narratives are presented with clear explanations that show how experienced clinicians think, enabling students to develop their own clinical reasoning and decision making. Clinical SBAs help with exam revision while Starter questions are a unique learning tool designed to stimulate interest in the subject.

Having biomedical principles and clinical applications together in one book will make their connections more explicit and easier to remember. Alongside repeated exposure to patients and practice of clinical and communication skills, we hope *Eureka* will equip medical students for a lifetime of successful clinical practice.

**Janine Henderson, David Oliveira, Stephen Parker**

# About the Series Editors

**Janine Henderson** is the MB BS undergraduate Programme Director at Hull York Medical School (HYMS). After medical school at the University of Oxford and clinical training in psychiatry, she combined her work as a consultant with postgraduate teaching roles, moving to the new Hull York Medical School in 2004. She has a particular interest in modern educational methods, curriculum design and clinical reasoning.

**David Oliveira** is Professor of Renal Medicine at St George's, University of London (SGUL), where he served as the MBBS Course Director between 2007 and 2013. Having trained at Cambridge University and the Westminster Hospital he obtained a PhD in cellular immunology and worked as a renal physician before being appointed as Foundation Chair of Renal Medicine at SGUL.

**Stephen Parker** is a Consultant Breast and General Paediatric Surgeon at St Mary's Hospital, Isle of Wight. He trained at St George's, University of London, and after service in the Royal Navy was appointed as Consultant Surgeon at University Hospital Coventry. He has a particular interest in e-learning and the use of multimedia platforms in medical education.

# About the Authors

**Paul Morris** is a Specialist Registrar in Cardiology. He enjoys teaching medical students and junior doctors and has extensive experience of writing exam questions and developing clinical assessment tools. He is also a Clinical Research Fellow in Cardiovascular Science at the University of Sheffield, working on the computational modelling of cardiovascular physiology.

**David Warriner** is a Specialist Registrar in Cardiology in South Yorkshire. He teaches undergraduates and postgraduates in lectures, tutorials and on the wards. He has developed novel interactive tools for understanding the pathophysiology of cardiovascular disease and still enjoys learning about cardiology as much as he does teaching it.

**Allison Morton** is a cardiologist in Bunbury, Western Australia. Previously she was a Consultant Cardiologist at Sheffield Teaching Hospitals, where she ran the clinical cardiology training for medical students, giving lectures and examining students on the MBChB course. She teaches candidates for the clinical PACES exam and is proud of her 100% pass rate!

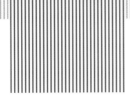

# Preface

The World Health Organization ranks cardiovascular disease as the leading cause of death, accounting for three in every ten deaths worldwide and frequently presenting as an emergency requiring immediate management. Irrespective of speciality, all doctors need to be confident in dealing with cardiovascular disease.

To achieve this, it is not enough to learn clinical medicine alone. One must also understand the scientific principles and mechanisms, including the relevant anatomy, physiology and pathology, which explain why and how things go wrong.

*Eureka Cardiovascular Medicine* integrates these core sciences, clinical medicine and surgery into one book. Our goal in writing was simple: to provide you with all the knowledge you need to bring you success in your exams and help you become a proficient doctor. The first two chapters are dedicated to cardiovascular anatomy and physiology, and the clinical principles and skills required to diagnose and manage cardiovascular presentations. The following chapters describe the important cardiovascular diseases, using cases and engaging graphic narratives. Next, we include chapters on emergencies and integrated care. Finally, a chapter of exam-style SBAs enables effective revision.

In short, *Eureka Cardiovascular Medicine* has everything you need from first year to finals and beyond. We have made every effort to include what we believe is relevant for preparing you for the demands of modern clinical practice.

We hope you enjoy this book and that it helps you to become a capable and confident doctor.

**Paul Morris, David Warriner, Allison Morton**
April 2015

# Contents

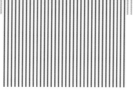

# Glossary

| | |
|---|---|
| AAo | aortic arch |
| AAo | ascending aorta |
| ABPI | ankle–brachial pressure index |
| ABPM | ambulatory blood pressure monitoring |
| ACE | angiotensin-converting enzyme |
| ACTH | adrenocorticotrophic hormone |
| ALP | alkaline phosphatase |
| ALT | alanine aminotransferase |
| Ao | aorta |
| ARB | angiotensin II receptor blocker |
| ASD | atrial septal defect |
| AST | aspartate aminotransferase |
| AV | aortic valve |
| aVF | augmented vector lead of the foot |
| aVL | augmented vector lead of the left arm |
| aVR | augmented vector lead of the right arm |
| | |
| BCT | brachiocephalic trunk |
| BP | blood pressure |
| | |
| CABG | coronary artery bypass graft |
| cAMP | cyclic AMP |
| CCB | calcium channel blocker |
| CCS | Canadian Cardiovascular Society |
| CCTA | coronary computed tomographic angiography |
| cGMP | cyclic guanosine monophosphate |
| COPD | chronic obstructive pulmonary disease |
| CRT | cardiac resynchronisation therapy |
| CT | computerised tomography |
| | |
| DAo | descending aorta |
| DCCV | direct current cardioversion |
| DCM | dilated cardiomyopathy |
| DVLA | Driver and Vehicle Licensing Agency |
| | |
| ECG | electrocardiogram |
| | |
| GMP | guanosine monophosphate |
| GP | general practitioner |
| GTP | guanosine triphosphate |
| | |
| HCM | hypertrophic cardiomyopathy |
| HDL | high-density lipoprotein |
| HFPEF | heart failure with preserved ejection fraction |
| HFREF | heart failure with reduced ejection fraction |

| | |
|---|---|
| HMG-CoA | hydroxymethylglutaryl-coenzyme A |
| | |
| ICD | implantable cardioverter defibrillator |
| ICS | intercostal space |
| INR | international normalised ratio |
| IVS | interventricular septum |
| | |
| LA | left atrium |
| LC | left carotid artery |
| LDL | low-density lipoprotein |
| LMWH | low-molecular-weight heparin |
| LPA | left pulmonary artery |
| LS | left subclavian artery |
| LV | left ventricle |
| | |
| M | muscarinic receptor |
| MRI | magnetic resonance imaging |
| MV | mitral valve |
| | |
| NO | nitric oxide |
| NSAID | non-steroidal anti-inflammatory drug |
| NSTEMI | non-ST elevation myocardial infarction |
| NYHA | New York Heart Association |
| | |
| PA | pulmonary artery |
| PDA | patent ductus arteriosus |
| PIP2 | phosphatidylinositol bisphosphate |
| PKC | protein kinase C |
| PLC | phospholipase C |
| PPAR | peroxisome proliferator-activated receptor |
| PPCI | primary percutaneous coronary intervention |
| PV | pulmonary valve |
| | |
| QTc | corrected QT interval |
| | |
| RA | right atrium |
| RPA | right pulmonary artery |
| RV | right ventricle |
| SSRI | selective serotonin reuptake inhibitor |
| STEMI | ST elevation myocardial infarction |
| | |
| TAVI | transcatheter aortic valve implantation |
| TGA | transposition of the great arteries |
| TV | tricuspid valve |
| | |
| VSD | ventricular septal defect |

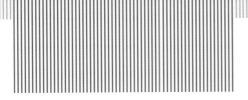

# Acknowledgements

Thanks to the following medical students for their help reviewing manuscripts: Jessica Dunlop, Aliza Imam, Roxanne McVittie, Daniel Roberts and Joseph Suich.

Figures 1.10, 1.26 and 1.28 are copyright of Sam Scott-Hunter and are reproduced from Tunstall R, Shah N. *Pocket Tutor Surface Anatomy*. London, JP Medical, 2012.

Figures 2.33, 3.1, 3.8, 3.11, 3.12, 5.1, 5.2a, 5.4a–d, 5.7, 10.1, 10.5, 12.1, 12.2, 12.3, 12.5, 12.6a–b, 12.8, 12.9 and 12.10 are reproduced from James S, Nelson K. *Pocket Tutor ECG Interpretation*. London: JP Medical, 2011.

Figures 8.2, 8.4, 8.6 and 8.7 are reproduced from Brugha R, et al. *Pocket Tutor Paediatric Clinical Examination*. London: JP Medical, 2013.

Figure 4.5a–b is reproduced from Sinha, R. *Pocket Tutor Abdominal Imaging*. London: JP Medical, 2011.

Figure 1.11a–b is reproduced from Darby M, et al. *Pocket Tutor Chest X-Ray Interpretation*. London: JP Medical, 2012.


We would like to acknowledge the contributions of Drs Abdallah Al-Mohammad, Chris Malkin, Andrew Narracott, Simon Nicholson, James Oliver, Paul Sheridan and Professor Patricia Lawford for their help reviewing the manuscript. We also wish to thank Drs Nachiketa Acharya, Pankaj Garg, Chris Malkin, Alex Rothman, Kim Suvarna and Professor Martin Rothman for their help providing several of the clinical images.

**PDM, DW, ACM**

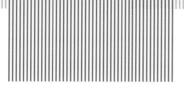

# Dedications

Dedicated to my parents, and to Tracey and Grace.

**PDM**

Dedicated to my parents and Bob.

**DW**

Dedicated to my parents, Phil, William and Archie.

**ACM**

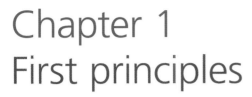

# Chapter 1
# First principles

## Overview of the cardiovascular system

### Starter questions

Answers to the following questions are on page 81.

1. Why are myocytes densely packed with mitochondria?
2. Why should blood from the right and left circulatory systems not mix?

The cardiovascular system comprises the heart, blood vessels and the lymphatics. It is the first system to function in the embryo, and cessation of its function defines death.

The main purpose of the cardiovascular system is to transport substances around the body. The heart beats from the 3rd week of embryonic life until the moment of death - more than 3 billion times in an average lifetime. Despite being only the size of a fist and weighing just 300 g, the heart pumps > 7,500 L of blood per day through nearly 100,000 km of blood vessels.

The cardiovascular system:

- distributes oxygen and nutrients
- removes carbon dioxide and other waste products
- transfers fluids and electrolytes
- transports hormones from glandular tissues to target organs
- aids thermoregulation
- aids immune function

The lymphatic circulation is also considered part of the cardiovascular system. It drains filtered tissue fluid back in to the circulating blood.

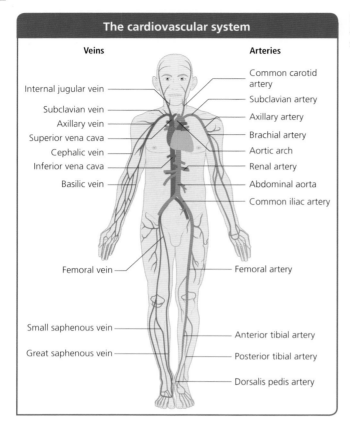

**Figure 1.1** The gross arrangement of the cardiovascular system.

# Circulation of blood

The average adult has a blood volume of about 5 L. Blood is composed of approximately:

- 55% plasma
- 44% red blood cells (erythrocytes)
- 1% white blood cells (leucocytes)

Plasma is about 92% water. The remaining 8% consists of dissolved substances, such as:

- nutrients
- respiratory gases
- proteins
- lipids
- electrolytes

The predominant plasma protein is albumin. Other proteins include antibodies, clotting factors and hormones.

Transport around the cardiovascular system is rapid. Even at rest, the entire blood volume circulates through the cardiovascular system once every minute. This rate of circulation can increase sixfold during strenuous exercise, when metabolic demands increase.

## The heart

Blood is pumped around the cardiovascular system by the heart (**Figure 1.2**). The heart is composed of two collecting chambers (the left and right atria) which fill, or prime, the two pumping chambers (the left and right ventricles). The junctions between the atria and the ventricles, and between the ventricles and the great arteries, are guarded by valves. These valves prevent blood flowing in the wrong direction.

The heart is a double pump.

- The right side of the heart pumps blood to the lungs (the pulmonary circulation)
- The left side pumps blood around the whole body (the systemic circulation)

The resistance to flow through the systemic circulation is about five times higher than that

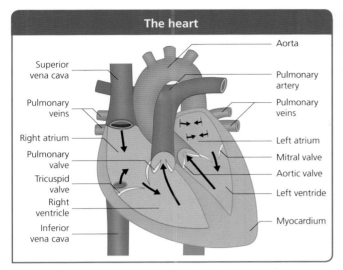

**The heart**

- Aorta
- Superior vena cava
- Pulmonary artery
- Pulmonary veins
- Pulmonary veins
- Right atrium
- Left atrium
- Pulmonary valve
- Mitral valve
- Tricuspid valve
- Aortic valve
- Right ventricle
- Left ventride
- Inferior vena cava
- Myocardium

**Figure 1.2** Gross anatomy of the heart and the major vessels. Blue indicates deoxygenated blood and red oxygenated blood.

of the pulmonary circulation. Consequently, the pressure required to drive systemic blood flow is also five times higher. Therefore the muscular left ventricular walls are significantly thicker than those of the right ventricle.

## Blood vessels

Blood flows away from the heart under high pressure through arteries, which distribute blood to all areas of the body. As the arteries undergo multiple generations of branching, the number of blood vessels increases but the calibre of individual vessels decreases. The smallest blood vessels are the capillaries, which have thin walls and a very high combined surface area.

In the tissues, the vast networks of capillaries are where substances are exchanged between the blood and the tissues. After this exchange has taken place, veins return blood to the heart under low pressure.

## Arrangement

The pulmonary and systemic circulations are arranged in series (end to end). This arrangement means that all the blood flowing through the left heart must also flow sequentially through the right heart.

The pulmonary artery carries deoxygenated blood from the right ventricle to the lungs, where gaseous exchange takes place. The pulmonary vein returns the blood, now oxygenated, to

the left atrium. From the left atrium, the blood passes through the mitral valve into the left ventricle, which then pumps blood through the aortic valve into the systemic circulation via the aorta.

The systemic arterial tree distributes blood to all organs and regions of the body. Systemic venous flow returns, deoxygenated, to the right atrium through the superior and inferior venae cavae. This blood passes through the tricuspid valve into the right ventricle, from which it is ejected into the pulmonary artery through the pulmonary valve. The pulmonary artery and aorta are known as the great arteries.

The systemic circulation is subdivided into organ-specific circulatory routes, each of which branch from the aorta. Through this parallel arrangement, each organ receives only a portion of the total cardiac output (**Table 1.1**).

## Control mechanisms

Blood flow through the cardiovascular system must meet the prevailing metabolic demands of the organs. These demands are dynamic; they increase and decrease according to the level of activity.

- If blood flow is too low, tissue ischaemia (oxygen and nutrient starvation) and infarction (cellular death) quickly ensue
- If blood flow is too high, vascular function becomes disrupted and vessels become damaged, with the development of oedema

## Distribution of cardiac output at rest

| Organ | Name of circulation | Percentage of cardiac output at rest |
|---|---|---|
| Lungs | Pulmonary | 100 |
| Kidneys | Renal | 22 |
| Gastrointestinal tract | Splanchnic | 18 |
| Skeletal muscle | Skeletal muscle | 15 |
| Brain | Cerebral | 12 |
| Other | Adipose tissue, adrenal, thyroid, etc. | 12 |
| Liver | Hepatic | 6 |
| Skin | Cutaneous | 6 |
| Bone | Bone | 5 |
| Heart | Coronary | 4 |

**Table 1.1** Distribution of cardiac output at rest

(fluid accumulation in the tissues, causing swelling)

The cardiovascular system closely regulates blood flow and blood pressure through a number of mechanisms. The blood vessels have inbuilt (intrinsic) mechanisms that control blood flow at a local level. Remote (extrinsic) mechanisms have a more global effect on the cardiovascular system. Overall control is coordinated by the cardiovascular centre in the medulla oblongata in the brainstem. The cardiovascular centre receives a variety of afferent signals from the body and coordinates its responses through the sympathetic and parasympathetic nervous systems, which richly innervate the heart and vasculature.

## Cardiac muscle

The heart is mainly muscle (myocardium) arranged around a framework of fibrous tissue. Cardiac myocytes are the predominant cell type (**Figure 1.3a**). They are branched, tubular cells (about 30 × 100 µm) with a central nucleus. Like the myocytes of skeletal muscle, cardiac myocytes are striated, but this appearance is less defined than in skeletal muscle.

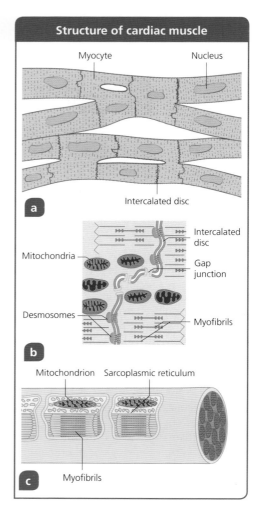

**Figure 1.3** Structure of cardiac muscle. (a) Cardiac myocytes are branched, nucleated, elongated, tubular cells joined at intercalated discs. (b) Intercalated discs. Desmosomes anchor the cells together, and gap junctions are intercellular junctions that allow ions to pass freely from cell to cell. (c) Cardiac muscle. Cardiac myocytes comprise multiple myofibrils.

Cardiac myocytes connect, end to end, at intercalated discs. The intercalated discs are folded providing a large surface area of contact between cells.

Intercalated discs contain desmosomes and gap junctions. Desmosomes anchor neighbouring cells together. Gap junctions allow ions to pass freely between cells (**Figure 1.3b**), thus waves of electrical depolarisation conduct rapidly across the myocardium.

Myocytes contain elongated fibres, myofibrils (**Figure 1.3c**), which are composed of repeating functional units called sarcomeres. The sarcomere is the basic contractile unit of the myocyte. Each sarcomere is bounded at each end by a Z line (**Figure 1.4a**) and contains contractile filaments made of the proteins actin and myosin.

■ Peripherally, actin thin filaments attach to the Z line
■ Centrally, myosin thick filaments interdigitate (overlap) with the actin filaments

This arrangement gives rise to the striated appearance of cardiac myocytes.

The cell membrane (sarcolemma) invaginates deeply into the myocyte around the Z lines to form T tubules. The T tubules are closely apposed to the sarcoplasmic reticulum, which contains intracellular stores of $Ca^{2+}$.

The sarcoplasmic reticulum forms cisternae close to the T tubules, which together form diads. The diads enable rapid coupling of membrane (T tubule) depolarisation with myofibril contraction, i.e. the release of $Ca^{2+}$ from the sarcoplasmic reticulum.

Thin filaments consist of actin, tropomyosin and troponin complexes (**Figure 1.4b**).

■ Troponin T attaches each troponin complex to the tropomyosin
■ Troponin I inhibits the binding of myosin heads to actin
■ Troponin C binds to $Ca^{2+}$

The binding of $Ca^{2+}$ to troponin C exposes the myosin binding site, allowing actin–myosin cross-bridges to form.

The myosin 'power stroke' pulls the filaments so that they slide in opposite directions; this action shortens the sarcomere. This ATP-dependent process repeats until $Ca^{2+}$ is cleared from the cell. Consistent with the high myocardial energy requirements, myocytes are rich in mitochondria and glycogen stores.

The space between the myocytes, the interstitium, comprises mainly collagen, elastin and fibrous connective tissue. It contains numerous blood and lymphatic vessels. The cellular arrangement of normal myocardium is demonstrated in **Figure 1.5.**

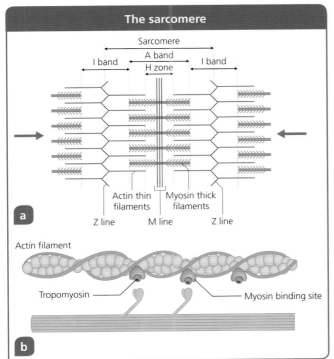

**The sarcomere**

Sarcomere

A band

I band

H zone

I band

Actin thin filaments

Myosin thick filaments

Z line

M line

Z line

a

Actin filament

Tropomyosin

Myosin binding site

b

**Figure 1.4** The sarcomere. (a) The sarcomere is bound by the Z lines. Thin actin filaments attach to the Z line, projecting towards the centre of the sarcomere, where they interdigitate with the thick myosin filaments. This arrangement gives rise to the striated appearance of cardiac myocytes, defined by the M line, the H zone and the A and I bands. The arrows indicate the how the sarcomere shortens during contraction. (b) Actin–myosin interaction.

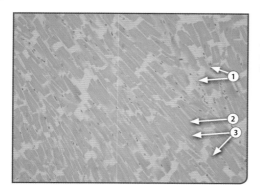

**Figure 1.5** Normal left ventricular myocardial histology with 'brick-like' myocytes. There is regular architecture and only minimal fibrosis. ① Loose interstitial cells and vasculature. ② Cardiac myocytes. ③ Myocyte nuclei. Courtesy of Dr K Suvarna.

# Development of the cardiovascular system

## Starter questions

Answers to the following questions are on page 81–82.

3. How do embryonic and fetal cells 'know' where to go and how to develop?
4. Why is blood shunting important in the fetal circulation?
5. Why might clinicians maintain blood shunting after birth?

The embryological development of the heart and circulation appears far removed from adult cardiology. However, an understanding of this topic is useful when appreciating the structure and function of the adult heart, especially the complex nature and array of congenital heart diseases.

## Development of the heart

The heart is the first functioning organ to develop in the embryo and starts beating just 3 weeks after fertilization. The initially single-chambered structure undergoes folding, looping and septation; these processes establish the cardiac chambers and major vessels. Subsequently, the valves, conduction tissues and coronary circulation develop.

In embryological nomenclature, the terms superior, inferior, anterior and posterior are replaced by **cranial, caudal, ventral** and **dorsal**, respectively.

## The heart tube

All three layers of cardiac tissue develop from the cardiogenic mesoderm at the cranial end of the embryo. In the embryonic disc, bilateral clusters of angiogenic cells (endothelial precursors) form paired heart tubes (angioblastic cords) laterally (around day 18). Embryonic folding aligns these tubes on the ventral surface, in the midline. The two tubes fuse to form the primitive, single-chambered heart tube (around day 21). The heart tube starts contracting from the 3rd week, pumping blood in a caudal to cranial direction.

The inner surface of the heart tube is lined with endocardium, which is separated from surrounding myocardium by an acellular matrix layer of cardiac jelly. Five distinct segments can be appreciated, each separated by one of four transitional zones (**Figure 1.6a**). The five segments develop into the chambers and great vessels, and the four zones become the connection points between the segments (**Table 1.2**).

| Eventual structure of the heart tube segments | |
|---|---|
| Segment | Eventual structure |
| Truncus arteriosus | Aortic and pulmonary outflow tracts |
| Bulbis cordis | Right ventricle |
| Ventricular | Left and right ventricles |
| Atrial | Left and right atria |
| Sinus venosus | Coronary sinus and right atrium |

**Table 1.2** Destiny of the individual heart tube segments (see **Figure 1.6**)

## Folding and looping

The venous (caudal) and arterial (cranial) ends of the heart tube are fixed dorsally. Therefore as the tube grows and elongates, it folds and loops (from day 23). The fold protrudes ventrally, with:

- the caudal segments (sinus venosus and primitive atria) moving dorsally
- the cranial segments (primitive ventricle and outflow tracts) moving ventrally

The folded heart tube also loops to the right in a clockwise fashion (**Figure 1.6b**). Throughout this process, the primitive ventricle comes to lie adjacent to the future atria, and the bulbus cordis (the future right ventricle) loops up towards the truncus arteriosus (the future outflow tracts). Looping is complete by day 28. The precision of this process is critical for the formation of the correct connections between the chambers and the vessels, and for the alignment of the valves.

## Septation and chamber formation

Once the segments of the heart are aligned, the atrial and ventricular segments begin to expand, differentiate and trabeculate. Externally, the heart starts to resemble the mature structure. However, internally it remains a relatively simple folded, looped tube. Septation separates and defines the chambers and outflow tracts.

## Ventricular septation

Around day 25, ventricular septation begins. From the apex of the cardiac loop, between the left ventricle and the bulbus cordis (the primary heart loop), the muscular interventricular septum starts to develop towards

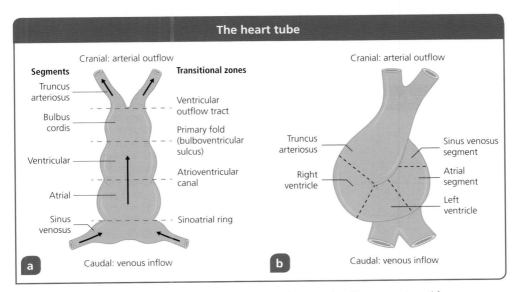

**The heart tube**

**Figure 1.6** Development of the heart tube. (a) The heart tube comprises five segments and four transitional zones. (b) Folding and looping of the heart tube, after which locations of the regions and zones start to resemble the mature heart (see **Table 1.2**).

the endocardial cushions. Until the septum is fully formed, there is an opening between the two sides of the ventricular cavity; this is called the interventricular foramen. The truncoconal septum (see pages 8–9) extends inferiorly into the ventricular cavity to form the membranous portion of the interventricular septum.

Ventricular septation is completed when the primary muscular septum, the truncoconal septum and the atrioventricular endocardial cushions fuse in the 7th week. This complex process eliminates the interventricular foramen. It also joins the ventricular and outflow tract septa, which connect the left and right ventricles to the aortic and pulmonary outflow tracts, respectively.

## Atrioventricular septation

From day 26, cells surrounding the atrioventricular canal start to infiltrate the cardiac jelly. This process forms endocardial cushions, which protrude inwardly. Fusion of these cushions completes septation of the atrioventricular canal (the septum intermedium).

The endocardial cushions serve as primitive atrioventricular valves; they eventually develop into the mature tricuspid and mitral valves. The endocardial cushions also project vertically becoming involved in the ventricular, atrial and conotruncal septa.

## Atrial septation

Around day 30, atrial septation starts with descent of the septum primum from the roof of the atrium towards the endocardial cushions. Fetal circulation depends on blood shunting between the atria (see page 10). Therefore once the septum primum fuses with the endocardial cushions, obliterating the orifice primum in the process, a second ostium develops: the ostium secundum.

The septum secundum then develops alongside, and to the right, of the septum primum. It also has a foramen in its posteroinferior portion: the foramen ovale. The two septa overlie each other, thus creating a flap valve that allows right-to-left blood flow in the fetus (**Figure 1.7**). The foramen ovale closes and fuses after birth, when left-sided blood pressure increases.

Dorsally, the left horn of the sinus venosus forms the coronary sinus, which empties into the right atrium. The right horn becomes incorporated into the structure of the right atrium.

## Outflow tract septation

Until this point, there is a common outflow tract: the truncus arteriosus. Along the length of the truncus, endocardial ridges form in a spiral arrangement. When these meet in the middle and fuse, they form a septum that separates the aortic outflow tract

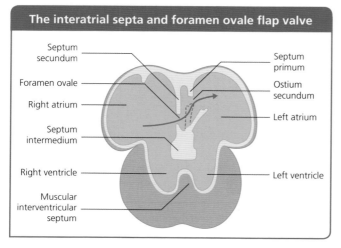

**The interatrial septa and foramen ovale flap valve**

- Septum secundum
- Foramen ovale
- Right atrium
- Septum intermedium
- Right ventricle
- Muscular interventricular septum
- Septum primum
- Ostium secundum
- Left atrium
- Left ventricle

**Figure 1.7** The interatrial septa and the foramen ovale flap valve (grey dashed line). The rigid septum secundum grows alongside the septum primum. In the embryo both septa have gaps: the foramen ovale of the septum secundum and the secundum in the septum primum. Fast flowing blood from the ductus venosus is directed across the atrial septa through the foramen ovale flap valve (red arrow). After birth, the valve closes when increased left atrial pressure forces the valve back against the septal wall.

(continuous with the left ventricle) from the pulmonary outflow tract (continuous with the right ventricle). The same process is responsible for development of the aortic and pulmonary semilunar valves, and is completed by week 9.

> Failure of septation results in septal defects between the cardiac chambers. This is a common type of congenital heart disease (see pages 288–289).

## The conduction tissue

The heart begins to contract regularly from day 22. However, the conduction tissues are not completely formed until much later. By the 7th week, cells in the primitive atrium start to differentiate into the specialised pacemaker cells of the sinoatrial node, and cells of the sinus venosus into the atrioventricular node. Cells of the conduction tissues develop from the transitional zones of the heart tube.

After chamber septation, the fibroannular ring of insulating tissue develops between the atria and the ventricles. The atrioventricular bundle of His is then the only electrical connection between the atria and the ventricles.

## Development of the blood vessels

Blood begins to circulate through a primitive network of blood vessels by the end of the third week. Although considerable further development will take place, the cardiovascular system is the first functioning system in the embryo.

## Vasculogenesis and angiogenesis

In early embryonic development, vascular and blood precursor cells (haemangioblasts) in the embryonic and extraembryonic mesoderm coalesce to form blood islands. Vasculogenesis occurs when vascular precursors (angioblasts) from adjacent blood islands extend and unite to form primitive vascular networks.

Angioblasts in these primitive vascular structures differentiate into endothelial cells, and a central lumen forms. Blood vessels then 'sprout' out and extend into the developing organs; this process is called angiogenesis. Blood cell precursors (haemocytoblasts) subsequently migrate to the liver, spleen and bone marrow.

## Arterial development

The arterial system develops from paired dorsal aortae, which receive blood from the heart through a series of aortic (or pharyngeal) arches. The paired dorsal aortae fuse to form the definitive (descending) aorta, from which arterial branches develop.

The arterial branches supply the body and lower limbs, and include the umbilical artery and the vitelline artery. The vitelline artery initially supplies the yolk sac but develops into the arteries supplying the adult gastrointestinal system.

The six, more ventral, paired aortic arches develop and regress according to the needs of the developing fetus (**Figure 1.8**).

- The first three arches develop into the arteries of the head and neck, including the internal carotid arteries
- The 4th pair develop into the aortic arch on the left and the subclavian artery on the right
- The 5th arches completely regress
- The 6th right arch develops into the right pulmonary artery, and the left arch develops into the left pulmonary artery and the ductus arteriosus

## Venous development

The venous system develops from the cardinal, umbilical and vitelline venous systems.

- The cardinal system drains the head and body
- The umbilical system supplies oxygen- and nutrient-rich blood from the placenta
- The vitelline system initially drains the yolk sac but develops into the hepatic, portal and superior mesenteric veins

All three systems drain into the sinus venosus.

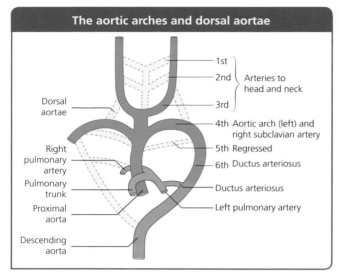

**The aortic arches and dorsal aortae**

- 1st ⎫
- 2nd ⎬ Arteries to head and neck
- 3rd ⎭
- Dorsal aortae
- 4th Aortic arch (left) and right subclavian artery
- 5th Regressed
- Right pulmonary artery
- 6th Ductus arteriosus
- Pulmonary trunk
- Ductus arteriosus
- Proximal aorta
- Left pulmonary artery
- Descending aorta

**Figure 1.8** The aortic arches and dorsal aortae. The six arches develop and (some) regress at different times. The 1st two arches regress but remnants form the adult maxillary and stapedial arteries. The 3rd pair persist forming the carotid arteries. The 4th pair form the arch of the aorta (left) and the right subclavian artery. The 5th pair regress. The 6th pair contribute to the right and left pulmonary arteries with the left also forming the ductus arteriosus. The dorsal aorta fuse in the midline forming the descending aorta.

# Fetal circulation

Prenatally, the systemic and pulmonary circulations exist in parallel, and the fetus is completely dependent on the placenta for respiratory function. On delivery, the baby breathes for the first time and the umbilical cord is cut. These two events trigger a quite remarkable series of events that, in seconds and minutes, reroute the two circulatory pathways into series and allow the baby to breathe and respire independently.

## Prenatal circulation

The placenta provides the fetus with oxygen and nutrients from the maternal circulation in exchange for carbon dioxide and other waste products. It connects the growing fetus to the mother's uterine wall through the umbilical cord, which contains the umbilical arteries and vein.

Deoxygenated fetal blood is delivered to the placenta through the umbilical arteries (**Figure 1.9**). In the placenta, these arteries branch radially into the chorionic and cotyledon arteries. These arteries terminate in arteriolar–capillary–venous complexes called villi, which are structurally akin to the alveolus.

The fetal villi project into the intervillous space and are completely surrounded by, and

bathed in, maternal blood. This ensures efficient gaseous exchange. Maternal and fetal blood are kept separate; they do not mix. Oxygen diffuses from the maternal blood to the fetal blood, and carbon dioxide diffuses from the fetal blood to the maternal blood.

## Oxygen-rich blood

Oxygenated blood (about 80% oxygen-saturated) is supplied to the fetus through the umbilical vein, which carries blood to the portal vein and the fetal liver. At this point, a shunt (a connection between the right and left circulations) called the ductus venosus diverts a significant proportion of the flowing blood away from the liver and into the inferior vena cava. In the vena cava, the diverted blood mixes with deoxygenated blood returning from the lower body. Therefore the inferior vena cava returns moderately oxygen-rich blood (about 70% saturated) to the heart.

Blood flow velocity through the ductus venosus is nearly five times that in the inferior vena cava. This difference creates two streams of blood:

- a fast posterior flow (of blood from the ductus)
- a slower anterior flow (of vena cava blood)

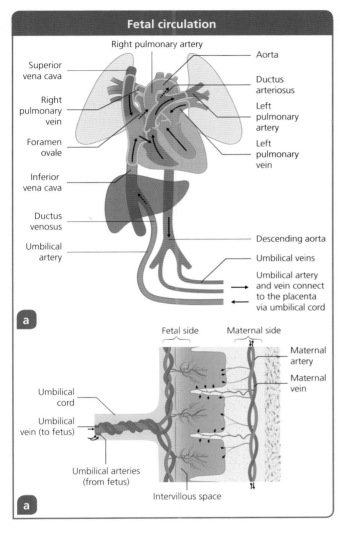

**Figure 1.9** (a) The prenatal circulation. Blood is shunted at the ductus venosus, the foramen ovale and the ductus arteriosus (dashed arrows). The colour of the blood differs according to location and shunting, reflecting variation in oxygen saturation through the circulation. (b) The placenta showing the anatomy of the fetal and maternal placental blood vessels. Villi of fetal blood vessels project into the intervillous space where they are bathed in maternal blood. Gaseous and nutrient exchange occurs here. This is enhanced by the opposite direction of venous blood flow on both the maternal and fetal sides.

At the point of entry into the right atrium, the Eustachian valve preferentially diverts the fast posterior stream of blood across the foramen ovale (**Figure 1.7**) into the left atrium. The slower anterior stream and blood from the superior vena cava flow through the right atrium into the right ventricle. Consequently, oxygen-rich blood passes into the left side of the heart and onwards, through the left ventricle and out through the aorta, to preferentially supply the head and arms with oxygenated blood. Only about one quarter of this blood continues to the descending aorta, where further mixing with deoxygenated blood from the ductus arteriosus occurs.

## Oxygen-depleted blood

Deoxygenated blood from the fetal tissues returns to the heart through the superior and inferior venae cavae. This blood enters the right ventricle, because it is not diverted across the foramen ovale. Until birth, the fetal lungs are filled with amniotic fluid and are collapsed. Consequently, pulmonary vascular resistance is high, and flow through the system is correspondingly low. Therefore blood is diverted from the pulmonary circulation into the descending aorta by a connecting vessel called the ductus arteriosus.

At this point, deoxygenated blood mixes with oxygen-rich blood, thus reducing the oxygen saturation of blood in the descending aorta. About half of this blood flows back to the placenta through the umbilical arteries, from which carbon dioxide and other waste products diffuse into the maternal circulation. The remaining blood continues onwards to supply the lower body with blood that is about 60% oxygen-saturated.

## Heart rate

Initially, the embryonic heart beats at a rate similar to that of the mother's. Heart rate peaks at the 9th week, at around 170 beats/min. From this point, the heart rate declines. The rate is about 140 beats/min at term and continues to decrease through childhood and into adolescence.

## Postnatal circulation

At the moment of birth, the baby takes its first breath. The lungs empty of amniotic fluid and expand. The rise in local oxygen tension induces pulmonary arterial dilation. Consequently, pulmonary vascular resistance and pressure decrease, and pulmonary arterial flow increases. This has several key effects.

1. Increased blood flow to the lungs reduces flow through the ductus arteriosus
2. Pulmonary venous return to the left atrium increases, therefore left atrial pressure increases
3. The increase in left atrial pressure and the decrease in right atrial pressure (see below) force the septum primum against the septum secundum, which closes the foramen ovale and prevents further interatrial blood flow

The rise in oxygen tension alters prostaglandin synthesis, which causes the ductus arteriosus to begin closing from the first day of life; the remnant becomes the ligamentum arteriosum. The ductus venosus also closes in response to altered prostaglandin synthesis over the 1st week of life.

Shortly after birth, the umbilical cord is tied off. This eliminates flow in the umbilical vein, thus reducing inferior vena cava pressure and right atrial pressure which also encourages the closure of the foramen ovale.

Formen ovale closure remains incomplete in up to a quarter of adults (patent foramen ovale). However, this is rarely of any haemodynamic or clinical significance.

# The heart

## Starter questions

Answers to the following questions are on page 82.

6. Why is normal coronary anatomy difficult to define?
7. Why does assessing coronary venous anatomy help treat heart failure?
8. Why is the mitral valve called the mitral valve?

The heart comprises four muscular chambers. Each chamber is connected to a great vessel, and each is separated from the adjoining chamber by one of four valves. Cardiac development (see page 6) results in a rather complicated, folded, rotated and asymmetrical three-dimensional arrangement in the thorax. The heart is surrounded by the pericardial sac and lies in the mediastinum.

## Surface, borders and position in the mediastinum

The heart is in the mediastinum, alongside the great vessels, the oesophagus and the trachea. Anatomically, the mediastinum is separated into four segments:

- anterior and posterior (relative to the heart)
- superior (relative to the manubrium sterni)
- middle (containing the heart)

In health, the heart is about the size of the fist, but it can dilate in disease. The heart is rotated and asymmetrical, so its base lies in the middle mediastinum and its apex points inferiorly and to the left. Anteriorly, the heart is adjacent to the sternum, costal cartilages and left lung pleura. Inferiorly, the heart is adjacent to the left diaphragm. The posterior surface of the heart is related to the thoracic vertebrae, the oesophagus and the descending aorta. The structures and borders of the cardiac surfaces are shown in **Table 1.3**.

An understanding of the surface anatomical relations of the heart helps during clinical examination (see page 101 and **Figure 1.10**). Knowledge of the borders is key to chest X-ray interpretation (see page 133 and **Figure 1.11**).

## Chambers and valves

The left atrium, left ventricle, right atrium and right ventricle make up the four cardiac chambers. The mitral valve, aortic valve, tricuspid valve and the pulmonary valve are the four cardiac valves. **Figure 1.12** shows the heart and its surrounding relations.

## Left atrium

During development, the four pulmonary veins are absorbed into the posterior left atrium. The left and right atria are separated by the interatrial septum. The left atrium continues into the left ventricle but is separated from it by the mitral orifice and the mitral valve. The left atrial myocardium usually receives its blood supply from the left circumflex coronary artery (see page 18). Also continuous with the left atrium is a muscular out-pouching known as the left atrial appendage or left auricle (**Figures 1.12, 1.13** and **1.14).**

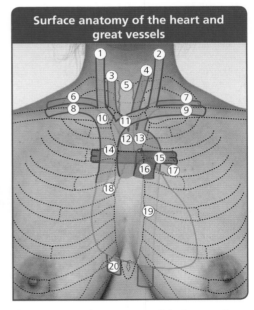

**Surface anatomy of the heart and great vessels**

**Figure 1.10** Surface anatomy of the heart and great vessels. ①, right internal jugular vein; ②, left internal jugular vein; ③, right common carotid artery; ④, left common carotid artery; ⑤, trachea; ⑥, right subclavian artery; ⑦, left subclavian artery; ⑧, right subclavian vein; ⑨, left subclavian vein; ⑩, right brachiocephalic vein; ⑪, left brachiocephalic vein; ⑫, brachiocephalic trunk; ⑬, arch of aorta; ⑭, superior vena cava; ⑮, left pulmonary artery; ⑯, pulmonary trunk; ⑰, left main bronchus; ⑱, right main bronchus; ⑲, descending aorta; ⑳, inferior vena cava.

| Structures and borders of the cardiac surfaces | | |
| --- | --- | --- |
| Cardiac surface | Main structure | Extracardiac relation |
| Anterior (sternocostal) | Right ventricle | Sternum |
| | | Costal cartilages |
| | | Left lung pleura |
| Posterior (base) | Left atrium | Thoracic vertebrae |
| | | Oesophagus |
| | | Descending aorta |
| Inferior | Left ventricle | Left hemidiaphragm |
| Apex | Left ventricle | Sternum |
| | | Costal cartilages |
| | | Left lung pleura |

**Table 1.3** The structures and borders of the four cardiac surfaces

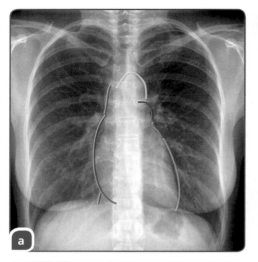

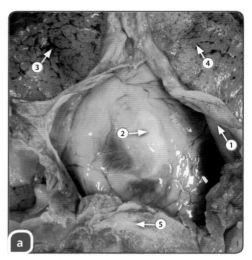

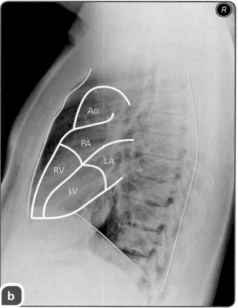

**Figure 1.11** Radiographs showing the borders of the heart and great vessels. (a) Frontal view. The right heart border (red) is formed mainly by the right atrium. The left heart border is formed mainly by the left ventricle (LV, green) and the left atrium (LA, blue). The inferior surface (against the diaphragm) represents the right ventricle (RV). The vena cava (pink) is above and below the right heart border, and the aortic arch (yellow) and pulmonary trunk (purple) are above the left atrium. (b) Lateral view. The anterior, posterior and inferior relations of the heart (orange) are formed by the sternum or left lung pleura, thoracic spine and diaphragm, respectively. Ao, aorta; PA, pulmonary artery.

**Figure 1.12** The heart and its surrounding structures. (a) The heart in situ. The pericardium ① has been reflected back to reveal the anterior aspect of the heart. ② The white area over the left ventricle is an area of fibrosis, where the heart rubs against the sternum. ③ Right lung. ④ Left lung. ⑤ Diaphragm. (b) Anterior view of the resected heart and the great vessels. ⑤ Aorta. ⑥ Left atrium (appendage). ⑦ Pulmonary artery. ⑧ Right atrium. ⑨ Right ventricle. ⑩ Left ventricle. Courtesy of Dr K Suvarna.

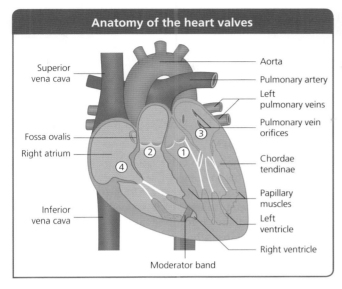

**Anatomy of the heart valves**

Superior vena cava

Fossa ovalis

Right atrium

Inferior vena cava

Aorta

Pulmonary artery

Left pulmonary veins

Pulmonary vein orifices

Chordae tendinae

Papillary muscles

Left ventricle

Right ventricle

Moderator band

**Figure 1.13** Anatomy of the heart valves. ① Aortic valve. ② Pulmonary valve. ③ Mitral valve. ④ Tricuspid valve.

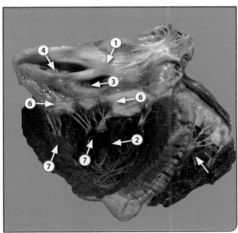

**Figure 1.14** An exploded view of the left atrium (LA) ① and left ventricle (LV) ②. The left atrial appendage ③ orifice and a pulmonary vein ④ are visible in the LA. Compare the finer LV trabeculations with the coarse trabeculations of the right ventricle ⑤. The mitral valve leaflets ⑥ are tethered to the papillary muscles ⑦ by the chordae tendinae. Courtesy of Dr K Suvarna.

In conditions such as atrial fibrillation and mitral stenosis, blood flow in the left atrial appendage becomes sluggish and stagnant, and clots may form. A piece of clot may break off and travel (embolise) to cause infarction in the brain (a stroke) or other systemic organs, hence the need for anticoagulation in patients with atrial fibrillation (see page 229).

## Mitral valve

The mitral valve separates the left atrium from the left ventricle. Its function is to prevent blood regurgitating back into the left atrium during ventricular systole.

The valve is bicuspid; it consists of two leaflets.

- The anterior mitral valve leaflet attaches to the anterior aspect of the mitral orifice
- The posterior leaflet attaches to the posterior orifice

The free edges of the leaflets are tethered to the ventricular walls by the chordae tendinae, which attach to the left ventricular papillary muscles (**Figure 1.13** and **1.14**).

The chordae tendinae and papillary muscles are collectively known as the subvalvular apparatus. During ventricular systole, the papillary muscles contract, preventing valve prolapse into the atria. Disruption of this function by dilatation of the ventricle or ischaemic damage to the papillary muscles results in regurgitation of blood into the atria (see page 270).

## Left ventricle

The left ventricle is an elongated inverted cone that is circular in cross-section. Its internal surface is heavily trabeculated, especially towards the apex. The medial wall forms the interventricular septum, which, apart from a slim superior membranous segment, is muscular (**Figure 1.14** and **1.15**).

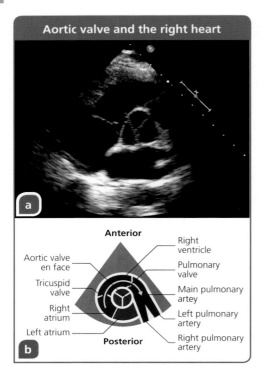

**Aortic valve and the right heart**

a

Anterior

Aortic valve en face — Right ventricle

Tricuspid valve — Pulmonary valve

Right atrium — Main pulmonary artey

Left atrium — Left pulmonary artery

Posterior — Right pulmonary artery

b

**Figure 1.15** The tricuspid aortic valve. (a) Transthoracic echocardiogram showing the tricuspid aortic valve in cross-section (end on). The three cusps form an upside-down Mercedes-Benz pattern. The right heart (atrium, ventricle and pulmonary artery) wrap around the left heart. (b) A stylised diagram showing the echocardiogram anatomy more clearly. The arrow indicates the direction of blood flow through the right heart.

The mitral valve chordae tendinae attach to two papillary muscles, one on the anterior wall and one on the posterior wall. The left ventricular walls are three times thicker (6–12 mm) than those of the right ventricle. This reflects the higher resistance and pressure of the systemic circulation compared with the pulmonary circulation (mean pressures, 120 mmHg versus 20 mmHg).

The inlet is bounded by the mitral valve and the outlet by the aortic valve. The outflow tract lies posterior to the right outflow tract, which 'wraps' around the aorta (**Figure 1.15**). The left ventricular myocardium blood supply is from the left anterior descending coronary artery and its diagonal branches (see page 18).

## Aortic valve and aortic root

The aortic valve has three semilunar cusps that in cross-section are arranged in a 'Mercedes-Benz' pattern (**Figure 1.15**). Immediately above the aortic valve, the aortic root dilates into three sinuses. From two of the sinuses the two coronary arteries originate.

The cusps are named according to the corresponding sinus: the right coronary cusp, the left coronary cusp and the non-coronary cusp (**Figure 1.16**). The ascending aorta continues superiorly and towards the right before bending leftwards and posteriorly, hooking over the hilum of the left lung (the arch).

## Right atrium

The right atrium (**Figure 1.17**) receives deoxygenated systemic venous blood from the superior and inferior venae cavae. It also receives coronary venous blood through the coronary sinus. The smooth posterior surface (which develops from the sinus venosus) is separated from the trabeculated anterior surface (which develops from the primitive atrium) by the crescent-shaped muscular band of the crista terminalis, marking the the junction between the heart and the sinus venosus from embryonic development.

The trabeculated right atrial appendage (the auricle) projects from the superior, anterior segment of the atrium. This has less clinical relevance than the left atrial appendage. The interatrial septum contains an oval ridge, the fossa ovalis, which represents the remnant of the antenatal foramen ovale (see pages 11–12).

## Tricuspid valve

The tricuspid valve (**Figure 1.17**) is so-named because it has three cusps: the anterior, posterior and septal leaflets. The bases of the leaflets are attached around the tricuspid orifice.

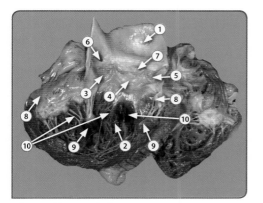

**Figure 1.16** An exploded view of the aorta ①, aortic valve and left ventricle ②. The aortic valve is trileafleted and the left ③, right ④ and non-coronary cusps ⑤ are visible. The left and right coronary arteries originate from the corresponding aortic sinuses ⑥ and ⑦ above the valve cusps.[311] The mitral valve ⑧ leaflets are tethered to the papillary muscles ⑨ by the chordae tendinae. ⑩ Right ventricle. Courtesy of Dr K Suvarna.

Similar to the leaflets of the mitral valve, the free edges of the tricuspid valve leaflets are attached to the ventricular walls by the chordae tendinae and papillary muscles. However, the right ventricular papillary muscles are less prominent than those on the left side.

## Right ventricle

The right ventricle, like the left ventricle, is an elongated inverted cone shape. However, it operates at a much lower pressure than the left ventricle. Therefore the higher pressure in the left ventricle causes the ventricular septum to bulge into the right ventricular cavity, indenting it (**Figure 1.18**). The right ventricle and pulmonary trunk effectively wrap around the left ventricle and around the aortic root.

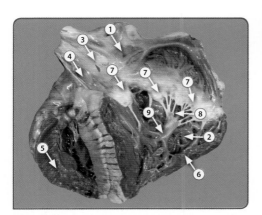

**Figure 1.17** An exploded view of the right atrium ① and the right ventricle (RV) ②. The fossa ovalis ③ and coronary sinus ④ are visible on the atrial septum. The myocardium of the left ventricle ⑤ is much thicker than that of the RV ⑥. ⑦ Tricuspid valve leaflets connecting with the chordae tendinae ⑧ and papillary muscles ⑨. Courtesy of Dr K Suvarna.

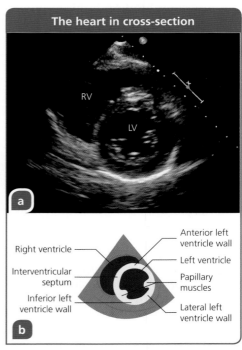

**Figure 1.18** The heart in cross-section. (a) Transthoracic echocardiogram showing the circular left ventricle (LV) with the papillary muscles. The low-pressure right ventricle (RV) accommodates the higher pressure left ventricle. The top of the image is anterior and the bottom is posterior in relation to the patient. (b) Anatomy shown on the echocardiogram.

The right ventricle contains a ridge of muscle that extends from the septum to the anterior ventricular wall at the base of the papillary muscle, traversing the right ventricular cavity. This ridge of muscle, the moderator band, can be visualised with echocardiography (**Figure 1.13**). It forms a part of the electrical conduction pathway ensuring early activation of the right-sided papillary muscles, which in turn ensures that the tricuspid valve is braced, ready for ventricular systole.

## Pulmonary valve

The pulmonary valve lies at the apex of the right ventricular outflow tract (the infundibulum). It is a tricuspid, semilunar valve, similar in structure to the aortic valve.

## Blood supply and drainage

The arterial blood supply and the venous drainage of the heart are highly relevant to clinical medicine. For example, the coronary arterial territories are important in the clinical presentation of myocardial infarction (see page 185) and in the interpretation of the electrocardiogram (see page 178).

## Arterial supply

Coronary arterial anatomy is naturally highly variable. However, most people have a left coronary artery originating from the left coronary sinus, and a right coronary artery emanating from the right coronary sinus.

Despite some minor anastomoses between the left and right systems, the coronary arteries are effectively end arteries. Therefore occlusion of a coronary artery (as happens in acute myocardial infarction; see page 185) quickly results in ischaemia and infarction of the myocardium supplied by that artery. The coronary arteries run along the epicardial surface of the heart until they branch into smaller arteries, which penetrate and supply the myocardium.

**Disease of the coronary arteries kills more people worldwide than any other disease.** Coronary artery disease occurs when an atherosclerotic plaque disrupts and occludes the coronary arterial lumen (see page 180).

## Left coronary artery

The left coronary artery (**Figure 1.19**) passes behind the pulmonary artery and onwards in the atrioventricular groove, where it divides. This artery arises as the left main stem, which divides into the left anterior descending artery and the circumflex arteries.

The left anterior descending artery descends down the anterior surface of the heart all the way to the apex, roughly following the line of the septum. The left anterior descending artery gives off diagonal branches laterally, to the left ventricle, and septal branches inferiorly, supplying the interventricular septum.

The circumflex artery winds around the left lateral surface of the heart in the atrioventricular groove towards the inferior surface. Distally, it anastomoses with right-sided vessels on the inferior surface of the heart. Along its length,

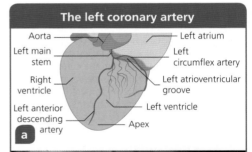

The left coronary artery

Aorta — Left atrium
Left main stem — Left circumflex artery
Right ventricle — Left atrioventricular groove
Left anterior descending artery — Left ventricle
— Apex
**a**

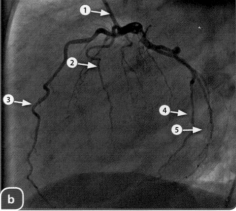

**b**

**Figure 1.19** The left coronary artery. (a) Relations with other cardiac structures. (b) Angiogram of the left coronary artery. A coronary catheter is sitting in the aortic root, where it injects dye into the left main stem. ①, coronary catheter; ②, diagonal artery; ③, left anterior descending artery; ④, obtuse marginal artery; ⑤, circumflex artery.

the circumflex artery supplies obtuse marginal branches that supply the high lateral wall of the left ventricle.

# Right coronary artery

The right coronary artery (**Figure 1.20**) travels in the right atrioventricular groove to the inferior surface of the heart. From here, it usually supplies the posterior descending artery (see box) lying along the line of the inferior interventricular septum. Proximally, the right coronary artery supplies a branch to the sinoatrial node. In its midsection, it provides a right ventricular branch.

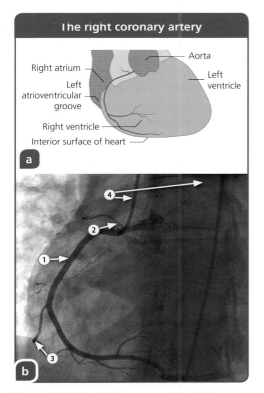

**Figure 1.20** The right coronary artery. (a) Relations with other cardiac structures. (b) The right coronary artery ① winds around the right atrioventricular groove, from which it branches to the sinoatrial node ② and right ventricle ③ before travelling down the inferior surface of the heart. A catheter ④ is visible in the descending aorta (right) and in the aortic root at the right coronary ostium (left).

**The consequences of coronary arterial occlusion (myocardial infarction)** can be predicted by knowing which parts of the heart an artery supplies.

- The left anterior descending artery supplies the left ventricle and septum; occlusion of this artery results in left ventricular failure
- In most people, the right coronary artery supplies the sinoatrial node, right ventricle, atrioventricular node and inferior surface of the left ventricle; occlusion can result in arrhythmias, heart block, right ventricular failure or inferior left ventricular wall dysfunction

# Arterial dominance

The coronary artery supplying the atrioventricular nodal branch determines arterial dominance. In practice, dominance is attributed to the artery supplying the posterior descending artery and thus the inferior cardiac surface. Not only is this clinically easier to deduce but the blood supply to the atrioventricular nodal branch is usually the same as that to the posterior descending artery.

- About 75% of people are right-dominant; the posterior descending artery and atrioventricular nodal branch are supplied by the right coronary artery
- About 10% are codominant; the supply is from the right and left systems
- About 15% are left-dominant; the supply is from the left coronary artery

# Venous return

The coronary veins accompany the arteries. Drainage of the anterior, posterior and lateral myocardial walls is through the great cardiac vein, which runs in the posterior, left atrioventricular groove. The blood finally drains into the right atrium through the coronary sinus.

The great cardiac vein accompanies the left anterior descending artery, and the middle cardiac vein accompanies the posterior descending artery. Many right ventricular veins drain through the small cardiac vein directly into the right atrium.

## Conducting tissues

Cardiac contraction is governed by cardiac conduction pathways (**Figure 1.21**).

The sinoatrial node is a collection of specialised pacemaker cells (see page 40) that lie in the superior posterior portion of the right atrium, close to its junction with the superior vena cava. It is richly innervated by sympathetic and parasympathetic nerves. The ventricles are insulated from the atria by fibrous tissue around the atrioventricular junction (the fibroannular rings). Waves of depolarisation spread across the right atrium and, through Bachmann's bundle (interatrial tract), into and across the left atrium. Inferiorly, the wave of electrical activity reaches the atrioventricular node.

The atrioventricular node is the only electrical connection between the atria and the ventricles. It is at the centre of an area known as Koch's triangle, bounded by the septal tricuspid leaflet, the membranous atrial septum and the coronary sinus. After a slight pause, the atrioventricular node conducts electrical activity onwards down the bundle of His.

The bundle of His descends in the ventricular septum and divides into a right bundle and a left bundle to supply the right and left ventricles, respectively. The left bundle further divides into an anterior and a posterior branch. The His fibres terminate in an extensive network of Purkinje's fibres.

The Purkinje's fibres innervate the myocardium such that ventricular contraction starts at the apex and spreads to the base. This pattern of contraction results in the efficient ejection of blood. It also ensures that the papillary muscles contract early, thus preventing tricuspid or mitral valve regurgitation.

**The space between the visceral and parietal pericardium is the pericardial cavity.** It normally contains only about 10–13 mL of serous fluid, but some diseases cause fluid or blood to accumulate as a pericardial effusion (see page 345). If the fluid collects under high pressure, the chambers of the heart can become compressed. This causes pericardial tamponade, an emergency requiring urgent drainage (see page 358).

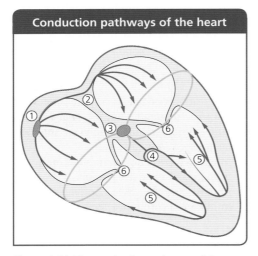

**Conduction pathways of the heart**

**Figure 1.21** The conduction pathways of the heart. The sinoatrial node ① is in the right atrium, close to the junction with the superior vena cava. Bachmann's bundle ② conducts electrical signals from the right atrium to the left atrium. The atrioventricular node ③ conducts electrical signals to the bundle of His ④, which divides into left and right bundle branches. Purkinje's fibres ⑤ rapidly conduct to the ventricles. Fibroannular rings ⑥ (shown in yellow) insulate the ventricles from the atria, and vice versa.

## The pericardium

The pericardial sac is analogous to the pleural membranes surrounding the lungs. The pericardium is a double-layered sac that envelopes the heart and the proximal segments of the great vessels. The pericardial fluid in the sac lubricates the heart, reducing motion friction as it beats and with breathing.

The pericardium fixes the heart to the mediastinum. It also contains lymphatic tissue so has a role in immune function. The outer fibrous pericardium consists of tough, fibrous and collagenous connective tissue. The inner layer, the serous pericardium, is composed of:

- a layer of mesothelial cells that line the inner surface of the fibrous sac (the parietal layer)
- a layer that lines the epicardial surface of the heart (the visceral layer)

The phrenic nerve innervates the fibrous and parietal layers of pericardium, whereas the visceral layer is innervated by the autonomic nervous system.

Inflammation of the pericardium (pericarditis; see page 343) increases friction between the visceral and parietal layers. This friction gives rise to a sharp, pleuritic type of chest pain.

# Circulatory routes

## Starter questions

Answers to the following questions are on page 82.

9. Why are blood clots in the legs potentially life-threatening?
10. Why are inpatients particularly prone to pulmonary emboli?
11. How do cardiologists gain access to the heart?

The systemic and pulmonary circulations are connected in series. The systemic circulation is subdivided into a number of parallel circulatory routes that perfuse and drain individual organ systems.

## Pulmonary circulation

The pulmonary circulation delivers deoxygenated blood to the lungs and returns oxygenated blood. It is a low pressure system driven by the right ventricle (**Figure 1.22**).

## Pulmonary arteries, capillaries and veins

From the pulmonary valve, the main pulmonary artery winds posteriorly and leftwards. It travels around the aortic root before bifurcating into the right and left pulmonary arteries, which pass to the right and left lung hila, respectively (**Figures 1.15, 1.22, 1.23 and 1.24**).

The main pulmonary artery is 2–3 cm in diameter and about 5 cm long. The pulmonary arteries carry deoxygenated blood to the lungs. These arteries follow and branch with the bronchi and pulmonary veins into the bronchopulmonary segments, undergoing multiple generations of branching before forming pulmonary capillaries.

The pulmonary capillaries form plexuses around the alveoli, where gaseous exchange occurs. Oxygenated blood is carried back to the heart through the pulmonary veins. Four pulmonary veins drain into the posterior wall of the left atrium (**Figure 1.25**).

## Bronchial arteries

The lungs also receive oxygenated blood from the bronchial arteries. Two left-sided bronchial arteries arise directly from the thoracic aorta. The right bronchial artery usually arises from either the aorta, a left bronchial artery or an intercostal artery. Drainage is mainly

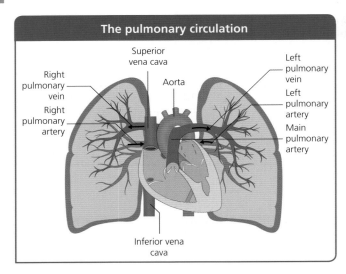

**The pulmonary circulation**

Superior
vena cava

Right
pulmonary
vein

Aorta

Right
pulmonary
artery

Left
pulmonary
vein

Left
pulmonary
artery

Main
pulmonary
artery

Inferior vena
cava

**Figure 1.22** The pulmonary circulation.

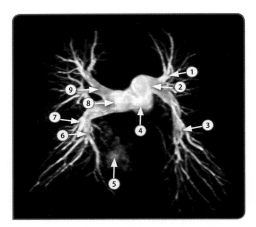

**Figure 1.23** Magnetic resonance angiogram of the pulmonary arterial system. The main pulmonary artery divides into right and left branches, which in turn divide and follow the bronchial and lobar anatomy of the lungs. ①, left superior lobar arteries; ②, left pulmonary artery; ③, left inferior lobar arteries; ④, main pulmonary artery; ⑤, residual contrast in the right ventricle; ⑥, right inferior lobar arteries; ⑦, right middle lobar arteries; ⑧, right pulmonary artery; ⑨, right superior lobar arteries. Courtesy of Professor Jim Wild.

through the pulmonary veins. Bronchial arteries also supply the visceral pleura.

## Intercostal arteries

The chest wall is supplied by the:

- anterior intercostal arteries (branches from the internal thoracic arteries, from the subclavian arteries)
- posterior intercostal arteries (segmental branches from the aorta)

The anterior and posterior intercostal arteries travel in the intercostal spaces (just below the corresponding rib in the neurovascular bundle), where they anastomose with each other.

> The right and left internal thoracic arteries are more traditionally known as the right and left internal mammary arteries. Cardiac surgeons reroute these vessels, anastomosing them with a coronary artery, as part of a coronary artery bypass graft operation. These vessels maintain patency longer than vein grafts.

## The azygos venous system

The right-sided azygos and left-sided hemiazygos and accessory hemiazygos veins make up the azygos venous system. This system lies on the posterior chest wall and drains the posterior intercostal veins.

The azygous venous system is continuous with the ascending lumbar veins, i.e. the thoracic and abdominal segmental veins. The anatomy of the system, especially the left-sided vessels, is highly variable. However, normally

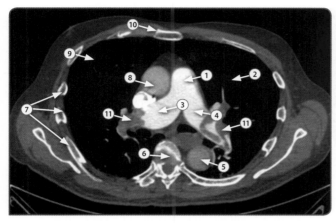

**Figure 1.24** Computerised tomography pulmonary angiogram showing the pulmonary arteries. ①, main pulmonary artery; ②, left lung; ③, right pulmonary artery; ④, left pulmonary artery; ⑤, descending aorta; ⑥, spine; ⑦, ribs; ⑧, ascending aorta; ⑨, right lung; ⑩, sternum. There are large clots (pulmonary emboli) obstructing the right and left pulmonary arteries ⑪. Courtesy of Dr Andrew Swift.

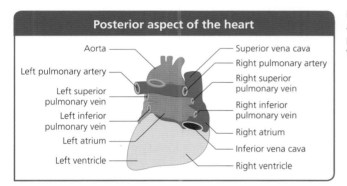

**Figure 1.25** The posterior aspect of the heart, showing the pulmonary arteries and veins along with the cardiac vessels.

the azygos vein drains into the superior vena cava after arching over the right lung hilum.

# The head and neck

The head and neck are supplied by the carotid and vertebrobasilar arterial systems, and are drained by the dural venous sinuses and internal jugular veins.

## Carotid arteries

The right common carotid artery is a branch of the brachiocephalic artery. The left emerges from the aortic arch directly. At the level of the upper border of the thyroid cartilage (the C3–C4 vertebrae), the common carotid arteries bifurcate into the internal and external carotid arteries (**Figure 1.26**).

The internal carotid artery does not provide any branches in the neck. It continues superiorly, entering the skull through the carotid canal. From here, it passes through the cavernous sinus and gives off the ophthalmic artery, which supplies the eye and the orbit. Its terminal branches are the middle and anterior cerebral arteries. The internal carotid artery is also integral to the circle of Willis (cerebral arterial circle) (**Figure 1.27**).

The external carotid artery initially lies medial (internal) to the internal carotid artery. Along its course, it has the following branches (inferior to superior):

- superior thyroid artery (supplying the larynx and thyroid gland)
- ascending pharyngeal artery (supplying the base of the skull)
- lingual artery (supplying the tongue and the floor of the mouth)
- facial artery (to the superficial face)
- occipital artery (supplying the back of the head and the sternomastoid muscles)

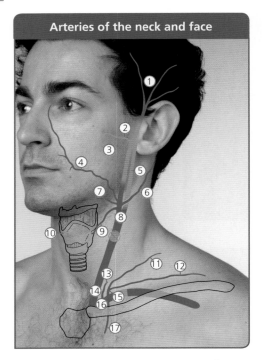

**Arteries of the neck and face**

**Figure 1.26** Arteries of the neck and face. ①, superficial temporal artery; ②, maxillary artery; ③, masseter muscle; ④, facial artery; ⑤, internal carotid artery; ⑥, occipital artery; ⑦, lingual artery; ⑧, carotid bifurcation; ⑨, superior thyroid artery; ⑩, thyroid cartilage (vertebral level C5); ⑪, transverse cervical artery; ⑫, suprascapular artery; ⑬, vertebral artery; ⑭, common carotid artery; ⑮, thyrocervical trunk; ⑯, subclavian artery; ⑰, internal thoracic artery. The best position to palpate the carotid artery is lateral to the larynx at the level of the thyroid cartilage ⊗.

- posterior auricular artery (to the scalp and ear)

The two terminal branches of the external carotid artery are the maxillary artery (to the meninges, maxilla and mandible) and the superficial temporal artery (to the scalp). The latter is palpable over the temples.

## Carotid sinus

The carotid sinus is a dilation in the carotid artery, just below the bifurcation of the common carotid artery. It contains numerous baro- and chemoreceptors, which have roles in blood pressure control (see page 74).

Because of disturbed (non-laminar) blood flow, the carotid sinus is prone to atherosclerosis and possible thromboembolism (causing strokes). Ultrasound of the carotid artery and sinus is used to assess for atherosclerosis and determine future risk of embolism in stroke patients (see page 133).

## Vertebrobasilar arteries

The vertebral arteries supply the cervical vertebrae and spinal cord. They arise from the subclavian arteries bilaterally, and ascend the neck in the vertebral transverse foramen from C6 to C1.

The vertebral arteries pass through the foramen magnum into the skull, where they pierce the meningeal membranes to enter the subarachnoid space. In the skull, they run anteriorly to the brain stem, which they supply (**Figure 1.27**). At the level of the pons, the right and left vertebral arteries unite to form the basilar artery.

The basilar artery supplies branches to the brain stem. It also anastomoses with the carotid system to form the circle of Willis, which lies under the base of the brain and supplies the brain with blood.

## Venous drainage of the neck

The internal jugular veins are the largest neck veins. They receive venous blood from the thyroid gland, pharynx and face, and run from the jugular foramen at the base of the skull. The internal jugular veins then terminate posterior to the sternoclavicular joint, where they drain into the subclavian veins to form the brachiocephalic veins (**Figure 1.28**). Along their course, they travel alongside the common carotid arteries in the right and left carotid sheaths.

The external jugular veins run more superficially and laterally. They travel from the angle of the mandible (the jaw) to drain into the subclavian veins at the mid-clavicular point.

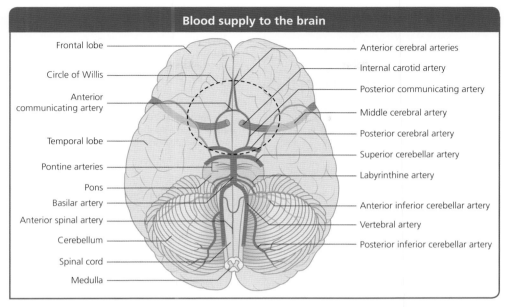

**Figure 1.27** Blood supply to the brain. The circle of Willis is formed by an anastamosis of the posterior cerebral, posterior communicating, internal carotid, anterior cerebral and anterior communicating arteries.

> The internal jugular vein is used to examine the jugular venous pressure as a part of the cardiovascular examination (see page 109) and as a site to gain central venous access.

# Brain

The brain receives arterial contributions from the internal carotid and vertebral arteries through the circle of Willis. The circle of Willis is a collateral circulation formed by the internal carotid, anterior cerebral, anterior communicating, posterior cerebral and posterior communicating arteries (**Figure 1.27**). If one part of the circle becomes occluded, cerebral perfusion can be preserved by flow through the adjacent segment. The anatomy and connections of the circle of Willis vary widely.

# Anterior cerebral arteries

The anterior cerebral arteries wind their way up in front of, and back over the corpus callosum, where they supply the corpus callosum and the (medial) frontal and parietal lobes. Close to their origin, the two arteries communicate with each other through the anterior communicating artery (**Figure 1.27**).

# Middle cerebral arteries

The middle cerebral arteries travel laterally in the lateral fissure (the sulcus), where they supply the parietal and the temporal lobes, along with the lateral surface of the frontal lobes and a portion of the occipital lobes.

# Basilar artery

The basilar artery branches to the cerebellum, labyrinth and pons. It terminates in the posterior cerebral arteries and the circle of Willis through the posterior communicating arteries.

# Posterior cerebral arteries

The posterior cerebral arteries travel laterally and posteriorly around the midbrain, where

## Superficial and deep veins of the neck and face

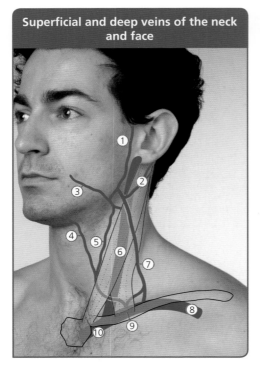

**Figure 1.28** Superficial and deep veins of the neck and face. ①, retromandibular vein; ②, posterior auricular vein; ③, facial vein; ④, anterior jugular vein; ⑤, communicating vein; ⑥, internal jugular vein; ⑦, external jugular vein; ⑧, axillary vein; ⑨, subclavian vein; ⑩, left brachiocephalic vein. The internal jugular vein passes deep to the sternocleidomastoid muscles (outlined), entering the subclavian vein (posteriorly) between the two heads of this muscle.

**Blood clotting in the dural venous sinuses (venous sinus thrombosis) causes severe headache or even stroke-like symptoms.** It is associated with thrombotic risk factors, including oral contraceptive use. Venous sinus thrombosis is diagnosed by computerised tomography or magnetic resonance imaging, and patients require anticoagulation treatment.

**Intracranial haemorrhages into different compartments have different mechanisms:**

■ extradural space: from rupture of meningeal arteries (often traumatic)

■ subdural space: from rupture of bridging veins spanning the subdural space (common in older patients after minimal trauma)

■ Subarachnoid space: from spontaneous rupture of an aneurysm or arteriovenous malformations

they supply most of the occipital cortex, including the visual cortex.

## Cerebral veins

The cerebral veins lie in the subarachnoid space. They drain into a network of venous sinuses, which are formed between layers of dura mater lined with endothelial cells. The dural venous sinuses also receive cerebrospinal fluid from the subarachnoid space. Ultimately, they drain into the internal jugular vein through the jugular foramen.

## The gut

Arterial supply to the gut is from branches of the abdominal aorta which enters the abdomen behind the diaphragm at the level of the T12 vertebra. It then descends, just to the left of the midline, and divides into the common iliac arteries at the level of the L4 vertebra. Along its descent, the abdominal aorta branches to multiple sites (**Table 1.4**).

Venous drainage is through veins draining, directly or indirectly (through the portal system), into the inferior vena cava. The inferior vena cava is formed by the confluence of the right and left common iliac veins. It then ascends the abdominal cavity, lying just to the right of the abdominal aorta, passing through the liver and into the thorax through the right hemidiaphragm at T8. Along its path, venous tributaries include the gonadal, renal, adrenal and hepatic veins.

| Branches of the abdominal aorta | |
|---|---|
| **Branches** | **Supplies** |
| Segmental arteries | Vertebrae |
| Coeliac and mesenteric arteries | Gastrointestinal tract |
| Renal arteries | Kidneys |
| Adrenal arteries | Adrenal glands |
| Gonadal arteries | Gonads |

**Table 1.4** Branches of the abdominal aorta

## Arterial supply

The gut is divided into three sections based on embryonic development.

- The foregut includes structures of the alimentary canal from the oesophagus to the proximal duodenum, including the liver, gall bladder, pancreas and spleen
- The midgut extends from the proximal duodenum to the transverse colon and includes small bowel, appendix and proximal large bowel
- The hindgut includes structures from the distal third of the transverse colon to the rectum

Collectively, the foregut, midgut and hindgut circulations are known as the splanchnic circulation.

## Foregut

This part of the gut is supplied with arterial blood from the coeliac trunk, the first major branch of the abdominal aorta (**Figure 1.29**). It emerges anteriorly at the level of the L1 vertebra and divides after a short course (about 1.4 cm) into three main divisions (**Table 1.5**).

> **The gastroduodenal artery** lies behind the first part of the duodenum (**Figure 1.29**). Posterior duodenal peptic ulcers erode into this artery resulting in a major haemorrhage.

The liver receives only about one quarter of its blood supply from the hepatic arteries. The remaining three quarters arrive through the portal venous system.

> **Systemic thromboembolic disease does not just cause stroke. Clots embolise to the legs** (causing acute limb ischaemia; see page 312) and to the gut. Occlusion of an intestinal artery quickly results in ischaemia and bowel infarction which requires emergency surgery.

## Midgut

The superior mesenteric artery supplies the midgut. The artery emerges from the

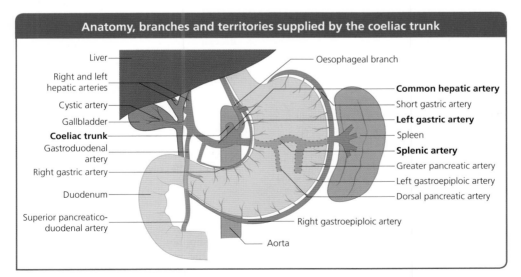

**Anatomy, branches and territories supplied by the coeliac trunk**

Liver — Oesophageal branch
Right and left hepatic arteries — **Common hepatic artery**
Cystic artery — Short gastric artery
Gallbladder — **Left gastric artery**
**Coeliac trunk** — Spleen
Gastroduodenal artery — **Splenic artery**
Right gastric artery — Greater pancreatic artery
— Left gastroepiploic artery
Duodenum — Dorsal pancreatic artery
Superior pancreatico-duodenal artery
Right gastroepiploic artery
Aorta

**Figure 1.29** The anatomy, branches and territory of the coeliac trunk. The left and right gastroepiploic and gastric arteries anastomose on the greater and lesser curves of the stomach.

| Branches, sub-branches and territories supplied by the coeliac trunk | | | |
| --- | --- | --- | --- |
| Branch | Arterial sub-branches | Territories supplied | Major anastomoses |
| Left gastric | Left gastric | Lesser curve of stomach | Right gastric artery on lesser curve of stomach |
| | Oesophageal branch | Lower third of oeosphagus | – |
| Common hepatic | Right gastric | Lesser curve of stomach | Left gastric artery on lesser curve of stomach |
| | Gastroduodenal | Duodenum, pancreas and greater curve of stomach (through right gastroepiploic artery) | Right and left gastroepiploic arteries, on greater curve of stomach |
| | Cystic | Gall bladder | – |
| | Right and left hepatic arteries (terminal branches) | Liver | – |
| Splenic artery | Dorsal pancreatic | Pancreas | – |
| | Short gastric arteries | Fundus of stomach | – |
| | Left gastroepiploic | Greater curve of stomach and greater omentum | Right and left gastroepiploic arteries, on greater curve of stomach |
| | Greater pancreatic | Most of pancreas | - |

**Table 1.5**  The branches, sub-branches and territories supplied by the coeliac

| Branches and territories supplied by the superior mesenteric artery | |
| --- | --- |
| Branch | Arterial territory |
| Inferior pancreatoduodenal | Pancreatic head and duodenum |
| Jejunal | Multiple jejunal arteries supply the jejunum |
| Middle colic artery* | Transverse colon |
| Ileal | Multiple ileal arteries supply the jejunum |
| Right colic* | Ascending colon |
| Ileocolic* | Ileum, caecum and appendix |

*The three branches supplying the colon anastomose with each other and the left colic (from the inferior mesenteric artery) on the inner curve of the colon to form the marginal artery.

**Table 1.6**  Branches and territories supplied by the superior mesenteric artery

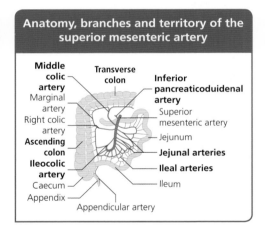

**Anatomy, branches and territory of the superior mesenteric artery**

**Figure 1.30**  The anatomy, branches and territory of the superior mesenteric artery. The marginal artery is formed by an anastomosis between the ileocolic, right colic and middle colic branches on the inner curve of the large bowel.

abdominal aorta anteriorly, about 1 cm below the coeliac trunk, at the level of the L1 vertebra. It branches extensively to supply all structures of the midgut (**Table 1.6** and **Figure 1.30**).

## Hindgut

This is supplied by the inferior mesenteric artery. This artery arises anteriorly from the abdominal aorta below the origin of the renal arteries, at the level of the L3 vertebra. It supplies three major branches: the left colic, sigmoid colic and superior rectal (**Table 1.7** and **Figure 1.31**).

## Venous drainage: the portal venous system

Venous blood is drained from the gut through the superior mesenteric, inferior mesenteric and splenic veins. These veins do not drain directly into the vena cava. Instead, they unite behind the neck of the pancreas to form the portal vein (**Figure 1.32**). At the porta hepatis, the portal vein divides into right and left branches.

Portal venous blood traverses the hepatic sinusoids to reach the hepatic veins, which drain into the inferior vena cava as it passes through the liver. This arrangement ensures that freshly digested nutrients (and any oral medications) are metabolised by the liver before they enter the systemic circulation. This is called first-pass metabolism.

**Liver disease (e.g. cirrhosis) obstructs portal venous blood flow causing portal venous hypertension.** When flow is obstructed, blood seeks the path of least resistance and bypasses the liver through portocaval anastomoses, naturally occurring connections between the portal and systemic venous systems. This causes distended blood vessels in the lower oesophagus (oeseophageal varices) and rectum (haemorrhoids) which can bleed. Oesophageal varices haemorrhage can be torrential and even fatal.

**Branches and territories supplied by the inferior mesenteric artery**

| Branch | Arterial territory |
|---|---|
| Left colic* | Descending colon |
| Sigmoid colic branches | Sigmoid colon |
| Superior rectal (terminal branch) | Rectum and upper anal canal |

*The left colic forms part of the marginal artery anastomosis.

**Table 1.7** Branches and territories supplied by the inferior mesenteric artery

**Anatomy, branches and territory of the inferior mesenteric artery**

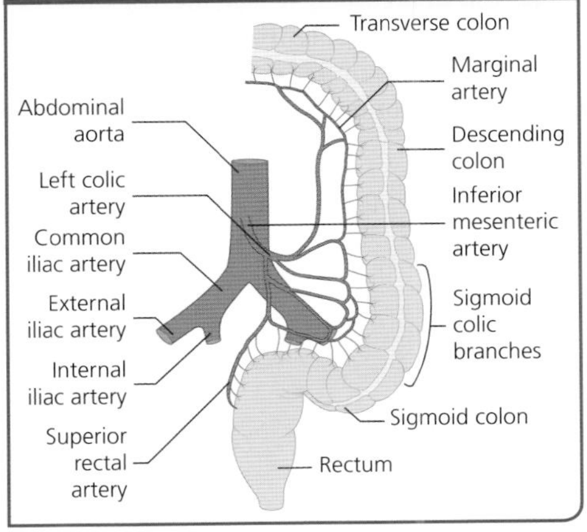

**Figure 1.31** The anatomy, branches and territory of the inferior mesenteric artery. The anastomotic marginal artery on the inner curve of the large bowel is continuous with the marginal artery supplied by the superior mesenteric artery.

## Renal and adrenal circulation

The renal arteries arise as lateral branches from the aorta at the level of the L1 vertebra.

**The portal venous system**

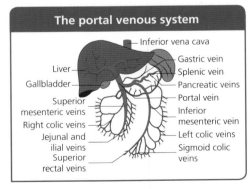

**Figure 1.32** The portal venous system. Venous blood from the foregut, midgut and hindgut drains to the portal vein and passes through the liver before entering the inferior vena cava through the hepatic veins.

Because of the position of the aorta, the right renal artery is slightly longer than the left, which passes posterior to the inferior vena cava along its course. The kidneys receive about a quarter of the total cardiac output, which explains the wide calibre of the vessels (0.5–1.0 cm). The renal arteries divide into segmental, lobar, interlobar and arcuate arteries before becoming the afferent arterioles supplying the glomeruli.

The renal veins mirror the arteries along their course. The left renal vein is longer than the right because of the position of the inferior vena cava (**Figure 1.33**).

The adrenal glands are supplied by three arterial branches: the superior, middle and inferior suprarenal arteries. The suprarenal arteries usually arise from the inferior phrenic artery, aorta and renal arteries, respectively. The right adrenal vein drains into the inferior vena cava, whereas the left drains into the left renal vein.

> **The renal arteries become narrowed by atherosclerosis or congenital diseases such as fibromuscular dysplasia.** Renal artery stenosis is a cause of resistant hypertension (see page 202). Ultimately, if the condition is uncorrected, the kidneys fail and become atrophied.

## Pelvis

The common iliac arteries divide into internal and external iliac arteries as they reach the pelvic rim. The pelvic walls, muscles and organs are supplied by branches of the internal iliac artery. The external iliac artery descends along the medial border of the psoas major muscle. Posterior to the midpoint of the inguinal ligament (the mid-inguinal point), the external iliac artery becomes the common femoral artery.

## Upper limb

## Arterial supply

Arterial blood to the upper limb is supplied by the axillary artery. The axillary artery is a continuation of the subclavian artery at the lateral border of the first rib. The axillary artery is surrounded by the brachial plexus and provides branches to the lateral chest wall, the axilla and the muscles and bones of the shoulder region.

At the lower border of the teres major muscle (a scapulohumeral muscle), the axillary artery becomes the brachial artery. The brachial artery descends the arm medial to the biceps muscle. Proximally, it supplies the profunda brachii branch that winds around the radius with the radial nerve, before descending into the forearm, anterior to the humeral lateral epicondyle. Finally, it anastomoses with the radial recurrent artery.

At the antecubital fossa (the region anterior to the elbow; **Figure 1.34**), the brachial artery divides into its terminal branches: the radial and ulnar arteries. The radial and ulnar

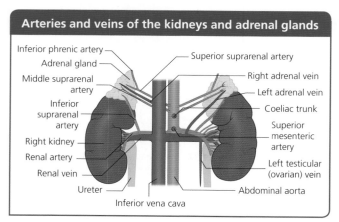

**Arteries and veins of the kidneys and adrenal glands**

Inferior phrenic artery
Adrenal gland
Middle suprarenal artery
Inferior suprarenal artery
Right kidney
Renal artery
Renal vein
Ureter
Inferior vena cava
Superior suprarenal artery
Right adrenal vein
Left adrenal vein
Coeliac trunk
Superior mesenteric artery
Left testicular (ovarian) vein
Abdominal aorta

**Figure 1.33** The arteries and veins of the kidneys and adrenal glands.

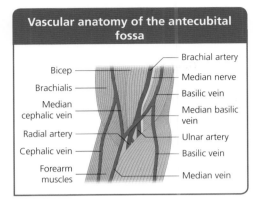

## Vascular anatomy of the antecubital fossa

- Bicep
- Brachialis
- Median cephalic vein
- Radial artery
- Cephalic vein
- Forearm muscles

- Brachial artery
- Median nerve
- Basilic vein
- Median basilic vein
- Ulnar artery
- Basilic vein
- Median vein

**Figure 1.34** The anatomy of the antecubital fossa. Venous anatomy in this region is highly variable. Some people have a single vein crossing the antecubital fossa connecting the cephalic and basilic veins (the median cubital vein) with no distinct median vein of the forearm.

arteries follow their respective sides of the forearm (**Figure 1.35**).

The ulnar artery provides the interosseal arteries, which supply the flexor and extensor muscle compartments of the forearm. Distally, the radial artery passes laterally and dorsally to pass through the anatomical snuffbox. The ulnar artery passes into the hand just superficial to the median nerve on the medial side of the wrist. In the palm, the radial and ulnar arteries form two anastomoses: the deep and superficial palmar (or volar) arches.

# Venous drainage

Venous drainage is through the deep veins, or venae comitantes (Latin for 'accompanying veins'), which accompany the corresponding arteries. The hands drain into the cephalic and basilic venous systems through the dorsal venous network. The superficial veins of the upper limb are commonly used for gaining peripheral venous access in clinical medicine.

- The cephalic vein runs along the lateral aspect of the forearm and lateral to the biceps muscle before entering the deltopectoral groove and emptying into the axillary vein
- The basilic vein ascends the medial aspect of the forearm and medial to the biceps muscle before joining the brachial vein to form the axillary vein

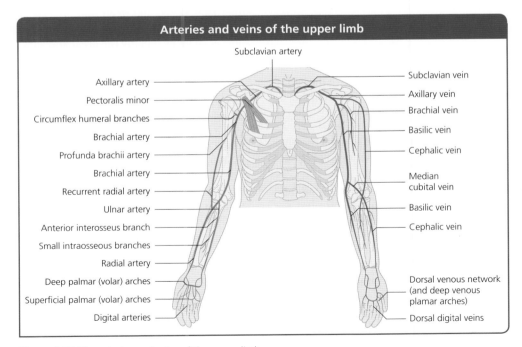

## Arteries and veins of the upper limb

Subclavian artery

- Axillary artery
- Pectoralis minor
- Circumflex humeral branches
- Brachial artery
- Profunda brachii artery
- Brachial artery
- Recurrent radial artery
- Ulnar artery
- Anterior interosseus branch
- Small intraosseous branches
- Radial artery
- Deep palmar (volar) arches
- Superficial palmar (volar) arches
- Digital arteries

- Subclavian vein
- Axillary vein
- Brachial vein
- Basilic vein
- Cephalic vein
- Median cubital vein
- Basilic vein
- Cephalic vein
- Dorsal venous network (and deep venous plamar arches)
- Dorsal digital veins

**Figure 1.35** The arteries and veins of the upper limb.

The basilic and cephalic veins are usually connected through the median cubital or median basilic veins at the antecubital fossa (**Figure 1.34**). This connecting vein is often used for peripheral venous access and phlebotomy. The precise distribution of the smaller veins is variable.

# Lower limb

Arterial supply to the lower limb is from the common femoral artery (**Figure 1.36**).

> **The arteries of the lower limb can normally be palpated at the following sites:**
>
> - the common femoral artery at the mid-inguinal point
> - the popliteal artery in the popliteal fossa
> - the posterior tibial and dorsalis pedis arteries at the foot
>
> Failure to palpate these pulses is a sign of peripheral vascular disease.

## Arterial supply

The common femoral artery enters the thigh posterior to the inguinal canal. It supplies the:

- superficial and deep external pudendal arteries (supplying the lower abdomen as well as the penis and scrotum or the labia)
- inferior epigastric artery (supplying the lower anterior abdominal wall)
- superficial circumflex iliac artery (supplying the femur and femoral head)
- descending genicular arteries (supplying the knee)

The largest branch of the common femoral artery is the profunda femoris, also known as the deep femoral artery. The profunda femoris supplies branches to the thigh muscles and the hip joint: the lateral circumflex branches (**Figure 1.36** and **1.37**).

After giving rise to the profunda, the femoral artery is known as the superficial femoral artery. It descends the thigh in the adductor canal before reaching the popliteal fossa (behind the knee) at the distal femur. At this point, it becomes the popliteal artery.

At the lower border of the popliteal fossa, the artery divides into the anterior tibial artery and the posterior tibial artery. These arteries descend the leg in the anterior and posterior compartments, respectively.

- The anterior tibial artery crosses the ankle joint to become the dorsalis pedis artery, which is palpable along the lateral border of the extensor hallucis longus (big toe) tendon
- The posterior tibial artery can be palpated posterior and inferior to the medial malleolus

> **The mid-inguinal point is the best place to palpate the femoral artery.** This point is halfway between the anterior superior iliac spine and the pubic symphysis. Lateral to the artery is the femoral nerve. The femoral vein lies medially. Remember 'NAVY': nerve, artery, vein and Y-fronts.

## Venous drainage

Similar to the upper limb, venous drainage is through deep venae comitantes and the superficial veins. The deep and superficial veins are connected by perforating veins. The superficial veins include the great and small saphenous veins (**Figure 1.36**).

The great saphenous vein runs from the dorsal venous arch of the foot and across the ankle (1 cm anterior to the medial malleolus). The vein then ascends the medial side of the leg and the thigh (**Figure 1.36** and **1.37**) before joining the deep common femoral vein at the saphenofemoral junction.

The small saphenous vein forms from the lateral dorsal arch of the foot. This vein ascends the leg in the posterior compartment. It drains into the popliteal vein at the popliteal fossa.

> **The great saphenous vein is occasionally used for gaining emergency venous access when other veins have collapsed as a result of shock.** Cardiothoracic surgeons harvest the saphenous vein for use as a conduit in a coronary artery bypass graft.

## Arteries and veins of the lower limb

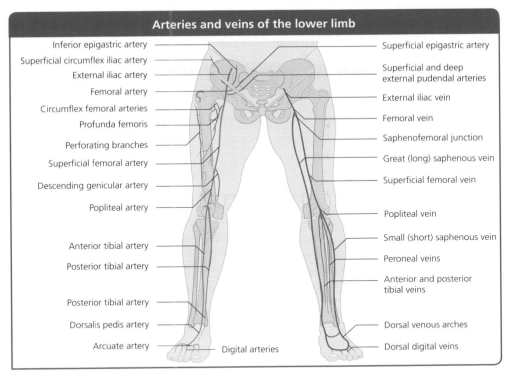

**Figure 1.36** The arteries and veins of the lower limb. The circumflex femoral arteries emanate from the profunda femoris and supply structures around, and including, the femoral head and hip. Arteries around the knee joint form a superficial and deep anastomotic plexus, which supplies collateral circulation to the knee; the genicular anastomosis.

## Anatomy of the femoral triangle

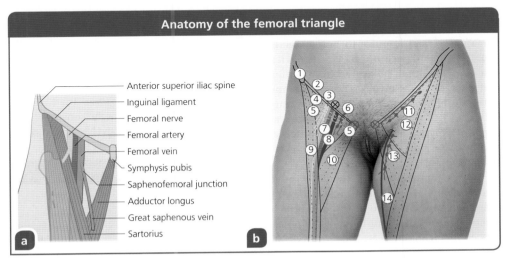

**Figure 1.37** The anatomy of the femoral triangle. (a) The femoral triangle is bordered superiorly by the inguinal ligament, laterally by the medial border of sartorius, and medially by the lateral border of adductor longus. It contains the femoral nerve, artery and vein. (b) ① Anterior superior iliac spine, ② inguinal ligament, ③ femoral nerve, ④ iliopsoas, ⑤ femoral sheath (grey hatch), ⑥ deep inguinal lymph nodes (Cloquet's node in femoral canal), ⑦ femoral artery, ⑧ femoral vein, ⑨ sartorius and subsartorial/adductor canal, ⑩ adductor longus, ⑪ superficial inguinal lymph nodes (proximal group), ⑫ femoral triangle border, ⑬ superficial inguinal lymph nodes (distal group), ⑭ long saphenous vein, ⊗ midinguinal point, ⊗ pubic tubercle.

# Cardiac electrophysiology

## Starter questions

Answers to the following questions are on page 82–83.

12. Why are most regions of the heart able to depolarise spontaneously?
13. Why is the resting membrane potential of pacemaker cells never completely stable?

Cardiac electrophysiology is the study of the heart's electrical activity in health and disease. Behind every heartbeat lies an intricate series of coordinated electrical and chemical processes. In concert, these processes result in the initiation and propagation of a wave of electrical activity that spreads throughout the heart to trigger myocardial contraction. An appreciation of the mechanisms and processes involved allows better understanding of the effects of antiarrhythmic drugs (see pages 150) and cardiac arrhythmia (see page 211).

## Resting membrane potential

For an electrical impulse to be conducted through the myocardium, an electrical charge (a potential, measured in mV) must first exist across the myocyte cell membrane. Relative to the extracellular space (assumed to be 0 mV), the innermost surface of the resting bilipid myocyte membrane is maintained at a negative potential (-90 mV); this is the resting membrane potential.

The resting membrane potential is generated by a combination of unbalanced ion concentrations and selective membrane permeability. The ions that contribute most to these concentration gradients are the cations $K^+$, $Na^+$ and $Ca^{2+}$. The generation and maintenance of the resting membrane potential is best understood if broken down into four stages (not to confused with the 4 phases of the action potential).

**Generation of the resting membrane potential is an active process.** This is why hypoxia and ischaemia can alter the electrochemical gradients across cardiomyocyte cell membranes, predisposing the heart to bradycardia and arrhythmia.

## Stage 1

Membrane-bound ion pumps generate concentration gradients by using active transport mechanisms to pump $K^+$, $Na^+$ and $Ca^{2+}$ cations against their concentration gradients. The major ion pumps (**Table 1.8**) are:

- $Na^+$–$K^+$ ATPase
- $Ca^{2+}$ ATPase
- $Na^+$–$Ca^{2+}$ exchanger

These active transport processes consume ATP, hence the name; ATPase. The $Na^+$–$Ca^{2+}$ exchanger does not directly consume ATP, but it is driven by the actively generated $Na^+$

| Major ion pumps | |
| --- | --- |
| Pump | Function |
| $Na^+$–$K^+$ ATPase | Pumps three $Na^+$ ions out of the cell and two $K^+$ ions into the cell |
| $Ca^{2+}$ ATPase | Pumps $Ca^{2+}$ out of the cell and into the sarcoplasmic reticulum |
| $Na^+$–$Ca^{2+}$ exchanger | Exchanges three $Na^+$ ions for one $Ca^{2+}$ ion |

**Table 1.8** Major ion pumps

| Intracellular and extracellular concentrations of important cations | | |
|---|---|---|
| Cation | Intracellular concentration (mmol/L) | Extracellular concentration (mmol/L) |
| $K^+$ | 150 | 4 |
| $Ca^{2+}$ | $10^{-4}$ | 2 |
| $Na^+$ | 15 | 145 |

**Table 1.9** Intracellular and extracellular concentrations of important cations

electrochemical gradient (i.e. secondary active transport). The net result is an imbalance between the intracellular and extracellular concentrations of $K^+$, $Na^+$ and $Ca^{2+}$ (**Table 1.9**).

The pumps move more positive charge out of the myocyte than into it, thus generating a slight negative electrical potential (**Figure 1.38**). This is not the primary mechanism driving the resting membrane potential, but it does contribute to a small degree.

When the myocyte is held at resting membrane potential, it is said to be polarised. Depolarisation triggers myocardial contraction and a heartbeat (the QRS complex on the electrocardiogram, ECG). Before another heartbeat can occur, the resting membrane potential must be restored through repolarisation (the T wave on the ECG).

Flow down electrical and chemical gradients is a passive process, but flow up such gradients is an active process. Substances flow down electrical and chemical gradients passively, in the same way that a ball rolls down a physical gradient (e.g. a hill). However, pushing substances up, i.e. against, their gradient is an active process which requires energy.

## Stage 2

The myocyte membrane is permeable to $K^+$ but not to other ions. The selectively permeable membrane allows $K^+$ to diffuse out of the cell (passively) through ion channels (membrane-spanning proteins) down its concentration gradient.

Every $K^+$ ion that diffuses out of the cell leaves one less positive charge intracellularly. The cell membrane is impermeable to larger negative ions such as proteins and sulphates. Therefore as the positive charge is lost, a negative charge develops inside the cell. If even 1 out of every 100,000 $K^+$ ions diffuses out of the cell, it is enough to generate a membrane potential of $-100$ mV.

## Stage 3

Opposing forces act on ion movement. The steep intracellular concentration continues to favour $K^+$ efflux. However, as electrical

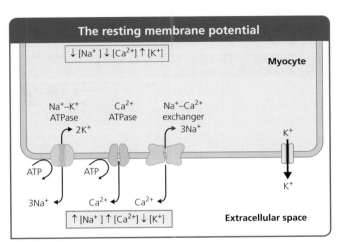

**Figure 1.38** The resting membrane potential. The three ion pumps (left) consume ATP to generate steep ionic concentration gradients. The myocyte membrane is permeable to $K^+$ but less permeable to other ions. Therefore $K^+$ diffuses passively down its concentration gradient (right), leaving less positive charge (i.e. a net negative charge) on the inside of the myocyte.

potential develops, it begins to oppose $K^+$ efflux, because the positive $K^+$ ion becomes attracted to the negative intracellular charge. There comes a point at which these forces balance: equilibrium. The potential at which this occurs is the equilibrium potential ($E$). The equilibrium point is determined by the charge on the ion and by the concentration gradient. It is calculated by using the Nernst equation:

Equilibrium potential =

$$\frac{-61}{\text{Charge on ion}} \cdot \log \frac{\text{Intracellular concentration}}{\text{Extracellular concentration}}$$

The intracellular concentration of $K^+$ is 150 mmol/L and is 4 mmol/L extracellularly. Each $K^+$ ion has only a single charge so the equilibrium potential for $K^+$ is –96 mV; this is written as $E_K = -96$ mV.

## Stage 4

The membrane potential ($E_m$) is equal to the sum of the equilibrium potentials of all the ions. Conductance (permeability) is another key factor. If $g$ is conductance, the membrane potential is calculated thus:

$$E_m = (g_k \times E_k) + (g_{Ca} \times E_{Ca}) + (g_{Na} \times E_{Na})$$

The membrane has a low conductance to other ions, so the other ions make only a small contribution towards the total membrane potential. Therefore the overall resting membrane potential is similar to the equilibrium potential for $K^+$ ($E_K$).

> **The Nernst equation explains why disturbances in serum concentrations of $K^+$ can be so dangerous.** If extracellular $K^+$ concentration, normally 4 mmol/L, increases to 10 mmol/L, then $E_K$ increases to 70 mmol/L. This high $E_K$ promoting depolarisation, which triggers dangerous cardiac arrhythmias.

In summary, the resting membrane potential is determined by the equilibrium potentials of the individual ions, the membrane's permeability to each of these ions (conductance) and the effects of the ion pumps.

The resting membrane potential is not uniform across all cardiac cell types. According to regional differences in tissue function, myocytes have different types and concentrations of ion channels. For example, pacemaker myocytes in the sinoatrial node have a less negative resting potential ($E_m = -60$ mV).

## Ion channels: gating

Membrane potential is dynamic and continually cycles through depolarisation and repolarisation with each heartbeat. This process is controlled by ion-specific channels that are activated (open) or inactivated (closed) depending on local factors such as electrical potential and the binding of ligands. The property of channels to alter their opening and closing is known as gating (**Table 1.10**).

Each of the various ion channels has specific properties, and each is differentially

| Gated ion channels | | |
|---|---|---|
| Gating mechanism | Response | Example |
| Voltage-gated channels | Activate or inactivate in response to variations in electrical potential | Generation of action potentials |
| Ligand-gated channels | Activate or inactivate in response to binding of a specific ligand | Ligands include hormones and neurotransmitters |
| Receptor-coupled channels | Activate or inactivate in response to a physical stimulus | Myocardial stretch |

**Table 1.10** Gated ion channels

| Ion channels | | |
|---|---|---|
| Channel | Current | Function |
| Fast Na+ channel | $I_{Na}$ | Rapid influx of Na+ during depolarisation |
| Slow Na+ channel | $I_b$ | Allows slow background influx of Na+ |
| 'Funny' Na+ channel | $I_f$ | Important factor in the generation of pacemaker potentials in pacemaker cells |
| Slow L-type Ca2+ channel | $I_{Ca-L}$ | Prolongs action potentials in non-pacemaker myocytes |
| | | important in initiating action potentials in pacemaker cells |
| Transient T-type Ca2+ channel | $I_{Ca-T}$ | Opens transiently during phase 4 of the action potential in pacemaker cells |
| | | Helps initiate action potentials |
| Inwardly rectifying K+ channel | $I_{ir}$ | Maintains resting membrane potential |
| Transient outward K+ channel | $I_{to}$ | Contributes to phase 1 of cardiac action potential |
| Delayed rectifier K+ channel | $I_{Kr}$ | Contributes to repolarisation in phase 3 of action potential |

**Table 1.11** Types of cardiac myocyte ion channel

expressed according to cell type (**Table 1.11**). For example, the voltage-gated fast Na+ channel is inactivated at the resting membrane potential (usually –90 mV) but becomes activated at a threshold potential of –45 mV. Consequently, Na+ ions flood into the cell along the steep concentration gradient.

When an ion moves through a channel, there is a flow of electrical charge (i.e. an electrical current, $I$). The electrical current ($I_{Na}$) produced by the inward movement of Na+ depolarises the cell membrane. Complete depolarisation inactivates the Na+ channel, which remains inactivated until the membrane has repolarised.

> **Mutations of rectifying K+ channels can cause delayed repolarisation.** This effect prolongs the duration of the action potential in the hearts of patients with long QT syndrome (see page 334).

There are numerous types of K+ ion channel. Inwardly rectifying K+ channels conduct K+ inwardly when the potential is more negative than $E_K$, and outwardly when the potential is higher than $E_K$. Thus these channels rectify (maintain) K+ concentration at $E_K$.

> **Na+, K+ and Ca2+ channels are the target for many antiarrhythmic drugs.** For example, drugs that block fast Na+ channels (e.g. flecainide and propafenone) delay phase 0 of the action potential (see page 38) and thus stabilise the membrane. The are used to treat certain arrhythmias (see Chapter 5).

# Action potential in non-pacemaker cardiac myocytes

The action potential is the cycle of depolarisation and repolarisation that triggers myocyte contraction. The action potential in cardiac myocytes is 100 times longer than that in skeletal myocytes: 300 ms versus 3 ms. This provides time for the heart to complete contraction (systole) and fill (diastole) before becoming excitable again.

In cardiac myocytes, the action potential occurs in five phases (**Figure 1.39**). The activation and inactivation of ion channels during these phases is summarised in **Figure 1.40**.

## Phase 4: resting

During the resting phase, the membrane is permeable to K+ and relatively impermeable to other ions. Therefore the membrane potential ($E_m$) approximates the K+ equilibrium potential ($E_K$), and myocytes are held at the resting membrane potential, polarised between -90 and –95 mV.

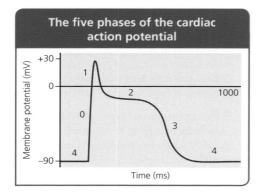

**The five phases of the cardiac action potential**

**Figure 1.39** The five phases of the cardiac action potential in a cardiac myocyte: 0, depolarisation; 1, transient partial repolarisation; 2, plateau; 3, repolarisation; and 4, resting.

The myocyte remains in phase 4 until a depolarising electrical stimulus is conducted to the myocyte from a neighbouring cell. If this stimulus increases the membrane potential to a threshold potential of about –60 mV, an action potential (phase 0) is triggered.

Phase 4 corresponds to diastole in the cardiac cycle.

## Phase 0: depolarisation

When the threshold potential is reached, fast Na⁺ channels activate. Na⁺ ions rush into the myocyte along the steep concentration gradient. The inward Na⁺ current ($I_{Na}$) rapidly increases the membrane potential to above zero (around +30 mV).

Increased Na⁺ conductance increases the potential moving it towards $E_{Na}$ (+60 mV). However, before this point is reached, at about +30 mV, the voltage-gated fast Na⁺ channels inactivate, $I_{Na}$ ceases and phase 0 ends abruptly.

## Phase 1: transient partial repolarisation

As the fast Na⁺ channels inactivate, voltage-gated, transient outward K⁺ channels activate. These open K⁺ channels allow a brief efflux of K⁺ ($I_{to}$). This K⁺ efflux causes a short-lived and only partial repolarisation, because the channels inactivate quickly.

## Phase 2: plateau

The phase 2 plateau is the result of several competing but balanced forces. Currents produced by the movement of Ca²⁺ and Na⁺ prolong repolarisation for about 250 ms. This effect is mediated by the current produced by an efflux of K⁺.

■ Voltage-gated L-type Ca²⁺ channels activate and inactivate slowly, which

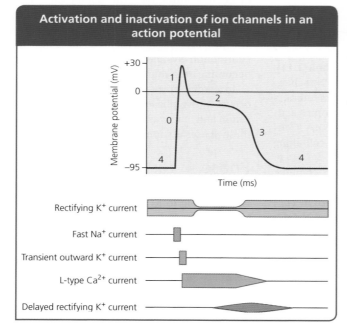

**Activation and inactivation of ion channels in an action potential**

**Figure 1.40** The activation and inactivation sequence of gated ion channels through an action potential in a cardiac myocyte. The phases are 0, depolarisation; 1, transient partial repolarisation; 2, plateau; 3, repolarisation; and 4, resting.

prolongs inward $Ca^{2+}$ current ($I_{Ca}$); this prolongs the action potential and triggers myocyte contraction
- Towards the end of phase 2, the $Na^+$–$Ca^{2+}$ exchanger allows $Na^+$ to enter the cell slowly; this $Na^+$ influx helps extend the plateau phase
- Outward rectifying $K^+$ currents oppose the $Ca^{2+}$ and $Na^+$ currents

Phases 1 and 2 correspond to systole and the QRS complex on the ECG.

> **Calcium channel blockers (e.g. verapamil and diltiazem) block L-type $Ca^{2+}$ channels shortening phase 2 plateau.** This reduces cardiac contractility, i.e. have a negative inotropic effect. $Ca^{2+}$ channels are also present in vascular smooth muscle and pacemaker cells. Therefore these drugs also reduce blood pressure (i.e. have antihypertensive effects) and slow the heart rate (i.e. have negative chronotropic effects).

## Phase 3: repolarisation

As the L-type $Ca^{2+}$ channels inactivate, delayed rectifying $K^+$ channels open. Therefore the membrane potential is brought close to $E_K$ again. The now unopposed $K^+$ efflux produces rapid repolarisation.

Phase 3 corresponds to the T wave on the ECG.

## Refractory periods

Activation of fast $Na^+$ channels is the trigger for phase 0 depolarisation. These channels inactivate quickly once the potential reaches about +30 mV and are not reactivated until the membrane repolarises during phase 3. No matter how strong the stimulus, another action potential cannot be initiated during phase 1 or 2; this is the absolute refractory period.

Fast $Na^+$ channels are increasingly reactivated during phase 3. During this phase, an electrical stimulus may trigger a further action potential. This is known as the relative refractory period, because the likelihood of further activation is relative to the magnitude of the stimulus and the number of reactivated fast $Na^+$ channels (**Figure 1.41**).

> **Drugs that block $K^+$ channels (e.g. amiodarone; see page 152) block the rectifying $K^+$ currents.** This effect prolongs phase 3 and therefore the refractory period. These drugs are useful for alleviating the symptoms of certain re-entry tachycardias.

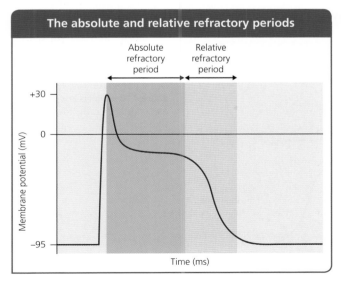

**Figure 1.41** The absolute and relative refractory periods of an action potential in a cardiac myocyte.

The absolute and relative refractory periods

# Action potential in pacemaker cells

Pacemaker cells are not dependent on an external stimulus to depolarise. They depolarise spontaneously and are capable of self-initiating the waves of depolarisation that propagate across the heart every heartbeat. This property is known as automaticity. Pacemaker cells are mainly clustered in the:

- sinoatrial node
- atrioventricular node
- conducting tissues

Automaticity is possible because pacemaker cells express different types of ion channel to those of non-pacemaker myocytes. Therefore pacemaker cells can produce action potentials in a different way (**Figure 1.42**).

## Phase 4

During phase 4, the membrane of pacemaker cells is less negative (about –60 mV) than that of non-pacemaker myocytes, because of a relative deficiency of rectifying K$^+$ channel activity. The potential is not static; pacemaker cells have no true resting membrane potential. Instead, the membrane potential spontaneously depolarises slowly towards threshold voltage. This property confers automaticity.

Constant upward drift in membrane potential is caused by the sequential activation

of 'funny' Na$^+$ channels ($I_f$), T-type Ca$^{2+}$ channels ($I_{Ca-T}$) and then L-type Ca$^{2+}$ channels ($I_{Ca-L}$). Activation of all these channels results in an inward cation current that gradually brings the membrane to threshold voltage (about –35 mV). These currents are known as pacemaker potentials.

> **The 'funny' Na$^+$ channel** is activated by polarisation, unlike regular Na$^+$ channels which are activated by depolarisation.

## Phase 0

Once threshold is reached, phase 0 depolarisation occurs. However, pacemaker cells are devoid of fast Na$^+$ channels; depolarisation occurs through L-type Ca$^{2+}$ channels instead. The L-type Ca$^{2+}$ current is slow, so the rate of depolarisation is also slow.

Because Na$^+$ channels have no role in action potentials in pacemaker myocytes, drugs that block fast Na$^+$ channels (e.g. flecainide and propafenone) have little effect on these cells.

## Phases 1 and 2

There is no transient partial repolarisation, nor is there a plateau phase, in pacemaker action potentials.

## Phase 3

During phase 3, the L-type Ca$^{2+}$ channels inactivate and K$^+$ channels open. The consequent

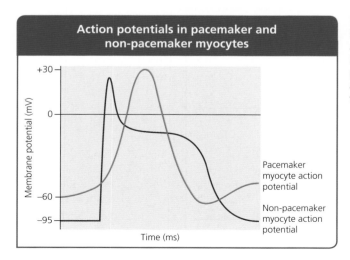

**Action potentials in pacemaker and non-pacemaker myocytes**

Membrane potential (mV)

+30
0
–60
–95

Time (ms)

Pacemaker myocyte action potential

Non-pacemaker myocyte action potential

**Figure 1.42** The action potential in a pacemaker myocyte and a non-pacemaker myocyte. In the pacemaker cell, the phase 4 potential is less negative and constantly drifts towards threshold.

K⁺ current ($I_K$) brings about repolarisation and phase 4.

## Pacemaker potentials

The rate at which action potentials are generated, and therefore the heart rate, is influenced by external factors, most importantly the autonomic nervous system (**Figure 1.43**). The rate of action potential generation is determined by the rate of inward Na⁺ and Ca²⁺ currents ($I_{Na}$ and $I_{Ca}$) during phase 4: the higher the rate, the steeper the increase in potential and the quicker the membrane reaches threshold. The quicker the membrane reaches threshold, the more frequently action potentials are generated. Factors that increase $I_{Na}$ and $I_{Ca}$ increase heart rate, whereas factors that reduce $I_{Na}$ and $I_{Ca}$ reduce heart rate.

## Effects of the autonomic nervous system

The autonomic nervous system is a division of the peripheral nervous system which controls involuntary functions of the internal (visceral) organs. The autonomic nervous system controls a wide range of body functions subconsciously (e.g. digestion, respiratory rate, heart rate, micturition, sexual arousal and many others) in order to match organ function with the prevailing environmental demands and maintain homeostasis. The autonomic nervous system is divided into sympathetic and parasympathetic divisions. Both systems comprise central neurones which synapse (connect) with more peripheral neurones which, in turn, innervate the viscera. These are known as pre- and post-ganglionic neurones, respectively.

Autonomic nervous control of the heart is coordinated by the cardiovascular centre in the medulla oblongata, which is located in the lower brain stem. The cardiovascular centre receives afferent (meaning towards the centre) sensory input from peripheral chemo- and baroreceptors, and control from

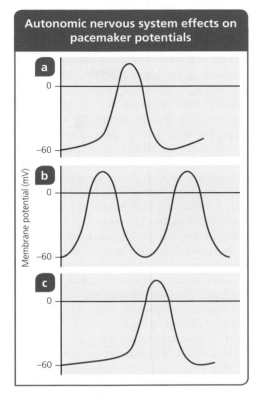

**Autonomic nervous system effects on pacemaker potentials**

**Figure 1.43** The effect of the autonomic nervous system on pacemaker potentials and heart rate. (a) Baseline pacemaker action potential. (b) The sympathetic nervous system causes a steeper rise in the phase 4 pacemaker potential. Threshold potential is reached quicker, so action potentials occur with greater frequency, resulting in a faster heart rate. (c) The parasympathetic nervous system reduces the pacemaker potential. Threshold potential is reached later, delaying the onset of action potentials and reducing heart rate.

the thalamus, hypothalamus and cerebral cortex.

## The sympathetic nervous system

Efferent (meaning away from the centre) sympathetic signals are transmitted from pre-ganglionic neurones in the lateral thoracic and lumbar spinal cord (levels T1-L2).

These neurones emanate from the spinal cord via anterior nerve roots and synapse with post-ganglionic neurones at one of several regions known as ganglia. Post-ganglionic neurones, destined for the heart, synapse with preganglionic neurones within ganglia located next to the thoracic vertebrae, i.e. the right and left paravertebral ganglia (sympathetic chains). Post-ganglionic cardiac innervation includes the atrial and ventricular myocardium, sinoatrial node, atrioventricular node and conduction tissues. Post-ganglionic neurones release noradrenaline (norepinephrine). Preganglionic sympathetic innervation of the adrenal medulla stimulates the release of adrenaline (epinephrine) into the bloodstream.

Noradrenaline and adrenaline bind to $\beta_1$ adrenoreceptors in the heart. These ligand-gated channels activate adenylate cyclase through a Gs-protein–coupled mechanism (see page 64–67). Activation increases cyclic AMP (cAMP) production and activates protein kinase A. cAMP activates $Na^+$ and $Ca^{2+}$ channels, which increases phase 4 pacemaker currents and thus increases heart rate. The same process augments:

- L-type $Ca^{2+}$ channels (increasing $Ca^{2+}$ influx and thus contractility)
- delayed rectifying $K^+$ channels (shortening action potential duration)
- $Ca^{2+}$ pumps (resulting in more rapid $Ca^{2+}$ clearance, which accelerates myocardial relaxation)

Therefore the effects of the sympathetic nervous system are to increase:

- heart rate, i.e. positive chronotropicity (Greek: *khronos*, time, and *trópos*, turn)
- contractility, i.e. positive inotropicity (Greek: *inos*, fibre)
- myocardial relaxation, i.e. positive lusitropicity (Greek: *lusi*, relax)
- conduction through the atrioventricular node, i.e. positive dromotropicity (Greek: *dromos*, running)

## The parasympathetic nervous system

Efferent parasympathetic innervation of the heart is through the right and left vagus nerves (the 10th cranial nerve), the axons of which emanate from the nucleus ambiguus of the medulla oblongata. Pre- and post-ganglionic neurones synapse very close to the heart. Post-ganglionic neurones primarily innervate the atrial myocardium, sinoatrial node and atrioventricular node.

Vagal activation releases acetylcholine, which binds to muscarinic $M_2$ receptors, thus antagonising cAMP production and protein kinase A activation. Vagal activation also results in $K^+$ channel activation and hyperpolarisation of the myocyte membrane. Therefore the parasympathetic nervous system reduces pacemaker potentials and heart rate. Parasympathetic innervation of the ventricles is scant, so contractility is unaffected.

> **Atropine blocks muscarinic acetylcholine receptors.** Thus atropine reduces parasympathetic activation of the heart and increases heart rate, i.e. it is a positive chronotrope.

The intrinsic rate of depolarisation depends on the location of the pacemaker cell. In the cells of the sinoatrial node, the intrinsic rate is about 110 depolarisations/min. However, the heart rate at rest is closer to 60 beats/min, and during exercise it may approach 200 beats/min. Therefore, at rest, the predominant influence is parasympathetic (vagal). Vagal tone is reduced during activity, and during exercise sympathetic activity dominates.

> **Digoxin acts centrally to increase parasympathetic activity through the vagus nerve, i.e. 'vagal tone'. This reduces atrioventricular node conductivity and limits the heart rate. Therefore digoxin is useful in treating tachycardias such as atrial fibrillation and flutter (see pages 224 and 229).**
>
> Digoxin also exerts a positive inotropic effect by inhibiting $Na^+$–$K^+$ ATPase function. This increases intracellular $Na^+$, which is exchanged for $Ca^{2+}$, leading to increased intracellular $Ca^{2+}$ and therefore increased myocyte contractility.

# Conduction of electrical activity

Each heartbeat is triggered by a wave of electrical depolarisation that spreads throughout the myocardium. As the wavefront extends through the conduction tissues, it sequentially triggers the phases of the cardiac cycle (see page 45). Haemodynamic efficiency is closely linked to the precision with which electrical activity is conducted.

## Pathway of conduction

In health, depolarisation is initiated by the sinoatrial node high in the posterior wall of the right atrium. The wavefront is conducted rapidly throughout the right atrium and, via Bachmann's bundle, through the left atrium. The atria and ventricles are electrically insulated from each other by the fibroannular rings surrounding the tricuspid and mitral valves. The only electrical connection is through the atrioventricular node in the inferior interatrial septum.

Conduction through the atrioventricular node is slow, because of prolonged phase 1, $I_{Ca-L}$ currents, and the electrical wavefront is briefly delayed (for about 0.1 s). Conduction velocity increases again, and continues, in the ventricular septum along the bundle of His.

The bundle of His divides into left and right branches. The left bundle branch subdivides into anterior and posterior hemibranches. At the cardiac apex, the bundle branch fibres branch into a vast network of Purkinje's fibres. These fibres rapidly conduct the wavefront throughout the ventricle, in an apex to base direction. This pattern of excitation and resulting contraction is optimal for the ejection of blood from the ventricles during systole.

## Cellular conduction

Cardiac myocytes are arranged longitudinally, connected end to end at intercalated discs. At these sites, anchoring proteins called desmosomes allow neighbouring cells to adhere to each other. Intercalated discs also contain gap junctions.

Gap junctions are small membrane-spanning pores (connexons) that allow the free flow of ions. Therefore they allow waves of depolarisation to spread from cell to cell, with little resistance. The gap junctions between myocardial cells enable them to act as a functional syncytium, i.e. a group of cells in continuity with each other and therefore capable of synchronised action.

The density and function of gap junctions determine the electrical resistance and speed of conduction. Cells that have just depolarised remain refractory for a short time. This refractory period ensures that wavefronts spread in an antegrade (forward) direction to polarised cells (phase 4), and not retrogradely (in reverse) in the conduction pathway.

## Pacemaker hierarchy

Automaticity is not confined to the sinoatrial node. Many areas of the heart can serve as potential pacemaker sites. This beneficial adaptation allows the heart to continue beating and thus prevent asystole even if the natural pacemaker fails, or if conduction is blocked at a particular location. However, if all the potential pacemaker tissues competed against each other, the cardiac cycle would become disorganised. A slower pacemaker is suppressed by a faster one, so the fastest pacemaker always assumes overall control and dictates heart rate.

The sinoatrial node has the highest inherent rate and therefore dictates heart rate. Subsidiary pacemaker sites are arranged hierarchically so that regions further down the conduction pathway have a slower inherent rate (Table 1.12). If the sinoatrial node fails, pacemaker cells in the atria or at the atrioventricular node assume control as the next

| Pacemaker hierarchy | |
| --- | --- |
| Pacemaker site | Intrinsic rate (depolarisations/min) |
| Sinoatrial node | 100 |
| Atrioventricular node | 40–60 |
| Bundle of His | 30–40 |
| Ventricles | ≤ 30 |

Table 1.12 Pacemaker hierarchy

fastest pacemaker site; an escape rhythm. If conduction is blocked completely, for example at the bundle of His, more distal pacemaker cells become the next fastest and assume control.

> **The heart has multiple potential pacemaker sites** as a fail-safe mechanism to prevent cardiac arrest (asystole) in the event of a conduction block. However, remember that the more distal the pacemaker, the slower the inherent 'escape' rate.

# Excitation–contraction coupling

An efficient and well-coordinated system of electrical activation and conduction is useless unless it triggers myocardial contraction. This occurs through the following process: excitation–contraction coupling.

1. During phase 2, inward $Ca^{2+}$ current through L-type channels increases intracellular $Ca^{2+}$ concentration, which activates ryanodine receptors in the sarcoplasmic reticulum membrane

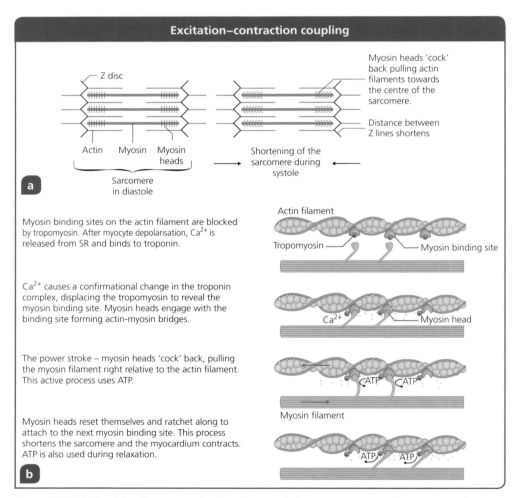

**Excitation–contraction coupling**

Z disc

Actin   Myosin   Myosin heads

Sarcomere in diastole

**a**

Shortening of the sarcomere during systole

Myosin heads 'cock' back pulling actin filaments towards the centre of the sarcomere.

Distance between Z lines shortens

Myosin binding sites on the actin filament are blocked by tropomyosin. After myocyte depolarisation, $Ca^{2+}$ is released from SR and binds to troponin.

Actin filament

Tropomyosin —    — Myosin binding site

$Ca^{2+}$ causes a confirmational change in the troponin complex, displacing the tropomyosin to reveal the myosin binding site. Myosin heads engage with the binding site forming actin-myosin bridges.

$Ca^{2+}$ — Myosin head

The power stroke – myosin heads 'cock' back, pulling the myosin filament right relative to the actin filament. This active process uses ATP.

ATP   ATP

Myosin filament

Myosin heads reset themselves and ratchet along to attach to the next myosin binding site. This process shortens the sarcomere and the myocardium contracts. ATP is also used during relaxation.

ATP   ATP

**b**

**Figure 1.44** (a) The sliding filament mechanism of myocardial contraction. Within the sarcomere, the central myosin thick filaments are surrounded by the actin thin filaments. Since myocardium is composed of many similar repeating units, the overall result is myocardial contraction causing the H band to disappear, the A band to increase and the I band to shorten. (b) Sliding filament mechanism of myocardial contraction.

2. The activation of ryanodine receptors triggers the release of $Ca^{2+}$ from sarcoplasmic reticulum stores ($Ca^{2+}$-induced $Ca^{2+}$ release)
3. The released $Ca^{2+}$ binds to troponin C molecules on the thin actin filaments (**Figure 1.44**)
4. The $Ca^{2+}$ also binds to troponin C molecules to induce a conformational change that exposes the myosin-binding site on each molecule and thus allows them to form cross-bridges with myosin
5. Binding causes a conformational change in actin that allows it to form cross-bridges with myosin (actin–myosin binding)
6. In an ATP-dependent process, the myosin heads 'cock' backwards, causing the actin filaments to slide ('ratchet') along each other
7. The sliding of actin filaments shortens the sarcomeres (systole)
8. When phase 2 ends and $Ca^{2+}$ influx ceases, $Ca^{2+}$ is pumped back into the sarcoplasmic reticulum, thus ending sarcomere shortening
9. Lengthening of the sarcomere (diastole) is also an ATP-dependent process

---

**Troponin is a complex of three protein subunits, each with a specific function.**

■ Troponin T attaches to tropomyosin in the actin filament

■ Troponin C has a $Ca^{2+}$-binding site

■ Troponin I inhibits the myosin-binding site

Troponin T and I are only found in cardiac myocytes and are used in the diagnosis of myocardial infarction or damage.

---

The process is also known as the sliding filament mechanism of myocyte contraction and is outlined in **Figure 1.44**. If the concentration of intracellular $Ca^{2+}$ increases, the number of actin–myosin cross-bridges increases and the force of contraction increases (positive inotropicity). Both sympathetic activation and increased myocardial stretch have a positive inotropic effect by increasing inward $Ca^{2+}$ currents and prolonging phase 2 of the action potential. Certain drugs have a similar effect and are known as inotropes (see page 51).

# The cardiac cycle

## Starter questions

Answers to the following questions are on page 83.

14. What would happen if there was no electrical connection between the atria and the ventricles?

To fulfil its primary function of pumping blood around the body, the heart must fill with venous blood and eject blood into the great arteries. Cardiac valves ensure that blood moves forwards and not backwards. Every heartbeat comprises a sequence of events that results in smooth and efficient cardiac function: the cardiac cycle (**Figure 1.45**).

The phases of the cardiac cycle overlap. For example, the end of atrial diastole (passive left ventricular filling) and the whole of atrial systole occur during ventricular diastole and early atrial diastole (atrial filling) occurs during ventricular systole.

The basic terms used to describe the cardiac cycle are shown in **Table 1.13**. The terms systole and diastole can refer to the ventricles or the atria. However, unless specifically stated, these terms are usually used to describe the state of the ventricles.

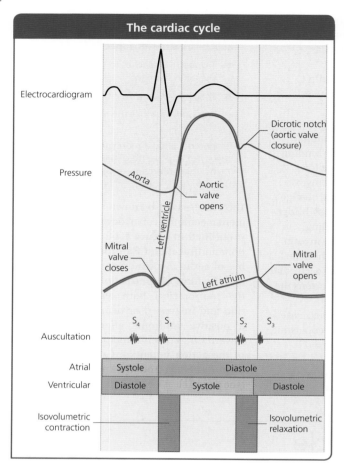

**The cardiac cycle**

Electrocardiogram

Pressure

Aorta

Left ventricle

Dicrotic notch (aortic valve closure)

Aortic valve opens

Mitral valve closes

Mitral valve opens

Left atrium

Auscultation    $S_4$    $S_1$    $S_2$    $S_3$

Atrial    Systole    Diastole

Ventricular    Diastole    Systole    Diastole

Isovolumetric contraction

Isovolumetric relaxation

**Figure 1.45** The phases of the cardiac cycle according to the electrocardiogram, pressure dynamics and heart sounds.

| Cardiac physiology terminology | |
|---|---|
| Term(s) | Definition |
| Diastole | Relaxation |
| Systole | Contraction |
| End-diastolic volume and end-systolic volume | Volume of blood in the ventricle at the end of diastole and systole, respectively |
| End-diastolic pressure and end-systolic pressure | Pressure inside the ventricle at the end of diastole and systole, respectively |
| Stroke volume | Volume of blood ejected in one cardiac cycle (normally 50–90 mL) |
| | Stroke volume = end-diastolic volume − end-systolic volume |
| Cardiac output | Volume of blood pumped by the heart in 1 min (normally 5–6 L/min at rest) |
| | Cardiac output = stroke volume × heart rate |
| $S_1$, $S_2$, $S_3$ and $S_4$ | 1st, 2nd, 3rd and 4th heart sounds |
| Atrioventricular valves | Mitral and tricuspid valves (between the atria and the ventricles) |
| Semilunar valves | Aortic and pulmonary valves |

**Table 1.13** Cardiac physiology terminology

# Atrial systole

During atrial systole, atria squeeze blood into the ventricles through the atrioventricular valves.

There are no valves between the veins and the atria. However, the sequence of electrical activation ensures that blood moves efficiently into the ventricles when the atria contract, with very little reflux into the pulmonary vein and vena cava. A small pressure wave is detectable in the veins during this phase; this is known as the a wave. Atrial systole follows a passive atrioventricular filling phase and augments ventricular filling.

Under resting conditions, atrial systole contributes about 10–20% of total end-diastolic volume. This contribution increases at higher heart rates because of the relative reduction in diastolic filling time. Ventricular stroke volume is proportional to end-diastolic volume, so atrial systole indirectly contributes to cardiac output. Atrial systole corresponds to the P wave on the ECG.

> The atrial systolic 'kick' is completely lost in atrial fibrillation because there is no coordinated atrial contraction. In an otherwise healthy heart, the haemodynamics of this do not compromise the cardiac output. However, output can be compromised in the presence of comorbid conditions, e.g. heart failure, which affect the haemodynamic function of the heart.

# Ventricular systole

During ventricular systole:

- ventricles contract
- atrioventricular valves close
- semilunar valves open
- blood is ejected

Ventricular systole causes an abrupt increase in ventricular pressure. When this pressure exceeds atrial pressure, the atrioventricular valves close. Closure of the atrioventricular valves is audible as the first heart sound ($S_1$; Table 1.14).

The atrioventricular valves bulge very slightly into the atria as they close. Therefore a small pressure wave (the c wave) can be detected in the veins by looking at the jugular venous pressure. The descent from the peak of the c wave is known as the x descent.

# Ventricular pressure increases

Until the ventricular pressure exceeds the aortic and pulmonary artery pressures, the semilunar valves remain closed. During this period, the ventricular pressure increases without any change in ventricular volume. Therefore it is known as the isovolumetric contraction time.

# The semilunar valves open and blood is ejected

The instant that ventricular pressure exceeds arterial pressure, the semilunar valves open

| Physiological basis of heart sounds | | | |
|---|---|---|---|
| Heart sound | Mechanism | Timing | Circumstance |
| 1st ($S_1$) | Atrioventricular valve closure | Immediately before the carotid pulse | Normal |
| 2nd ($S_2$) | Semilunar valve closure | Immediately after the carotid pulse | Normal |
| 3rd ($S_3$) | Rapid early (passive) ventricular filling | Shortly after $S_2$ | Can be normal in young fit people but is also a sign of increased end-diastolic pressure, which occurs in heart failure |
| 4th ($S_4$) | Atrial systole against stiffened ventricle | Shortly before $S_1$ | Indicates stiffened (hypertrophied) ventricular walls |

**Table 1.14** The physiological basis of the heart sounds

and blood flows into the pulmonary artery and aorta. The open semilunar valves offer little resistance to blood flow. Therefore, during this period, the pressure in the ventricles remains only slightly higher than the arterial pressures; the gradient across the valves is minimal. Towards the end of ventricular systole, the myocardium begins to repolarise.

On the ECG, ventricular systole corresponds to the QRS complex, and repolarisation corresponds to the T wave. Atrial repolarisation is not visualised by electrocardiography, because it occurs during ventricular systole and is hidden in the QRS complex.

During ventricular systole, venous blood flows into the atria (atrial diastole). As blood fills the atria, there is a corresponding increase in atrial pressure that corresponds to the v wave in the venous pressure trace.

> **Disease of the valves may result in stiffness, i.e. stenosis** (see Chapter 7). Stenosis increases resistance to the flow of blood resulting in greater pressure loss across the valve. The magnitude of this drop indicates the severity of valve disease, and is calculated from the flow velocity through the valve (measured with Doppler echocardiography), using the simplified Bernoulli equation:
>
> $$\Delta P = 4V^2$$
>
> $\Delta P$ is the difference in pressure and V is the blood flow velocity.

## Ventricular diastole

During ventricular diastole:

- ventricles relax
- semilunar valves close
- atrioventricular valves open

As ventricular systole ends, ventricular pressure decreases to a point at which it is less than the pulmonary and aortic pressures. At this point, the momentum of the blood allows forward flow to continue for a very short time.

Arterial blood flow very briefly reverses, which closes the semilunar valves. Closure of the semilunar valves is heard as the second heart

sound ($S_2$; **Table 1.14**). The 'rebound' of blood closing the valves is detectable in the aortic pressure signal as the dicrotic notch (or incisure).

## Ventricular pressure decreases

After the semilunar valves close, ventricular pressure continues to decrease. During this period, the volume of the ventricular cavity is unchanged until the atrioventricular valves open. Therefore this short period is known as the isovolumetric relaxation time.

Ventricular relaxation is not a passive process. Furthermore, active recoil of the ventricles effectively helps to suck in blood during the next phase.

> **Venous pressure waves normally comprise:**
>
> - a wave
> - v wave
> - x descent
> - y descent
>
> These waves are visible in the jugular vein in the neck. They are assessed during clinical examination of the cardiovascular system to help diagnose various diseases (see page 109).

## The atrioventricular valves open

As soon as atrial pressure exceeds ventricular pressure, the atrioventricular valves open. Immediately before this event is the point of peak atrial filling and pressure. This peak corresponds to the v wave in the venous pressure trace.

As the atrioventricular valves open, atrial pressure decreases rapidly. This drop in atrial pressure corresponds to a drop in the venous pressure trace: the y descent.

At first, the ventricles fill rapidly. As ventricular filling proceeds, the atrioventricular pressure gradient declines and the process continues but at a reduced rate.

Towards the end of atrial diastole, the atria contract (atrial systole) and the cycle starts again.

Myocardial contraction and relaxation are both energy-dependent processes. Impairment of either can result in heart failure. To operate as an efficient pump, the heart must eject and fill with blood. Failure to do so is the basis for 'systolic' and 'diastolic' heart failure (see page 241).

## Heart sounds

The heart sounds are the noises caused by cardiac valve closure (first and second heart sounds) or, more rarely, by turbulent blood flow during ventricular filling (third and fourth heart sounds). The clinical relevance of heart sounds is outlined in more detail in chapter 2 (page 114). **Table 1.14** outlines the physiological basis behind each of the heart sounds and **Figure 1.45** demonstrates the timing of each of the heart sounds in relation to the ECG and pressure dynamics that characterise the cardiac cycle.

# Cardiac output

## Starter questions

Answers to the following questions are on page 83.

15 Why must the cardiac output of the right and left ventricles balance?

Cardiac output is the volume of blood pumped by the left and right ventricles in 1 min (expressed as L/min). The same volume should be pumped by each ventricle.

Cardiac output is the product of stroke volume and heart rate, therefore:

cardiac output = stroke volume × heart rate

In an average-sized person under resting conditions, stroke volume is about 75 mL and heart rate is about 70 beats/min. Therefore cardiac output can be calculated thus:

cardiac output = 0.075 L × 70 beats/min = 5.25 L/min

Cardiac output increases and decreases in line with the body's metabolic demands. During strenuous exercise, output can increase fivefold. In a highly trained athlete, it may increase eightfold to > 40 L/min.

Because cardiac output is determined by stroke volume and heart rate, it can be controlled by regulating these two variables.

The average circulating blood volume is just under 5 L, and the average cardiac output is just over 5 L/min. Therefore the entire blood volume is pumped by ventricular every minute. During strenuous exercise, the entire blood volume circulates through the heart about every 10 s.

## Control of stroke volume

Stroke volume is the volume of blood ejected with each heartbeat. It is the difference between the end-diastolic volume and the end-systolic volume:

stroke volume = end-diastolic volume – end-systolic volume

Stroke volume is influenced by preload, myocardial contractility and afterload.

The ejection fraction is the percentage of blood ejected from the ventricle with each heart beat:

$$\text{ejection fraction} = \frac{\text{stroke volume}}{\text{end-diastolic volume}} \times 100$$

> In healthy people, ejection fraction is normally 50–70%. However, ejection fraction is reduced in patients with systolic heart failure. In this condition, the reduced contractility of the heart results in decreased stroke volume and increased end-diastolic volume.

## Cardiac preload

Cardiac preload is a measure of the volume and pressure of blood in the ventricle just before systole. Therefore preload is a function of both end-diastolic volume and end-diastolic pressure. Preload is the key factor influencing stroke volume.

## The Frank–Starling law of the heart

To accommodate an increase in preload, the ventricular myocardium becomes stretched. As the myocardium stretches:

- the number of active actin–myosin cross-bridges increases
- the affinity between $Ca^{2+}$ and troponin C increases

The result is a more forceful contraction and a greater stroke volume. The opposite is also true: a decrease in preload results in a reduced stroke volume. These phenomena are the basis for the Frank–Starling law of the heart, which states that 'the mechanical energy discharged during ventricular systole is a function of the initial fibre length'.

The Frank–Starling relationship (**Figure 1.46**) ensures that the output of the left and right ventricles is balanced. If the cardiac output of one ventricle increases, venous return to the other must also increase. This results in a greater end-diastolic volume and thus, according to the Frank–Starling relationship, augments stroke volume. The net result is an equalisation of left and right cardiac output.

A more detailed haemodynamic description would be:

1. Venous return to the right atrium increases (e.g. in response to exercise, increased

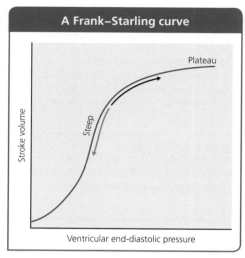

**A Frank–Starling curve**

Stroke volume

Steep

Plateau

Ventricular end-diastolic pressure

**Figure 1.46** A Frank–Starling curve. An increase in end-diastolic pressure results in a greater stroke volume (black arrow). Conversely, a decrease in end-diastolic pressure causes a reduced stroke volume (red arrow). In the physiological range, the curve is steep, indicating that the ventricles are particularly sensitive to changes in end-diastolic volume and pressure. Beyond the physiological range, the curve plateaus; further increases in end-diastolic pressure do not increase stroke volume.

blood volume or increased venous tone)
2. Increased right ventricle end-diastolic pressure causes an increase in stroke volume and cardiac output
3. Venous return to the left atrium increases
4. Increased left ventricular end-diastolic pressure results in an increase in stroke volume and cardiac output

The opposite is true of a decrease in venous return to the right atrium, for example in response to assuming an upright position, a reduction in blood volume or a reduction in venous tone. Therefore a change in the cardiac output of one ventricle influences the other so that the two outputs equalise.

The Frank–Starling relationship also explains the increase in cardiac output during exercise (increased venous return to the right ventricle) and why conditions associated with reduced venous return (e.g. haemorrhage) result in a depressed cardiac output. **Tables 1.15** and **1.16** summarise some of the factors influencing preload.

## Central venous pressure

This is the pressure of blood in the thoracic vena cava, which is continuous with the right atrial pressure. Central venous pressure reflects venous return to the heart. An increase in central venous pressure is analogous to an increase in right ventricle end-diastolic pressure (i.e. preload).

| Factors increasing preload | |
| --- | --- |
| Factor | Mechanisms |
| Central venous pressure ↑ | Exercise |
| | Increased blood volume |
| | Sympathetic venoconstriction |
| Heart rate ↓ (bradycardia) | Prolongs diastole, causing ↑ in ventricular filling time |
| Afterload ↑ | Reduces stroke volume, causing ↑ in end-systolic volume and ↑ in end-diastolic volume |
| Ventricular compliance ↑ | Ventricle accommodates greater end-diastolic volume |
| Atrial contraction | Augments filling of left ventricle, causing ↑ in end-diastolic volume |

**Table 1.15** Factors increasing preload

| Factors decreasing preload | |
| --- | --- |
| Factor | Mechanisms |
| Central venous pressure ↓ | Low blood volume (e.g. dehydration and haemorrhage) |
| Heart rate ↑ (tachycardia) | Shortens diastole, causing ↓ in ventricular filling time |
| Afterload ↓ | Increases stroke volume, causing ↓ in end-systolic volume and ↓ in end-diastolic volume |
| Ventricular compliance ↓ | Lower end-diastolic volume caused by stiffening of the myocardium |
| Loss of atrial contraction | Reduces filling of left ventricle, causing ↓ in end-diastolic volume |

**Table 1.16** Factors decreasing preload

## Influence of venous return

The veins act like a reservoir for blood volume. Fluctuations in venous tone (degree of vascular smooth muscle contraction) have similar effects to changes in circulating blood volume. An increase in venous tone reduces the volume of blood held in the venous system. This displaces blood towards the heart, which results in greater venous return and central venous pressure. Therefore an increase in venous tone is analogous to an increase in blood volume.

Conversely, a decrease in venous tone increases the volume of blood in the veins. This reduces venous return and central venous pressure, and is therefore analogous to a reduction in blood volume.

Sympathetic activation increases venous tone and therefore increases right ventricular preload. The result is an increase in stroke volume and cardiac output.

## Contractility

Contractility is the force of myocardial contraction, independent of the effects of cardiac preload. Agents that affect contractility are called inotropes (**Table 1.17**).

■ Agents that increase cytoplasmic $Ca^{2+}$ concentration increase contractility; they are called positive inotropes
■ Agents that decrease cytoplasmic $Ca^{2+}$ decrease contractility; they are negative inotropes

| Positive and negative inotropes | |
| --- | --- |
| Positive inotropes | Negative inotropes |
| Hormones, e.g. adrenaline (epinephrine) and thyroxine | General ill health (e.g. myocardial ischaemia, acidosis and hypoxia) |
| Serum ions ($Ca^{2+}$) | $\beta_1$-antagonist (beta-blockers) |
| $\beta_1$-agonist (e.g. dobutamine, isoprenaline and adrenaline) | Calcium channel blockers |
| Phosphodiesterase inhibitors (e.g. milrinone) | |

**Table 1.17** Positive and negative inotropes

Contractility is influenced by the sympathetic nervous system (see page 66). Ventricular myocytes express $\beta_1$ adrenoreceptors, which, through Gs protein coupling, activate adenylate cyclase. Adenylate cyclase, in turn, catalyses the production of cAMP. cAMP activates protein kinase A, which opens L-type $Ca^{2+}$ channels. $Ca^{2+}$ enters the myocytes through these channels, thus increasing cytoplasmic $Ca^{2+}$ concentration. Thus activation of $\beta_1$ adrenoreceptors increases contractility and heart rate.

Parasympathetic activation reduces heart rate but has no effect on contractility, because of the sparse ventricular innervation. Systolic heart failure (see page 241) is the state of reduced contractility.

An increase in contractility or a reduction in afterload shifts the Frank–Starling curve upwards (**Figure 1.47**). Conversely, a reduction in contractility or an increase in afterload shifts the curve downwards. In this example, under resting conditions, a left ventricular end-diastolic pressure of 10 mmHg corresponds to a stroke volume of 75 mL. Given an identical left ventricular end-diastolic pressure, the upper curve corresponds to a stroke volume of 100 mL, whereas the lower curve corresponds to a stroke volume of only 50 mL.

## Cardiac afterload

Afterload is the tension (force) that the ventricles must develop to eject blood. In health, afterload is determined by the pulmonary and aortic pressures, against which the ventricles contract.

- An increase in afterload increases end-systolic volume and reduces stroke volume
- An increase in preload increases end-diastolic volume and increases stroke volume

Factors increasing afterload include arterial hypertension (pulmonary and systemic) and aortic stenosis. Tension is a factor of pressure and volume (**Figures 1.45** and **1.48**). Therefore conditions associated with ventricular dilatation (e.g. dilated cardiomyopathy) are also associated with increased afterload.

A transient increase in afterload first decreases stroke volume and cardiac output. This reduction causes an increase in ventricular volume that, by the Frank–Starling mechanism, increases cardiac output, coun-

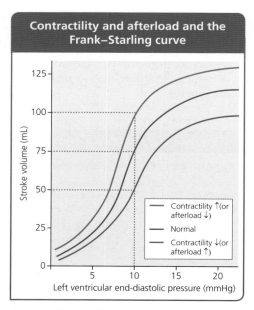

**Figure 1.47** The effect of contractility and afterload on the Frank–Starling curve.

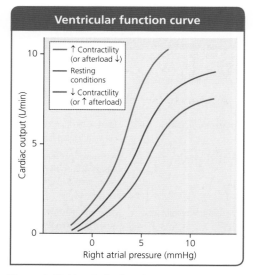

**Figure 1.48** Ventricular function curve. An increase in venous pressure (analogous to venous return) causes an increase in cardiac output, and vice versa. The curve is almost identical to the Frank–Starling curve, because of the relationships between stroke volume and cardiac output, and between right atrial pressure and end diastolic pressure.

teracting the initial reduction. However, in chronic pathological states (e.g. hypertension, valve disease and heart failure), there comes a point at which the heart can no longer compensate and cardiac output falls.

## Control of heart rate

Heart rate is a key determinant of cardiac output, especially in conditions that impair stroke volume regulation, such as heart failure and low blood volume. Heart rate is controlled by a number of integrated mechanisms.

The autonomic nervous system is the most significant influence on heart rate (see pages 41 and 66). It comprises the sympathetic system and the parasympathetic system, which act reciprocally so that activation of one is associated with inhibition of the other. If heart rate alone increases, diastolic filling time and therefore end-diastolic volume (preload) decrease. However, sympathetic activation also causes an increase in contractility that prevents a decline in stroke volume.

The principal sensory input to the cardiovascular centre is from baroreceptors. An increase in pressure results in vagal activation, which decreases heart rate, and vice versa.

Chemoreceptors also influence the cardiovascular centre. Hormones such as thyroxine and its metabolites increase heart rate. Extreme cold causes a reduction in heart rate, and higher body temperatures result in an increase in heart rate.

The mechanisms involved in heart rate control are integrated with those controlling blood pressure (see page 74).

> **Increased central venous pressure increases cardiac output by increasing cardiac preload and also through Bainbridge's reflex.** Bainbridge's reflex is the phenomenon of right atrial stretch receptors detecting the increase in pressure and responding by augmenting sympathetic activation to the heart.

# Blood circulation: vascular haemodynamics

## Starter questions

Answers to the following questions are on page 83.

16. Why are electrical circuits a good model for the circulatory system?
17. Why is the Bernoulli equation helpful for assessing valve disease?
18. Why is the difference between laminar and turbulent blood flow useful in clinical examinations?

Vascular haemodynamics (the physical laws governing vascular blood flow) can be a complicated field. However, a basic grasp of the principles governing blood flow through blood vessels is important for understanding vascular physiology and the clinical features of cardiovascular disease.

## Pressure, flow and resistance

The heart is an intermittent pump. It generates pressure that drives blood flow through the circulation. The relationship between pressure and flow is analogous to Ohm's electrical law, where $V$ is voltage (potential difference), $I$ is current and $R$ is resistance:

$$V = IR$$

In a hydraulic system such as the human circulation, potential difference is analogous to pressure difference ($\Delta P$), and current is analogous to blood flow ($Q$). Therefore the relationship between pressure, flow and resistance ($R$) can be described as:

$$\Delta P = QR$$

Rearranging the equation shows that flow equals the ratio of the pressure difference ($\Delta P$) to the resistance.

$$Q = \frac{\Delta P}{R}$$

This is logical, because an increase in driving pressure, or a reduction in the resistance to flow, would both be expected to increase blood flow.

In the circulatory system:

- the pressure difference is the difference between the mean arterial pressure generated by the heart, and the central venous pressure of blood returning to the heart
- blood flow is the cardiac output
- resistance is the total peripheral resistance

Therefore:

$$\text{Cardiac output} = \frac{\text{Mean arterial pressure – central venous pressure}}{\text{Total peripheral resistance}}$$

Cardiac output can therefore be increased by generating higher pressures by increasing cardiac contractility. However, the principal mechanism by which blood flow is regulated through the cardiovascular system is changes to peripheral arterial resistance (see pages 53–54, 63).

# The importance of vessel radius: Poiseuille's law

In haemodynamics, resistance is determined by the viscosity ($\eta$) of the flowing fluid, the length ($L$) of the vessels and the radius ($r$) of the vessel. For a straight tube, this relationship is described by the Poiseuille's equation:

$$R = \frac{8\eta L}{\pi r^4}$$

Substituting the previous equation into Poiseuille's equation produces:

$$Q = \frac{\Delta P}{L} \cdot \frac{\pi r^4}{8\eta}$$

Because blood viscosity and vessel length remain relatively constant, this equation simplifies to:

$$Q \propto \Delta P \cdot r^4$$

The key principle here is the $r^4$ term. Flow through the circulatory system increases linearly with increases in pressure but by the 4th power of the radius. This means that very small alterations in radius have a profound effect on resistance and flow. The regulation of peripheral resistance, and hence regional blood flow, is achieved by adjusting the tone of vascular smooth muscle to produce constriction and dilatation. This occurs chiefly in the arterioles (see below).

> **Poiseuille's law** means that doubling the radius of a blood vessel allows blood flow to increase 16-fold.

It is not essential to remember all the haemodynamic equations by rote. However, it is important to understand the key principles.

- Blood flow increases when blood pressure increases
- Blood flow decreases when vascular resistance increases
- Arterioles are the chief resistance vessels
- Vascular resistance is extremely sensitive to changes in the calibre of the resistance vessels (because of Poiseuille's law, $Q \propto r^4$).

# Series or parallel?

Along the length of the arterial system, arteries, arterioles, capillaries, venules and veins are arranged in series. The pulmonary circulation is in series with the systemic circulation (end to end). In contrast, through the aorta, circulation to individual organs is arranged mostly in parallel (**Figure 1.49**).

## Circulation in series and in parallel

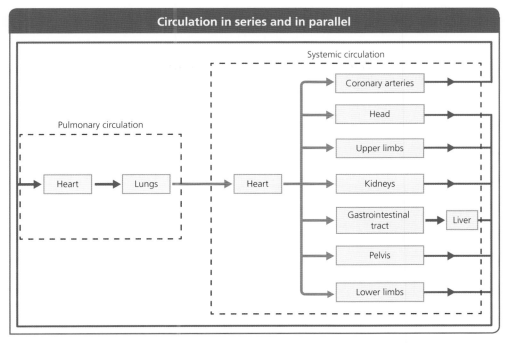

**Figure 1.49** Circulation in series and in parallel. The pulmonary and systemic circulations are arranged in series. The circulation of blood to the individual systemic organs is arranged in parallel. The gastrointestinal tract circulation drains into the portal venous system before the vena cava. The coronary circulation drains into the right atrium via the coronary sinus.

In a series arrangement, the total resistance is equal to the sum of all the individual resistances:

$$R_{total} = R_1 + R_2 + R_3 + R_n$$

In a parallel arrangement, all individual circulations experience the same systemic mean arterial pressure, and all drain to the same central venous pressure. Therefore the pressure drop across each parallel system is identical and:

$$\frac{1}{R_{total}} = \frac{1}{R_1} + \frac{1}{R_2} + \frac{1}{R_3} + \frac{1}{R_n}$$

This is significant, because the total resistance in a parallel arrangement is less than any of the individual resistances.

The parallel arrangement of organ systems in the cardiovascular system is an advantage, because it allows individual organs to receive fully oxygenated blood at a constantly high pressure. It also enables independent regulation of regional blood flow through each organ system, which would not be possible if the routes were arranged in series.

## Flow velocity

The overall rate of flow, i.e. the volume of fluid flowing per unit of time, is consistent at all levels of the systemic and pulmonary circulation. For example, all the blood volume flowing out of the left ventricle must pass through all levels of the systemic vascular tree and back to the right atrium. Therefore venous return equals cardiac output, i.e. there is continuity of flow.

Unlike the overall rate of flow, flow velocity varies throughout the circulation. Flow velocity is inversely proportional to the cross-sectional area of the system through which it flows. The total cross-sectional area of all the capillaries is far greater than that of vessels at any other level of the vascular tree. Therefore flow through the capillaries is slow and transit time prolonged. Slow flow through the capillaries allows

## Laminar and turbulent blood flow

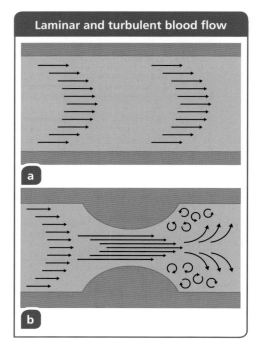

**Figure 1.50** Flow through blood vessels. (a) Laminar flow. Friction between the vessel wall and flowing blood causes a parabolic velocity profile with the highest flow velocity centrally and the slowest at the periphery. (b) Turbulent flow : acceleration through narrowed segment causes flow separation and vortex formation in the post-stenosis region.

sufficient time for the exchange of gases, nutrients and waste products (see pages 71–74).

## The effect of viscosity

Poiseuille's equation also explains why an increase in blood viscosity results in greater peripheral resistance and higher blood pressure. Blood plasma has low viscosity, similar to that of water. However, circulating erythrocytes (red blood cells) increase the viscosity of blood significantly. Therefore anaemia (a reduction in the number of erythrocytes) is associated with a reduction in total peripheral resistance, which leads to an increase in blood flow to maintain a similar blood pressure. Polycythaemia (an excess of erythrocytes) has the opposite effect.

## Laminar or turbulent?

Flow through blood vessels is normally laminar: concentric layers of fluid move parallel to the axis of the vessel (**Figure 1.50a**). Friction between the vessel wall and the flowing blood causes a parabolic velocity profile, with the highest flow velocity in the centre of the vessel and the slowest at the periphery.

However, laminar flow may become turbulent (disturbed and chaotic; **Figure 1.50b**) if:

- blood flow velocity increases (as it goes through narrower spaces)
- blood viscosity reduces
- vessel diameter increases

When blood flow is turbulent, the relationship between pressure and flow is no longer linear, and more pressure (energy) is required to affect an equivalent flow. Therefore turbulent flow is less efficient than laminar flow.

# Blood vessels

## Starter questions

Answers to the following questions are on page 83–84.

19. Why does the pressure in the arterial system not fall to zero during diastole?
20. Why do women who have undergone mastectomy often suffer from lymphoedema?

Blood vessels are not passive conduits through which blood flows. They are highly specialised, dynamic structures adapted to serve local physiological requirements. The arrangement of the vasculature allows blood to be distributed to all regions of the body to exchange gases, nutrients and waste products with the tissues, and to be returned to the heart.

# General vessel structure

Aside from the capillaries, the walls of all blood vessels consist of three layers called tunicae (**Figure 1.51**):

- tunica intima
- tunica media
- tunica externa

## Tunica intima

The tunica intima is the thinnest and innermost layer. It is composed of a single layer of endothelial cells, supported by a thin layer of connective tissue and a longitudinal arrangement of elastic fibres. The connective tissue is called the lamina propria and the elastic fibres are known as the internal elastic lamina. The luminal surface of the endothelial cells is in contact with flowing blood.

## Tunica media

The middle layer, the tunica media, is made up of smooth muscle cells and elastic fibres in a circumferential arrangement. The smooth

muscle is innervated by the sympathetic nervous system to control tone, i.e. vessel diameter. The external elastic lamina provides additional support

## Tunica externa

Also known as the tunica adventitia, the tunica externa is the outermost layer and comprises mainly collagenous connective tissue. This supporting layer fuses with surrounding connective tissue to anchor vessels in place.

The tunica externa contains its own blood and nerve supply through the vasa vasorum ('vessels of the vessels') and nervi vascularis ('nerves of the vessels'), respectively.

---

**Understanding the structure of blood vessel walls** is aided by a brief lesson in Latin.

- *Tunica*: shirt or coat
- *Intima*: inmost
- *Media*: middle
- *Externa*: outward or external
- *Lamina*: thin sheet or layer
- *Adventitia*: outside, foreign or arrived from afar
- *Propria*: to own or to possess special characteristics

---

Each type of artery and vein serves a different function according to its location and position in the vascular tree (**Table 1.18**). This is reflected in modifications to the structure and composition of the three layers (**Figure 1.52**). Arteries have a prominent tunica media. Veins have a much thinner tunica media, with the tunica externa being the principal layer. The exception is the capillary, which consists of just a single layer of endothelial cells with minimal supporting connective tissue.

# Types of vessel and their functions

Blood ejected from the left heart enters the large elastic arteries, the first of which is the aorta. As the blood advances through the system, it enters smaller muscular arteries and still smaller arterioles before enter-

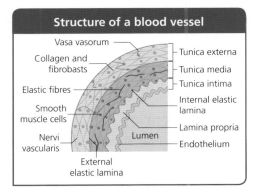

**Structure of a blood vessel**

Vasa vasorum
Collagen and fibrobasts
Elastic fibres
Smooth muscle cells
Nervi vascularis
External elastic lamina

Tunica externa
Tunica media
Tunica intima
Internal elastic lamina
Lamina propria
Endothelium
Lumen

**Figure 1.51** The general structure of a blood vessel.

## Structure and function of major vessels

| Vessel(s) | Major function | Modification |
| --- | --- | --- |
| Aorta and large elastic arteries | Compliance: distensibility and elasticity convert pulsatile to continuous flow | Thick media layer, rich in elastic fibres, collagen and smooth muscle |
| Muscular arteies | Distribution of blood to the arterioles | Thick media layer, rich in smooth muscle |
| Arterioles | Provision of resistance: regional blood flow control | Layers of smooth muscle |
| | | Richly innervated by the autonomic nervous system |
| Capillaries | Exchange of gases, nutrients and waste products with the tissues | Single layer of endothelial cells |
| Venules | Collection of capillary blood | Thin, poorly developed tunica media |
| Veins | Acts as capacitance vessel | Thin media layer, with scant elastic and smooth muscle fibres |
| | | Compliant and contains valves |
| Vena cava | Returns blood to the right atrium | Very large vein in which flow is influenced by action of respiratory and cardiac pumps |

**Table 1.18** Function and structural modifications of major vessels

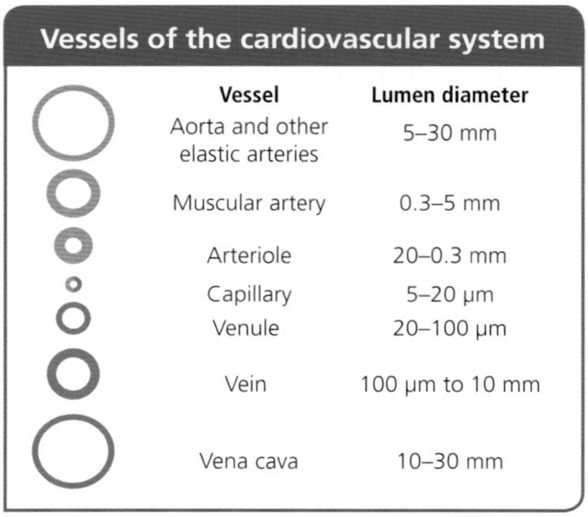

### Vessels of the cardiovascular system

| Vessel | Lumen diameter |
| --- | --- |
| Aorta and other elastic arteries | 5–30 mm |
| Muscular artery | 0.3–5 mm |
| Arteriole | 20–0.3 mm |
| Capillary | 5–20 μm |
| Venule | 20–100 μm |
| Vein | 100 μm to 10 mm |
| Vena cava | 10–30 mm |

**Figure 1.52** The vessels of the cardiovascular system. The composition of the vessel tunicae and the size of the lumen vary according to function.

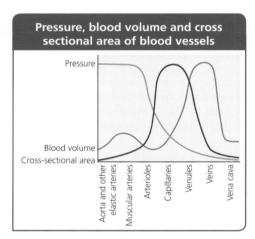

### Pressure, blood volume and cross sectional area of blood vessels

**Figure 1.53** Pressure, blood volume and cross-sectional area at each level of circulation. The largest pressure drop occurs at the resistance vessels (arterioles). The veins (capacitance vessels) hold the most blood volume. The capillaries have the largest surface area.

ing the capillaries. The capillary is where the exchange of nutrients and gases occurs. From the capillaries, blood returns to the heart through venules, veins and finally the vena cava, which empties into the right atrium.

Each vessel type has a specific function, adapting to variability in pressure, volume and surface area through the vascular tree from the aorta to the vena cava (**Figure 1.53**).

## Elastic arteries

The major proximal arteries (the aorta and the brachiocephalic, carotid, subclavian, iliac and pulmonary arteries) are elastic arteries. They contain high numbers of elastic fibres in the tunica media. Elastic arteries are also rich in smooth muscle, but this remains relatively quiescent.

Most (about two thirds) of the cardiac cycle is spent in diastole, yet blood flow though the peripheral circulation is continuous. This is necessary in order to maintain constant organ perfusion.. The conversion of pulsatile to continuous flow is made possible by the compliance of the elastic arteries.

When a ventricle contracts, high pressure is generated in the proximal arteries; this drives blood flow. However, the elastic arteries distend under the pressure, thus absorbing some of the energy. During diastole, they recoil and discharge the stored energy. Therefore the elastic arteries act as a hydraulic capacitor (or hydraulic filter): they absorb (store) energy during systole and discharge energy during diastole. The net result is continuous blood flow through the arterial system.

## Muscular arteries

Elastic arteries branch into the next generation of arteries, the smaller muscular arteries. Muscular arteries are also known as distributing arteries, because their primary function is to distribute blood to the resistance vessels. They contain multiple layers of smooth muscle. Examples of muscular arteries are the radial, mesenteric and femoral arteries.

## Arterioles

Muscular arteries branch into smaller arteries and arterioles. The arterioles are known as the resistance vessels, because they contribute the most resistance to blood flow. Arterioles contain one or two layers of vascular smooth muscle and are able to regulate their tone, i.e. the residual tension that controls vessel diameter.

Arteriolar tone directly influences flow through the distal capillary bed, as well as blood pressure and vascular resistance. Flow is equal to pressure divided by resistance; if the tone is reduced (vasodilation), resistance decreases and flow increases. Only small changes in the diameter of the resistance vessels result in significant alterations in blood flow (see page 53–54).

Arterioles are richly innervated by the sympathetic nervous system and are subject to hormonal regulation.

## Capillaries

The capillaries are composed of just a single endothelial cell layer. They are the smallest of all blood vessels in the body, being 5–20 µm in diameter and about 1 mm long. However, together they have a very large cross-sectional area, which results in a slow transit time.

The capillaries are known as exchange vessels, because it is at their level that the primary function of the cardiovascular system is carried out: the exchange of gases, nutrients and waste products between the blood and the tissues. The thin walls, large combined surface area and slow transit time of the capillaries make them well suited for their role.

There are three main types of capillary (**Table 1.19**):

- continuous
- fenestrated
- discontinuous (or sinusoidal)

In the brain, there is a high density of endothelial cells tightly connected by tight junctions and other structural proteins. Thus capillary endothelium is rendered impermeable to even small molecules; this is the basis for the blood–brain barrier.

## The microcirculation

The microcirculation comprises the:

- terminal arterioles (resistance vessels)
- capillaries (exchange vessels)
- post-capillary venules (drainage vessels)

Flow through the microcirculation is regulated extrinsically and intrinsically (see page 63–68).

- Extrinsic regulation is provided chiefly by the sympathetic nervous system, which innervates the proximal arterioles
- Intrinsic control is through autoregulation of the terminal arterioles

The precise architecture of the microcirculation varies; specific patterns reflect the functional demands of the tissue. Terminal arterioles divide into capillaries, which form a network of interconnected vessels draining into the post-capillary venule (**Figure 1.54**).

| The main types of capillary | | | |
|---|---|---|---|
| Type | Typical location | Endothelial structure | Notes on function |
| Continuous | Skeletal muscles and skin | Uninterrupted layer bound incompletely by tight junctions that leave small clefts in the capillary wall | Permit small molecules and ions to diffuse across the endothelium |
| Fenestrated | Kidneys, gut and glandular tissue | Contain fenestrations (pores) covered loosely by a membrane | More permeable than continuous capillaries to hydrophilic molecules |
| | | | Present in vascular beds where rapid diffusion of hydrophilic molecules is necessary |
| Discontinuous (or Sinusoidal) | Liver, bone marrow and spleen | Lack tight junctions, so the endothelium is interrupted by gaps between cells | Permits large proteins and blood cells (erythrocytes and leucocytes) to cross the capillary wall |
| | | | Well suited to the hepatic and haemopoietic tissues, where this ability is necessary |

**Table 1.19** The main types of capillary

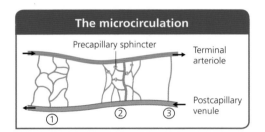

**Figure 1.54** The microcirculation. ① The simple branched microcirculation architecture present in most tissues. ② Central metarteriole, a thoroughfare channel with branching capillaries. ③ Direct atrioventricular anastomosis found in cutaneous tissues.

In some tissues, for example the splanchnic circulation, capillaries branch from metarterioles. Metarterioles provide a direct thoroughfare from the arteriole to the post-capillary venule.

Rings of vascular smooth muscle encircle the entrance to the capillaries. These precapillary sphincters control whether blood flows through the capillaries or shunts directly into the post-capillary venules through the metarteriole. Direct, unbranched arteriovenous anastomoses serve a key role in controlling cutaneous blood flow and thermoregulation.

Blood flow through the microcirculation is not constant. Even under stable, resting conditions, terminal arterioles undergo slow rhythmic contraction and relaxation. This is called capillary vasomotion and results in oscillating flow.

# Venules and veins

Distally, the post-capillary venules join to form venules, which join to form veins. Venules and veins contain smooth muscle but have a much thinner medial layer. In contrast to arteries, veins are thin, compliant and lack elastic recoil. Consequently, they accommodate large increases in blood volume with minimal increase in pressure. These factors account for the significantly lower pressure in the venous system. However, the overall cross-sectional area of the venous compartment is large, so it offers little resistance to flow. Low resistance means that the low pressures in the venous compartment are sufficient to return blood to the heart.

**Varicose veins are caused by incompetent venous valves.** Valvular incompetence causes reversed venous flow and increased venous pressure (venous hypertension). Clinically, this results in chronically distended, tortuous superficial veins. These are not just cosmetically displeasing; they may also cause aching, eczema and chronic skin changes (see page 319).

Compared with the arteries, veins accommodate a far greater proportion of circulating blood at any one time. Therefore veins are known as capacitance vessels. The capacity to act as a reservoir for large volumes of blood is regulated by the autonomic nervous system.

Sympathetic activation, for example in response to decreased blood pressure, results in venous constriction. The constriction displaces blood volume towards the heart, increasing venous return (and central venous pressure). These changes result in a homeostatic increase in cardiac output through the Frank–Starling mechanism.

## Venous return

The effect of gravity is such that venous pressure depends on posture.

- In the supine position, all veins are at about the level of the heart, and venous pressure is uniformly close to zero
- In the upright posture, venous pressure in the feet can be as high as 100 mmHg

The pressure at the level of the heart remains close to zero. In the head, there is negative venous pressure.

Gravity affects arterial pressure in a similar manner to its effects on venous pressure. This ensures that a local arterial–venous pressure gradient is maintained. Although high venous pressures in the lower extremities encourage blood pooling, this phenomenon is limited by reflex vasoconstriction, which maintains venous return to the right heart. Reverse blood flow in the veins is prevented by valves that allow blood to pass in the anterograde direction only.

Venous return is driven by the arterial–venous pressure gradient, which forces flow to the veins from behind (vis a tergo). This effect is aided by three additional mechanisms, which act as pumps: the cardiac pump, the respiratory pump and the muscle pump.

## The cardiac pump

As the tricuspid valve opens, the right ventricle expands and blood is drawn in. This action draws (sucks) blood into the right atrium from the vena cava.

## The respiratory pump

Inspiration causes a decrease in intrathoracic pressure but an increase in intra-abdominal pressure, because of the movement of the diaphragm. This augments the pressure gradient driving blood towards the heart. The opposite effect occurs on expiration. A prolonged Valsalva manoeuvre (forced expiration against a closed glottis) reduces venous return to a point at which syncope may occur.

> **Standing upright for prolonged periods causes blood to pool in the legs.** Blood pooling reduces venous return and is a trigger for vasovagal syncope, otherwise known as fainting (see page 94). In vasovagal syncope, sympathetic activation is followed by reflex parasympathetic (vagal) activation and sympathetic inhibition. This triggers cardioinhibition (reduced heart rate and contractility) and vasodepression (widespread vasodilation). Cardiac output decreases and effective blood volume is reduced (because of increased venous capacity). The net effect is a drop in blood pressure, causing loss of consciousness.

## The muscle pump

Contraction of skeletal muscle displaces blood in the veins and drives it back to the heart (**Figure 1.55**). The skeletal muscle pump

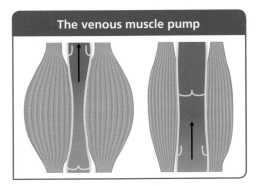

**Figure 1.55** The venous muscle pump. (a) Muscular contraction compresses the vein, displacing the blood within. (b) When the muscles relax, the vein re-expands, drawing in blood from the distal compartment.

is augmented by even light exercise, such as walking.

## Lymphatic system

The lymphatic system forms an additional circulatory system. Lymphatic vessels clear tissue fluid (lymph) from the extracellular space.

The capillaries filter about 20 L of fluid (plasma) per day. However, they reabsorb only 15–18 L (see page 72). Therefore the lymphatic vessels collect the extra fluid and transport it back into the bloodstream to prevent its accumulation in tissue. The lymphatic system is an arrangement of capillaries and vessels that transport lymph through lymphoid tissues back to the bloodstream via the subclavian veins (**Figure 1.56**). Lymphatic vessels also transport digested fatty acids from the gut to the bloodstream.

**Lymphadenopathy is the local or generalised swelling of lymph nodes.** It can be caused by infection, autoimmunity or malignancy. Lymphadenopathy can also represent metastatic spread of a tumour or lymphoma, a cancer of the lymphoid tissue itself.

## Lymphoid tissue

Lymphoid tissues include lymph nodes and mucosa-associated lymphoid tissue, (e.g. lymph follicles) in regions such as the tonsils, spleen, intestines and adenoids.

The function of these lymphoid tissues is to detect and process antigens. These tissues contain a high concentration of lymphocytes, which are activated by antigen processing. Activation of lymphocytes causes their clonal expansion. This effect is essential for triggering a prompt antibody-mediated immune response to any microbes or foreign materials that arrive at lymphoid tissues in the afferent vessels. The inguinal, axillary and cervical lymph node groups are superficial and can be palpated during clinical examination.

**If lymphatic drainage is disrupted, tissue fluid accumulates. The result is significant swelling (oedema) in the distal tissues: lymphoedema (see 73 and 96).** The skin acquires the appearance of orange peel, a phenomenon referred to by the French term peau d'orange. Lympoedema has many causes, a common one being lymph node resection as part of breast cancer surgery to prevent lymphatic spread of a tumour.

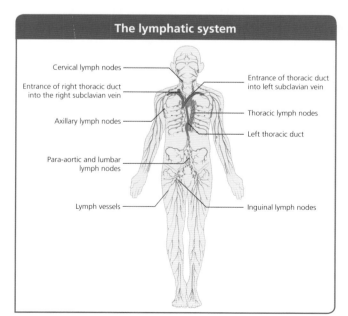

**The lymphatic system**

Cervical lymph nodes

Entrance of right thoracic duct into the right subclavian vein

Axillary lymph nodes

Para-aortic and lumbar lymph nodes

Lymph vessels

Entrance of thoracic duct into left subclavian vein

Thoracic lymph nodes

Left thoracic duct

Inguinal lymph nodes

**Figure 1.56** The lymphatic system.

## Lymphatic circulation

Lymph capillaries are blind-ending, thin-walled vessels present in most body tissues. They consist of a single layer of overlapping endothelial cells. Areas of cell overlap act like valves that permit extracellular fluid, proteins and microbes to enter but do not allow outward flow.

During conditions that increase the volume of extracellular fluid (oedema or inflammation), the surrounding tissue volume expands. This physically stretches the endothelial cells apart. The stretching increases lymphatic permeability and fluid flow, which helps to clear the excess tissue fluid (**Figure 1.57**).

Lymph capillaries join to become collecting vessels. These vessels contain smooth muscle and internal valves. External muscular compression, local arterial pulsation and intrinsic smooth muscle contraction each displace lymph fluid forwards, in a similar way to the venous muscle pump. Some lymph is reabsorbed

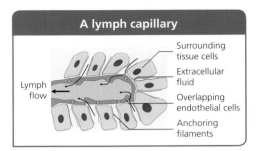

**A lymph capillary**

Surrounding tissue cells

Extracellular fluid

Lymph flow

Overlapping endothelial cells

Anchoring filaments

**Figure 1.57** A lymph capillary.

into the blood in the lymph nodes. The remaining fluid re-enters the bloodstream.

- Lymph from the right side of the head and neck, and from the right arm and upper torso, drains into the right subclavian vein
- Lymph from all other regions of the body drains into the abdominal cisterna chyli and onwards through the thoracic duct, which carries lymph to enter the circulation via the left subclavian vein

# Local and regional blood flow control

## Starter questions

Answers to the following questions are on page 84.

21. Why does coronary atherosclerosis only limit blood flow to the myocardium when it occludes ≥50% of the arterial diameter?
22. Why do systemic and pulmonary arterioles react in opposite ways to hypoxia?

Blood flow must:

- be continuous to avoid ischaemia
- match metabolic demands

Blood flow ($Q$) through the vasculature is determined by the driving blood pressure ($P$) and the resistance to flow ($R$):

$$Q = \frac{P}{R}$$

Resistance is determined by the vascular smooth muscle tone in the arterioles. Because mean arterial blood pressure is maintained at a relatively constant level by homeostatic mechanisms (see pages 74–91), blood flow is regulated by controlling the diameter of the arterioles feeding the capillary beds.

The mechanisms controlling blood flow can be divided into:

- extrinsic control mechanisms, which have a more generalised effect on the circulation
- intrinsic control mechanisms, which control localised blood flow

# Vascular smooth muscle

Contraction in vascular smooth muscle, in a similar way to in cardiac muscle, results from actin and myosin filaments sliding over each other (see page 44), a process triggered by an increase in intracellular $Ca^{2+}$. Unlike cardiac muscle, which undergoes rapid, transient contraction, vascular smooth muscle exerts a slow, sustained, tonic contraction that consumes significantly less ATP. Furthermore, vascular smooth muscle lacks the troponin complex, and its cells are not arranged in striations

Vascular smooth muscle contracts in response to:

- electrical stimulation (membrane depolarisation)
- mechanical stimulation (stretch)
- chemical stimulation (receptor binding)

All three mechanisms increase intracellular $Ca^{2+}$, which enters the cytoplasm from the extracellular space and is released from intracellular sarcoplasmic reticulum stores.

The mechanism of excitation–contraction coupling is distinct from that in cardiac myocytes. In vascular smooth muscle, $Ca^{2+}$ binds to the protein calmodulin. The $Ca^{2+}$–calmodulin complex activates myosin light chain kinase, which in turn phosphorylates myosin light chains, allowing actin–myosin cross-bridges to form. Vascular smooth muscle contraction then proceeds. $Ca^{2+}$ is actively removed from the myocyte by $Ca^{2+}$ ATPase pumps and the $Na^+$–$Ca^{2+}$ exchanger.

Vascular smooth muscle always has some degree of tone. However, the magnitude of tone is proportional to the intracellular $Ca^{2+}$ concentration. Therefore vascular smooth muscle tone is determined by the balance between $Ca^{2+}$ influx and $Ca^{2+}$ removal mechanisms.

# Extrinsic control of blood flow

Vascular smooth muscle tone is regulated extrinsically through a host of chemicals that act through signal transduction pathways, as well as the autonomic nervous system.

Therefore extrinsic control of vascular tone is determined by:

- vasoconstricting and vasodilating chemicals in the blood
- the activity of the autonomic nervous system
- variations in the distribution of different receptor types

# The inositol triphosphate–diacylglycerol pathway

This pathway causes vasoconstriction when activated by:

- the catecholamines adrenaline (epinephrine) and noradrenaline (norepinephrine) (through $\alpha_1$ receptors)
- angiotensin II
- thromboxane $A_2$
- endothelin 1
- vasopressin

Binding of these molecules to a membrane-bound receptor activates a G protein ($G_q$)–coupled mechanism that activates phospholipase C (**Figure 1.58**). Phospholipase C converts phosphatidylinositol bisphosphate into inositol triphosphate and diacylglycerol. Inositol triphosphate stimulates the release of $Ca^{2+}$ from the sarcoplasmic reticulum. Diacylglycerol activates protein kinase C, which, through a further pathway, promotes myosin light chain phosphorylation, augmenting contraction. Further effects include membrane depolarisation (by opening L-type $Ca^{2+}$ channels) and $Ca^{2+}$ sensitisation, which amplifies the contractile response relative to the cytoplasmic $Ca^{2+}$ concentration.

# The adenylate cyclase (cAMP) pathway

Adenylate cyclase converts ATP into cAMP (**Figure 1.59**). Unlike in cardiac myocytes, an increase in cAMP reduces vascular smooth muscle contractility, because cAMP inhibits myosin light chain kinase.

Receptor binding triggers one of two things.

- Inhibit adenylate cyclase through the $G_i$ protein–coupled mechanism, resulting in a reduction in cAMP, which leads to vasoconstriction; catecholamines activate this pathway via $\alpha2$ receptors,

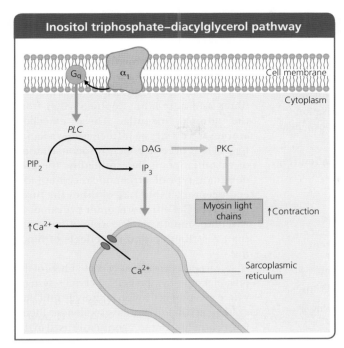

**Figure 1.58** The $\alpha_1$ adrenoreceptor, $G_q$-coupled to the inositol triphosphate ($IP_3$)–diacylglycerol (DAG) pathway. Receptor binding activates these pathways. The net effect is a rise in intracellular Ca2+, increased smooth muscle contraction and vasoconstriction. $PIP_2$, phosphatidylinositol bisphosphate; PKC, protein kinase C; PLC, phospholipase C.

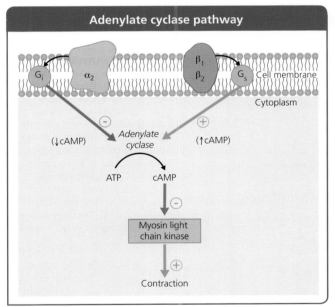

**Figure 1.59** The adenylate cyclase pathway and the $\alpha_2$, $\beta_1$ and $\beta_2$ receptors. cAMP, cyclic AMP. Adenylyl cyclase is inhibited by the $G_i$ coupled $\alpha_2$ receptor and stimulated by the Gs coupled $\beta_1$ and $\beta_2$ adrenoreceptors. Inhibition of adenylyl cyclase reduces cAMP which reduces inhibition of MLCK resulting in vasoconstriction. Stimulation of adenylyl cyclase increases cAMP levels which results in vasodilatation.

■ Stimulate adenylate cyclase through the $G_s$ protein–coupled mechanism, resulting in an increase in cAMP, which leads to vasodilatation; catecholamines (acting through $\beta_2$ receptors), adenosine and acetylcholine cause vasodilatation through this pathway

## Nitric oxide–cyclic GMP pathway

This pathway is triggered by nitric oxide. Nitric oxide is synthesised by vascular endothelial cells. It diffuses through the vascular smooth muscle cell membrane and activates guanylate cyclase, which generates cyclic guanosine monophosphate (cGMP) from guanosine triphosphate (GTP). cGMP:

- inhibits $Ca^{2+}$ influx
- reduces intracellular $Ca^{2+}$
- reduces inositol triphosphate synthesis
- inhibits cell membrane depolarisation
- causes dephosphorylation of myosin light chains

All these effects result in vasodilation (**Figure 1.60**).

> **Cyclic GMP is broken down by the enzyme phosphodiesterase**. A specific phosphodiesterase (type 5) is present in vascular smooth muscle cells of the corpus cavernosum in the penis. Sildenafil (Viagra) and similar drugs inhibit this enzyme, causing the prolonged vasodilation that sustains an erection.

# The sympathetic nervous system

Activation of the sympathetic nervous system triggers the release of noradrenaline (norepinephrine) from the postganglionic fibres and adrenaline (epinephrine) from the adrenal medulla. These catecholamines have a strong influence on vascular tone. Their precise effect, vasoconstriction or vasodilation, is determined by the predominant type of adrenergic receptor (adrenoreceptor). **Table 1.20** outlines the three main types of adrenoreceptor prevalent in vascular smooth muscle cells along with their distribution and the effects of binding.

$\alpha_2$ receptors are also present in fibres of the preganglionic sympathetic nervous system, where receptor activation is strongly inhibitory. Their activation causes vasodilation. Therefore centrally acting $\alpha_2$ agonists are used in the treatment of hypertension.

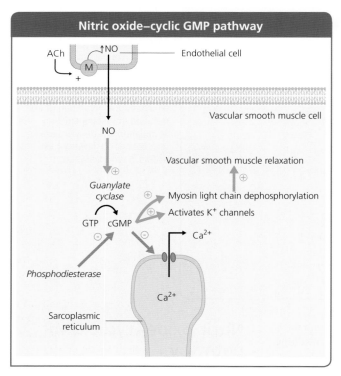

**Nitric oxide–cyclic GMP pathway**

ACh
↑NO
M
Endothelial cell
+
Vascular smooth muscle cell
NO
Vascular smooth muscle relaxation
⊕
Guanylate cyclase
⊕
Myosin light chain dephosphorylation
⊕
Activates K⁺ channels
GTP   cGMP
⊖
⊖
$Ca^{2+}$
Phosphodiesterase
$Ca^{2+}$
Sarcoplasmic reticulum

**Figure 1.60** The nitric oxide–cyclic GMP pathway. NO is produced by endothelial cells (in this case, in response to acetyl choline via a muscaranic receptor). NO diffuses through the vascular smooth muscle cell membrane and activates guanylyl cylcase which converts GTP to cGMP. cGMP has several effects, all of which promote vasodilatation. cGMP is broken down by phosphodiesterase. ACh, acetylcholine; cGMP, cyclic guanosine monophosphate; GTP, guanosine triphosphate; M, muscarinic receptor; NO, nitrous oxide.

| Vascular smooth muscle adrenoreceptors | | | | |
|---|---|---|---|---|
| Receptor | Effect of catecholamine binding | Transduction mechanism | Site | Major ligand |
| $\alpha_1$ | Vasoconstriction | $G_q$-coupled activation of phospholipase C (increases inositol triphosphate and diacylglycerol) | Splanchnic, renal and cutaneous circulations | Binds adrenaline (epinephrine) and noradrenaline (norepinephrine) equally |
| $\alpha_2$ | Vasoconstriction | $G_i$-coupled inhibition of adenylate cyclase (decreases cyclic AMP) | Veins | Binds adrenaline with greater affinity than noradrenaline |
| $\beta_2$ | Vasodilation | $G_s$-coupled activation of adenylate cyclase (increases cyclic AMP) | Skeletal muscle and coronary circulation | Binds noradrenaline and adrenaline equally |

**Table 1.20** Adrenoreceptors in vascular smooth muscle

$\beta_1$ receptors are mainly present in the myocardium, where binding increases heart rate and contractility. Vascular smooth muscle $\beta_1$ receptors also cause vasodilation, but this effect is less significant.

## The parasympathetic nervous system

The parasympathetic nervous system releases acetylcholine. In vascular smooth muscle, acetylcholine binds to muscarinic receptors, which induces vasoconstriction through the inositol triphosphate–diacylglycerol pathway. However, in the vasculature, acetylcholine is predominantly a vasodilator, because it binds to endothelial receptors, triggering the synthesis and release of nitric oxide (**Figure 1.60**). The vasodilator effect of acetylcholine overpowers its vasoconstricting effect.

The vasodilating influence of the parasympathetic nervous system on vascular smooth muscle cells is significant only in a limited number of regions including the genitals, salivary glands and bladder. In the penis, parasympathetic nervous system–mediated vasodilation of vessels in the corpora spongiosum and cavernosa induce erection.

> Clinically, $\alpha_1$ agonists are used in conditions such as septic shock. These drugs augment systemic blood pressure through vasoconstriction of peripheral blood vessels.

## Intrinsic control of blood flow: autoregulation

Autoregulation:

- maintains constant tissue perfusion (blood flow) despite fluctuations in blood pressure
- matches blood flow to metabolic demands, which vary according to activity

Autoregulation controls blood flow at a local level. It is an automatic process, intrinsic to the blood vessels themselves. Autoregulation involves myogenic control and metabolic adaption.

## Myogenic control

Myogenic control is a process by which vascular smooth muscle responds directly to variations in blood pressure. Ordinarily, an increase in perfusion blood pressure would result in an increase in flow. However, increased pressure stretches vascular smooth muscle, which responds by increasing its tone and vasoconstricting. The corresponding increase in resistance opposes the increase in flow, and this maintains a constant flow. Reduced hydrostatic pressure results in reflex vasodilation. Thus myogenic control maintains constant blood flow in situations of fluctuating mean arterial blood pressure (**Figure 1.61**).

## Myogenic control of blood flow

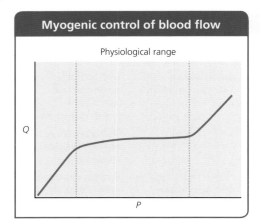

Physiological range

Q

P

**Figure 1.61** Myogenic control ensures that flow (*Q*) remains constant in a physiological range of blood pressure (*P*). Beyond this range, myogenic control fails and flow is affected.

## Metabolic control of blood flow

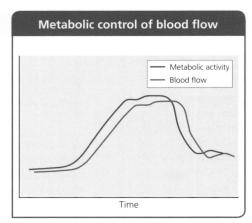

— Metabolic activity
— Blood flow

Time

**Figure 1.62** Metabolic adaptation ensures that blood flow corresponds with prevailing metabolic demands over time.

## Metabolic adaptation

When an organ or a region of tissue becomes more active, it requires increased blood flow to deliver more oxygen and nutrients and to remove more carbon dioxide and waste products. Increased cellular metabolism produces an increase in metabolites, which diffuse into the interstitial space, local to the arterioles. Arterioles are sensitive to a range of metabolites and respond by vasodilating, which increases local flow. When tissue is less active, fewer metabolites are produced and arteriolar tone increases again, bringing flow back to baseline. Thus local blood flow is closely matched to prevailing metabolic demands (**Figure 1.62**).

Key metabolic factors include:

- $K^+$ ions
- adenosine
- carbon dioxide

A reduction in blood flow to a tissue region, for example when a tourniquet is applied, causes ischaemia and an increase in metabolic factors. Restoration of flow, for example by removal of a tourniquet, results in vasodilation and increased flow.

- When hyperaemia (increased flow) is a response to increased metabolic activity, it is known as metabolic hyperaemia or functional hyperaemia

- When it occurs secondary to transient hypoperfusion or ischaemia (cessation and restoration of flow), it is termed reactive hyperaemia

## Regional blood flow control

Some organs require a dynamic blood flow to reflect fluctuations in metabolic activity; other organs, such as the brain, require a very constant blood flow. The body is adapted to divert blood flow to the areas where it is needed. For example, during strenuous exercise blood flow is increased to the skeletal muscle, heart and skin but reduced to the gut and kidneys. However, such diversions in blood flow do not occur at the expense of cerebral and myocardial perfusion, which must be preserved at all times.

Blood flow is tightly controlled and maintained in the brain, kidneys and heart, by precise autoregulatory control. This is less relevant in the skeletal muscle, gut, liver and cutaneous circulation, where autoregulation is less well developed.

**Left-sided heart failure causes pulmonary venous pressure to increase.** Eventually, the increased pressure causes fluid to filter from the capillaries into the interstitial space and alveoli. This produces pulmonary oedema, which is a medical emergency (see page 249).

# Pulmonary circulation

The pulmonary circulation receives the total cardiac output. The pulmonary arteries are large in diameter and thin walled. They are structurally similar to veins and offer little resistance to flow. Therefore blood flows through the pulmonary circulation at much lower arterial pressures (20/10 mmHg) than in the systemic circulation (120/80 mmHg). Reduced hydrostatic pressure means that there is no significant net filtration out of the pulmonary capillaries (see pages 71–73).

Autoregulatory response in the pulmonary circulation is the opposite of that in the systemic circulation, in that hypoxia causes vasoconstriction, and vice versa. This ensures that blood perfusion is directed to well-ventilated areas of lung and bypasses poorly ventilated areas. Good ventilation–perfusion coupling ensures optimal gaseous exchange.

> The low perfusion pressures of the pulmonary circulation make it particularly sensitive to the effects of gravity, with lower pressures in the lung apices and higher pressures in the basal segments. This is why patients with pulmonary oedema are helped by sitting upright. This position reduces their apical and midzone perfusion pressures and helps relieve their symptoms.

# Cerebral circulation

The cerebral circulation is regulated by the most precise autoregulatory system in the body. The brain is positioned inside a rigid skull and is intolerant to ischaemia. Therefore a cerebral blood flow that is slightly too high or low can have devastating consequences.

Myogenic control maintains total cerebral blood flow at a constant rate (about 750 mL/min) at all times. However, metabolic adaptation is particularly sensitive to increases in carbon dioxide and pH, which induce vasodilation and allow regional variations in brain activity to be matched by local variations in flow. Hypocapnia (low carbon dioxide, which occurs with hyperventilation) induces cerebral vasoconstriction and occasionally transient loss of consciousness (syncope).

Myogenic control protects the brain from fluctuations in blood pressure. However, it cannot compensate with extremely high (mean > 160 mmHg) or low (mean < 55 mmHg) blood pressures when, cerebral oedema and ischaemia develop respectively.

## Cushing's reflex

The brain lies inside a rigid skull. Therefore any abnormal increase in intracranial pressure, for example from a brain tumour, causes vascular compression, threatening cerebral perfusion. As a response to increased intracranial pressure, the autonomic nervous system becomes activated. This results in:

- increased systemic blood pressure (sympathetic activation)
- reduced heart rate (parasympathetic activation)

This combined response helps maintain cerebral perfusion and is known as Cushing's reflex.

# Coronary circulation

Myocardium has a high capillary density, and cardiac myocytes are densely packed with mitochondria. Consequently, the heart extracts more oxygen from the blood than any other organ (about 70%), even during resting conditions. Therefore increasing blood flow is the only way of providing more oxygen during exercise. At rest, the heart receives blood at a rate of about 200–250 mL/min, but this coronary blood flow can increase fourfold during exercise, secondary to metabolic adaptation.

Uniquely, coronary blood flow is impaired during systole and enhanced during diastole.

- In systole, the small coronary vessels that penetrate the myocardium are compressed as the myocardium contracts under high pressure
- During diastole, these vessels are no longer compressed and flow is restored

This effect is more pronounced in the left coronary system than in the right; this is a reflection of the higher left ventricular pressures (**Figure 1.63**).

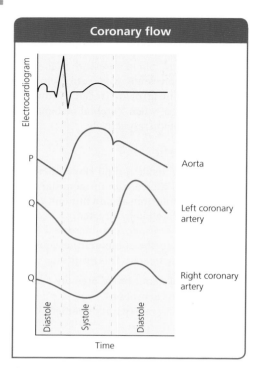

**Coronary flow**

P — Aorta

Q — Left coronary artery

Q — Right coronary artery

Diastole | Systole | Diastole

Time

**Figure 1.63** Coronary flow. Aortic pressure (P) peaks in systole; left coronary arterial flow (Q) peaks in diastole, due to high systolic resistance caused by compression of vessels in the left ventricular wall. This effect is less pronounced in the right coronary artery, due to the lower right ventricular systolic pressures.

## Coronary flow reserve

The ratio of maximal flow velocity in a coronary artery to resting flow is the coronary flow reserve. Coronary flow velocity is measured with an intracoronary Doppler wire during coronary angiography. The velocity is measured at rest and during pharmacologically induced maximal flow. Hyperaemic flow velocity divided by baseline velocity is the coronary flow reserve. Coronary flow reserve is reduced in patients with significant, flow-limiting coronary artery disease.

## Skeletal muscle circulation

Blood flow to the skeletal muscle is about 1000 mL/min at rest but can increase more than tenfold during exercise. Under resting conditions, skeletal muscle arterioles maintain a high basal tone and are mainly under myogenic control. During exercise, the effects of metabolic adaptation and the sympathetic nervous system dominate. Adrenaline (epinephrine) and noradrenaline (norepinephrine) cause vasodilatation through $\beta_2$ adrenoreceptors. During strenuous exercise, blood is diverted away from non-vital areas, such as the gut and skin, to optimise flow to the muscles.

At the limits of physical exercise, very high levels of sympathetic activation cause vasoconstriction through activation of a adrenoreceptors. This protective mechanism is triggered when muscle oxygen delivery diminishes despite maximal flow. It protects blood flow to vital organs such as the brain and kidneys.

> **The body diverts blood to where it is most needed.** During strenuous exercise, blood flow to the heart and skin increases, and flow to skeletal muscles increases more than tenfold. These changes are achieved by increasing cardiac output and diverting blood from less vital areas, such as the gut.

## Cutaneous circulation

The skin does not have a high metabolic demand. Under basal conditions, the cutaneous circulation receives only about 2–3% of total cardiac output. Cutaneous vessels play a key role in thermoregulation.

- Cutaneous vasodilation allows more blood to flow close to the skin surface, which increases heat loss and cools the circulating blood
- Cutaneous vasoconstriction limits superficial blood flow, thus promoting heat conservation

A decrease in body temperature is detected by central and peripheral thermoreceptors. This causes sympathetic activation and cutaneous vasoconstriction through a adrenoreceptors. Increased body temperature results in a reduction in cutaneous sympathetic activity. Local skin temperature also influences cutaneous vascular tone through an intrinsically mediated nitric oxide–dependent mechanism.

## Renal circulation

Despite their modest size, the kidneys receive 20% of cardiac output. The glomerulus (network of renal capillaries where renal filtration takes place) is unique in that its capillary bed has both an afferent arteriole and an efferent arteriole. As resistance vessels, these arterioles allow the glomerular microcirculation to maintain a constantly high capillary pressure. This maintains glomerular filtration over a wide range of systemic perfusion pressures. However, in severe hypotension, autoregulation fails and urine production decreases.

The efferent arterioles form the peritubular capillaries, and the vasa recta capillaries are intertwined with the loops of Henle. These capillaries function at a lower hydrostatic pressure and are well adapted for absorption.

> In hypotensive patients, use of an indwelling urinary catheter allows close monitoring of urine output. Urine output is used as a marker of end-organ perfusion and glomerular filtration.

## Mesenteric circulation

The intestinal microcirculation is the site of absorption of digested substances. The mesenteric circulation is connected, in series, to the portal venous system that perfuses the liver. Mesenteric and portal vein autoregulation is not well developed. However, mesenteric arterioles dilate when food is ingested (functional hyperaemia) in response to:

- fatty acids
- glucose
- gut hormones (e.g. gastrin and cholecystokinin)
- parasympathetic nervous (vagal) activity

Therefore in the post-prandial period, blood flow to the intestines and through the portal venous system increases.

The hepatic arterial system autoregulates. Autoregulation allows flow in the portal venous system and the hepatic arterial system to fluctuate reciprocally so that overall blood flow to the liver is preserved. During exercise, $\alpha$ receptor stimulation reduces blood flow to the gut.

# Capillary exchange

## Starter questions

Answers to the following questions are on page 84.

23. Why do patients with liver disease develop oedema?
24. Why do bed-bound heart failure patients develop sacral swelling?

The main purposes of the cardiovascular system are to:

- deliver oxygen and nutrients to the tissues
- remove carbon dioxide and waste products

This exchange occurs at the level of the capillary. In capillaries, fluids and solutes are continually being exchanged between intravascular (plasma) and extravascular (interstitial) fluid compartments, across the capillary endothelium. This process is called capillary exchange.

Blood flow through capillary beds is dynamic. The process is controlled by autoregulation, vasomotion and extrinsic mechanisms. Capillary exchange occurs through three mechanisms: diffusion, filtration and transcytosis.

## Diffusion

Diffusion is the key mechanism by which substances are exchanged between capillaries and the tissues. The process is passive and always occurs along a concentration gradient.

Substances that diffuse across the capillary wall are:

- respiratory gases (oxygen and carbon dioxide)
- nutrients (glucose, lipids and amino acids)
- many other small molecules (electrolytes)

Oxygen and nutrients are concentrated in the blood. However, they have a low concentration in the interstitial space as a result of consumption by tissue metabolism. The opposite is true of carbon dioxide and waste products. Therefore oxygen and nutrients diffuse from the capillary into the interstitial space, and carbon dioxide and waste products diffuse from the interstitial space into the capillary. Small water-soluble molecules diffuse through clefts and fenestrations (pores) between endothelial cells in the capillary wall. Lipid-soluble molecules such as oxygen and carbon dioxide diffuse freely through the membrane (lipid bilayer).

## Filtration and absorption

Fluid is constantly filtered out of the capillary to the interstitial space, and constantly absorbed from the interstitial space into the capillary. Hydrostatic pressure drives fluid out of the capillary, whereas colloid osmotic pressure draws fluid back into it. The balance between these opposing Starling forces determines net fluid movements.

## Hydrostatic pressure

Hydrostatic pressure is the force exerted by flowing fluid against the capillary wall. This pressure is greatest at the entrance to the capillary (about 30–40 mmHg) but declines along the length of the capillary to its lowest value at the venous end (about 10–20 mmHg).

Hydrostatic pressure in the interstitial space is usually about 0 mmHg. Therefore the hydrostatic pressure gradient favours fluid filtration along the entire length of the capillary but is greatest at the arteriolar end.

## Colloid osmotic pressure

Large molecules, such as proteins, which cannot diffuse across the capillary wall exert a force called colloid osmotic pressure. This pressure draws water molecules towards them by osmosis. The colloid osmotic pressure, considered negative, opposes the hydrostatic force.

Colloid osmotic pressure in the interstitial space is only about 1 mmHg, because of the relative absence of proteins. In contrast to hydrostatic pressure, colloid osmotic pressure is relatively constant along the length of the capillary.

## Net fluid movements

Hydrostatic forces exceed colloid osmotic pressure at the arteriolar end of the capillary, favouring filtration (**Figure 1.64**). As hydrostatic pressure declines along the length of the capillary, there comes a point at which colloid osmotic pressure exceeds hydrostatic pressure; from this point, fluid is absorbed. Therefore fluid is filtered out at the arterial end and absorbed into the capillary at the venous end.

Net fluid movement is determined by the sum of these opposing forces at each point along the capillary. The Starling equation allows net flow ($J_v$) to be calculated. Where $\Delta P$ and $\Delta \pi$ are the hydrostatic and colloid osmotic pressure differences, respectively, between the capillary and interstitial space:

$$J_v = K_f (\Delta P) - \sigma (\Delta \pi)$$

$K_f$ is the filtration coefficient, which reflects capillary permeability. $\sigma$ is the reflection coefficient, which corrects for protein movement into the interstitial space; this varies according to location and is given a value between 0 and 1. According to the Starling equation:

- if net hydrostatic pressure exceeds net colloid osmotic pressure, more fluid is filtered than is absorbed
- if net colloid osmotic pressure exceeds net hydrostatic pressure, more fluid is absorbed than is filtered

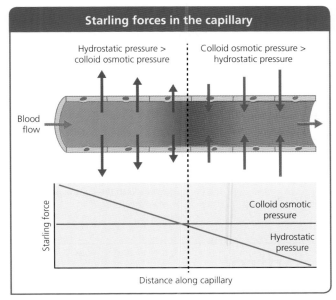

**Starling forces in the capillary**

Hydrostatic pressure > colloid osmotic pressure

Colloid osmotic pressure > hydrostatic pressure

Blood flow

Starling force

Colloid osmotic pressure

Hydrostatic pressure

Distance along capillary

**Figure 1.64** Starling forces in the capillary. At the arterial end, hydrostatic pressure exceeds colloid osmotic pressure and fluid is filtered out. Hydrostatic pressure declines along the length of the capillary but colloid osmotic pressure remains constant. At the venous end colloid osmotic pressure exceeds hydrostatic pressure and fluid is absorbed.

- if net colloid osmotic pressure is equal to net hydrostatic pressure, fluid is filtered and absorbed in equal measure
- highly permeable capillaries (with a high value of $K_f$) favour net filtration

Under normal conditions, net flow is positive: fluid flows into the interstitial space. Each day, the body filters about 2–5 L more fluid than it absorbs. This fluid is taken into the lymphatic system, from which it is returned to the systemic circulation (see page 62).

Arteriolar dilation increases capillary hydrostatic pressure, favouring net filtration. Vasoconstriction reduces hydrostatic pressure, favouring net absorption. Higher venous pressures increase capillary hydrostatic pressure. Higher venous pressures occur in heart failure (see page 241). They can also occur more locally, secondary to deep vein thrombosis and venous insufficiency (see pages 316 and 319), as well as in pregnancy and obesity (because of abdominal venous compression).

**Oedema is the accumulation of fluid in tissue interstitium (see pages 73 and 96).** The Starling equation explains why oedema develops in certain pathological situations.

- Heart failure: oedema is caused by increased intravascular hydrostatic pressures (increased $\Delta P$)
- Low protein states (as occur in liver disease): oedema results from reduced intravascular colloid osmotic pressure (decreased $\Delta\pi$)
- Local tissue infection or inflammation: oedema is caused by increased interstitial colloid osmotic pressure (decreased $\Delta\pi$) and increased capillary permeability (increased $K_f$)

Lymphatic obstruction or dysfunction also results in oedema because of reduced clearance of filtered tissue fluid.

## Transcytosis

Some large water-soluble molecules, such as proteins, are absorbed into endothelial cells by endocytosis; they are transported across the cell by vesicular transport and exit the other side of the cell by exocytosis. This is transcytosis (**Figure 1.65**).

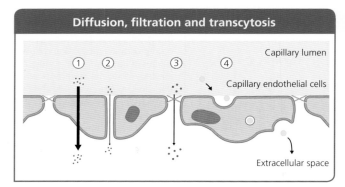

**Figure 1.65** Diffusion, filtration and transcytosis. ① Lipid soluble molecules can diffuse directly through the lipid membrane. ② Water soluble molecules cross the epithelium through pores, fenestrations or gap junctions between endothelial cells ③. ④ Larger protein molecules such as hormones and immunoglobulins are transported across endothelial cell layer by transcystosis. Proteins are absorbed (endocytosis) into the cells inside vesicles and are released to the contralateral side via exocytosis.

# Blood pressure control

## Starter questions

Answers to the following questions are on page 84.

25. Why is it unsafe to palpate both carotid arteries at the same time?
26. Why does eating too much salt cause increased blood pressure?

Blood pressure is the force that the blood exerts on the vascular walls. The heart is an intermittent pump, so blood pressure increases and decreases with each cardiac cycle. Maximum blood pressure is reached during systole; this is the systolic blood pressure. During diastole, no pressure is generated and blood pressure decreases. Elastic recoil of the large arteries maintains pressure during this period (see page 59). The minimum blood pressure reached is the diastolic blood pressure.

Blood pressure is expressed as the systolic value over the diastolic value, for example 120/80 mmHg. Mean arterial pressure is the average blood pressure over the period of the cardiac cycle (**Figure 1.66**). In this section, blood pressure refers to systemic blood pressure.

Blood pressure is routinely measured with a sphygmomanometer using the brachial artery at the antecubital fossa (the elbow), using the brachial artery (see page 107). Pressure declines distally through the circulation,

so the pressure here is lower than that in the aorta (see page 58).

Blood pressure equals the sum of the arterial and venous pressures. However, central venous pressure is usually discounted, because it is close to zero (normally 2-5 mmHg). Recall the following relationship:

$$\text{Pressure } (P) = \text{flow } (Q) \times \text{resistance } (R)$$

Flow is equivalent to cardiac output:

$$\text{cardiac output} = \text{stroke volume} \times \text{heart rate}$$

Resistance equals the sum of all the resistances in the systemic circulation, i.e. the total peripheral resistance. Therefore:

$$\text{Mean arterial pressure} = \text{stroke volume} \times$$
$$\text{heart rate} \times \text{total peripheral resistance}$$

This relationship shows that an increase or a decrease in stroke volume, heart rate or total peripheral resistance will cause a corresponding increase or decrease in mean arterial

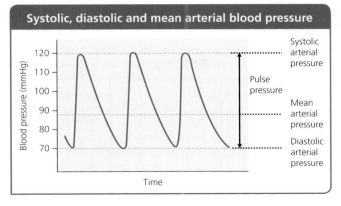

**Figure 1.66** Systolic, diastolic and mean arterial blood pressure. The pulse pressure is the difference between the systolic pressure and the diastolic pressure.

pressure. Stroke volume is closely related to blood volume (see page 49). Therefore the major determinants of mean arterial pressure are:

■ total peripheral resistance
■ cardiac output (stroke volume × heart rate)
■ blood volume

Any factor that affects these variables will influence blood pressure.

The body has multiple homeostatic mechanisms designed to maintain blood pressure. Some respond rapidly to effect short-term control, and others influence long-term control.

■ Systolic blood pressure is determined mainly by stroke volume and compliance: an increase in stroke volume increases systolic blood pressure; reduced arterial compliance also increases systolic blood pressure, because less energy is absorbed in systole
■ Diastolic blood pressure is determined mainly by total peripheral resistance: elastic arterial recoil pushes blood through the peripheral resistance vessels, and an increase in resistance increases diastolic blood pressure
■ Mean arterial blood pressure is determined mainly by total peripheral resistance, cardiac output and blood volume

## Short-term blood pressure control

Pressure drives blood flow through the circulation. Cessation of flow for even a minute or two has disastrous consequences.

Autoregulation ensures adequate blood flow through the tissues provided the perfusing blood pressure remains in the physiological range (see page 67). It is vital that the body carefully regulates blood pressure so that it remains in this range. Any deviation from the physiological range must be corrected quickly to ensure appropriate tissue perfusion and organ function (**Figure 1.67**).

If a deviation in total peripheral resistance, cardiac output or blood volume alters mean arterial pressure, the body aims to correct it by effecting changes in the other variables. Overall control of blood pressure is coordinated in the cardiovascular centre in the medulla oblongata through regulation of the sympathetic and parasympathetic nervous systems.

Activation of the sympathetic nervous system increases blood pressure by increasing:

■ heart rate (which increases cardiac output)
■ contractility (which increases stroke volume and thus cardiac output)
■ arterial vascular tone (which increases total peripheral resistance)
■ venous tone (which increases central venous pressure and thus cardiac output)

The sympathetic nervous system also triggers secretion of adrenaline (epinephrine) from the adrenal medulla and renin from the kidneys (see page 78).

Activation of the parasympathetic nervous system decreases blood pressure by reducing:

■ heart rate
■ arterial vascular tone
■ venous tone

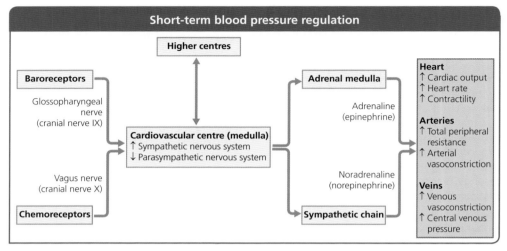

**Figure 1.67** The main short-term mechanisms controlling blood pressure. A decrease in blood pressure (hypotension) is detected by baroreceptors and chemoreceptors. The cardiovascular centre coordinates the activation of the sympathetic nervous system and inhibition of the parasympathetic nervous system. The result is a compensatory increase in blood pressure.

**At rest, diastole constitutes about two thirds of the cardiac cycle and systole one third.** This means that mean arterial blood pressure can be approximated by:

mean       = 1/3 systolic blood
arterial      pressure + 2/3
pressure     diastolic blood pressure

## Baroreceptors and the baroreflex

Baroreceptors are pressure-sensitive stretch receptors in the walls of the larger upper body arteries. They are mainly found in the carotid sinus and aortic arch. Afferent signals from the baroreceptors are carried to the medulla by nerve fibres in the glossopharyngeal nerve (cranial nerve IX) and the vagus nerve (cranial nerves X).

A decrease in pulse pressure or mean arterial blood pressure reduces baroreceptor stretch. Baroreceptors respond by reducing their firing rate. In the medulla, this activates sympathetic nervous system outflow and inhibits parasympathetic nervous system outflow.

An increase in blood pressure has the opposite effect.

**The baroreflex does not correct chronic changes in blood pressure.** In essential hypertension (see page 195), the baroreflex threshold becomes reset to a higher point.

This baroreflex is rapid (occurring in seconds). It protects the body from acute alterations in blood pressure, such as those in response to changes in posture, acute haemorrhage and shock. The baroreflex threshold, i.e. blood pressure values that trigger the reflex, can be modified by higher brain centres. For example, during exercise a higher blood pressure is desirable; it is tolerated because of the influence of afferent signals to the medulla from higher centres.

**Carotid sinus massage stimulates the baroreceptors, resulting in increased vagal (parasympathetic nervous system) activity and a reduction in heart rate.** Carotid sinus massage is used as a first-line treatment for terminating supraventricular tachycardias (see page 225).

# Chemoreceptors

As well as baroreceptors, peripheral chemo-receptors are in the aortic arch. These receptors are sensitive to changes in blood oxygen, carbon dioxide and pH. Afferent nerve fibres from the chemoreceptors accompany the baroreceptor fibres to the medulla.

Chemoreceptors mainly influence the respiratory centre in the medulla. The respiratory centre controls the concentration of respiratory gases and pH through regulation of respiratory rate and tidal volume, i.e. the rate and depth of breathing.

> **Carotid sinus hypersensitivity results in an exaggerated baroreflex in response to manual stimulation of the carotid body.** This hypersensitivity causes syncope in some people.

In the cardiovascular centre, chemoreceptor activation in response to decreased oxygen, decreased pH and increased carbon dioxide produces a mixed response: an increase in vascular tone increases blood pressure, but heart rate is reduced. However, concurrent activation of stretch receptors in the lungs (in response to increased tidal volume and respiratory rate) increases heart rate through an indirect pathway involving the sympathetic nervous system. The overall effect is an increase in vascular tone and heart rate, with a corresponding increase in blood pressure.

## Muscle receptors

Skeletal muscle contains receptors that are sensitive to increases in metabolic activity (decreased pH or increased $K^+$) and mechanoreceptors that detect contractile activity. Activation of these receptors stimulates the sympathetic nervous system through the cardiovascular centre. The response is an increase in blood pressure and cardiac output, which are appropriate during exercise.

## Higher centre influence

Blood pressure control is coordinated by the cardiovascular centre in the medulla oblongata. Higher brain centres, including the thalamus, hypothalamus and cerebral cortex, can modify homeostatic blood pressure responses. This occurs in certain conditions, including temperature changes (through the hypothalamus), exercise (through the cerebellum), pain (through the thalamus) and emotion (through the cerebral cortex).

The fight-or-flight response is a good example of such control. This acute stress response is triggered by the perception of threat.

- Blood pressure increases
- Tachycardia and tachypnoea occur
- Blood is diverted to skeletal muscles and becomes more coagulable
- The pupils dilate
- The bladder relaxes
- Digestion slows
- Energy is released from stores

The response originates in the amygdala and hypothalamus. It triggers a host of physiological reactions that prepare the body for physical attack. The principal physiological response is a sudden increase in sympathetic nervous system discharge, causing increased heart rate, blood pressure, contractility and venous tone. Arterial vascular tone increases, especially in less vital areas (e.g. the splanchnic circulation), but vessels in the skeletal muscles vasodilate.

The fight-or-flight response occurs in situations of perceived threat. Therefore it can be triggered by emotional stimuli such as fear and anxiety. In such cases, the response may become maladaptive and detrimental, for example when it causes panic attacks.

## Hormones and chemicals

In addition to the autonomic system, a host of circulating hormones influence blood pressure. Clinically, the most significant of these are adrenaline (epinephrine), angiotensin II, antidiuretic hormone and atrial natriuretic peptide.

### Adrenaline

Stimulation of the sympathetic nervous system causes the adrenal medulla to release adrenaline (epinephrine) into the bloodstream. This is a non-selective adrenoreceptor agonist that has similar physiological effects to those of noradrenaline (norepinephrine), which is also released from sympathetic nerves.

## Angiotensin II and antidiuretic hormone

Hypotension triggers synthesis of angiotensin II and antidiuretic hormone (vasopressin). Both hormones increase blood pressure by causing vasoconstriction and renal retention of salt and water (see page 79).

## Atrial natriuretic peptide

This powerful vasodilator (see page 79) is released by atrial cells in response to increased atrial stretch (increased central venous pressure). Atrial natriuretic peptide augments renal sodium and water clearance, thus reducing blood volume and blood pressure.

**Adrenaline (epinephrine) is synthesised by some tumours, for example phaeochromocytoma.** The resulting excess of adrenaline causes (secondary) hypertension (see page 206).

## Long-term blood pressure control: regulating blood volume

The processes described so far are effective in correcting short-term variations in blood pressure. Over longer periods of time, blood pressure is regulated by altering blood volume. Blood volume homeostasis is determined by how much sodium and water are reabsorbed by the kidneys of blood volume (**Figure 1.68**).

**Osmolality is a measure of the balance between electrolytes and water in the blood plasma.**

■ Concentrated plasma (high electrolyte and low water concentration) has high osmolality
■ Dilute blood plasma (high water and low electrolyte concentration) has low osmolality

## Antidiuretic hormone

Osmoreceptors in the hypothalamus are sensitive to fluctuations in serum osmolality.

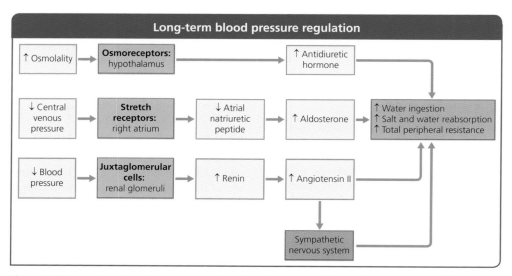

**Figure 1.68** Long-term blood pressure regulation through control of blood volume. The overall effect is a reflex increase in blood pressure by increasing both blood volume and total peripheral resistance.

If osmolality increases, the hypothalamus causes antidiuretic hormone to be secreted from the posterior pituitary gland. Antidiuretic hormone causes peripheral vasoconstriction and induces thirst. It also up-regulates the number of effective aquaporins (membrane spanning water pores) in the collecting ducts and distal convoluted tubules of the nephron. This effect increases water reabsorption from the nephron into the blood.

The resulting increase in the water content of the blood homeostatically corrects the initial change in osmolality while increasing blood volume. Therefore antidiuretic hormone increases blood pressure by increasing both total peripheral resistance and blood volume. A reduction in plasma osmolality has the opposite effect.

The primary determinant of plasma osmolality is the plasma concentration of sodium. An increase in sodium causes an increase in blood volume, and vice versa. Therefore a low salt (NaCl) diet is advised for hypertensive patients.

> **Antidiuretic hormone secretion is inhibited by alcohol.** Alcohol ingestion leads to increased diuresis and more frequent visits to the toilet.

## Atrial natriuretic peptide

Atrial natriuretic peptide is secreted by atrial cells in response to increased blood volume (increased central venous pressure). A natriuretic is any agent which increases the elimination sodium in the urine (natriuresis). Atrial natriuretic peptide reduces blood pressure by:

- acting as a peripheral vasodilator, which decreases total peripheral resistance
- increasing glomerular filtration (atrial natriuretic peptide dilates afferent and constricts efferent glomerular arterioles), which decreases blood volume
- reducing reabsorption of sodium and water (reducing blood flow in the vasa recta), which decreases blood volume
- inhibiting renin and aldosterone synthesis (see page 78), which decreases total peripheral resistance and blood volume

Therefore the effects of atrial natriuretic peptide are to reduce blood pressure by decreasing blood volume and total peripheral resistance.

> **The renin–angiotensin–aldosterone system is a key determinant of blood volume and blood pressure.** This explains the efficacy of angiotensin-converting enzyme inhibitors and angiotensin II receptor blockers in the treatment of hypertension.

## Renin–angiotensin–aldosterone system

The renin–angiotensin–aldosterone system is shown in **Figure 1.69**. A reduction in blood pressure is detected in the renal juxtaglomerular cells in the kidneys. The cells respond by secreting renin enzyme. Renin converts angiotensinogen (secreted in the liver) into angiotensin I. Angiotensin I is converted to angiotensin II by angiotensin-converting enzyme, mainly in the lungs.

Angiotensin II increases blood pressure because it:

- is a powerful vasoconstrictor (vasoconstriction increases total peripheral resistance)

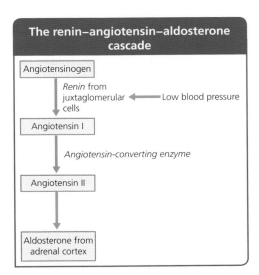

**Figure 1.69** The renin–angiotensin–aldosterone cascade.

- increases sodium and water reabsorption in the nephron (which increases blood volume)
- stimulates the sympathetic nervous system
- stimulates aldosterone secretion from the adrenal cortex (which increases blood volume)
- stimulates release of antidiuretic hormone (which increases total peripheral resistance and blood volume)

Aldosterone (a mineralocorticoid hormone) also increases sodium and water retention by its actions on the distal convoluted tubule and collecting ducts.

> **The renal juxtaglomerular (or granular) cells are specialised vascular smooth muscle cells in the afferent glomerular arterioles.** Their membranes contain ß1 adrenoreceptors, which increase renin secretion when stimulated. In addition to their direct effects on the cardiovascular system, beta-blocking drugs also reduce blood pressure by reducing renin secretion.

## Blood pressure and shock

Shock is when blood pressure falls below the effective autoregulatory range and thus blood flow is not sufficient to meet the metabolic demands of the tissues. It is an acute condition which, if not corrected rapidly, quickly results in multi-organ failure, cardiac arrest and death. Because MAP = CO × TPR, shock is caused by reduced cardiac output or increased total peripheral resistance. When shock occurs secondary to pump failure, it is known as cardiogenic shock (**Table 1.21**).

When thinking about shock, imagine a fluid-filled central heating system. If there is not enough fluid in the system there will be insufficient pressure and the system will fail. This is analogous to hypovolaemic shock. If the volume of fluid remains constant but you double the number of radiators (increased volume/capacity), the effect is the same and the system will fail. This is analogous to hyporesistive shock where profound vasodilation increases the capacity of the system.

| Causes of shock | | |
|---|---|---|
| Type of shock | Mechanism | Causes |
| Cardiogenic | ↓ Cardiac output | Heart failure |
| | | Acute myocardial infarction |
| | | Arrhythmia |
| | | Valve disease |
| Hypovolaemic | ↓ Blood volume | Haemorrhage |
| | | Profound dehydration (gastroenteritis, diabetic ketoacidosis) |
| | | Burns |
| Hyporesistive (distributive) | ↓ Total peripheral resistance ↑ Capacity | Sepsis Anaphylaxis |
| Obstructive | ↓ Cardiac output | Pulmonary embolus |
| | | Cardiac tamponade |
| | | Dissecting aortic aneurysm |
| | | Severe aortic stenosis |

**Table 1.21** Causes of shock

## Hypovolaemic shock

In hypovolaemic shock, the cardiovascular system attempts to compensate for the loss of blood pressure via reflex activation of the sympathetic, and inhibition of the parasympathetic nervous systems resulting in:

- tachycardia (increased heart rate)
- arterial vasoconstriction (increased total peripheral resistance)
- venous vasoconstriction (central venous pressure)
- increased contractility (stroke volume)

> **Hypovolaemic shock is a medical emergency that requires rapid intravenous fluid resuscitation.** Patients are given boluses of either crystalloid, colloid, or cross-matched blood (depending upon the cause of the hypovolaemia) while the cause of the hypovolaemia is corrected and until the patient has stabilised.

Sympathetic activation also induces sweating. Patients with hypovolaemic shock are therefore pale (peripheral vasoconstriction), clammy (sweating) and tachycardic. Shock also results in renal hypoperfusion which activates the renin–angiotensin system promoting salt and water retention (increases blood volume)) and vasoconstriction (increases total peripheral resistance).

## Hyporesistive shock

Septic shock results from profound vasodilatation induced by infection. Anaphylactic shock is caused when exposure to an allergen causes a significant release of histamine (a powerful vasodilator). Unlike hypovolaemic shock, septic and anaphylactic shock are both associated with vasodilation.

**The principles of treating shock are:**

1. Correct the cause (e.g. antibiotics, cessation of haemorrhage, removal of allergen)
2. Rapid intravenous fluids
3. Careful administration of a peripheral vasoconstrictor (e.g. noradrenaline or adrenaline) in a specialist environment

## Obstructive shock

In obstructive shock, blood pressure is reduced by a mechanical obstruction, such as occlusion of the aorta (e.g. aortic stenosis), pulmonary artery (e.g. pulmonary embolism) or external compression of the heart (cardiac tamponade, see page 358).

## Answers to starter questions

1. The myocardium has a high energy demand and requires a blood supply to match. Mitochondria are the main energy producers of any cell; highly active cells like myocardium contain high numbers of them. Unlike skeletal and smooth muscle the myocardium is active continuously from before birth until death, meaning its energy requirements (in the form of ATP) are high and sustained. In addition, the heart increases its cardiac output fivefold during times of physiological stress (e.g. exercise). To cope with these demands, the heart extracts more oxygen from the blood and has a higher mitochondrial density than any other organ.

2. The right (pulmonary) and left (systemic) circulatory systems are separate but are connected to each other in series. Occasionally, blood from the right and left systems mix via abnormal connections called shunts . Because the systemic circulation operates at a higher pressure a shunt will usually cause blood to pass from the left circulation into the right. This increases blood flow through the right side of the heart and causes oxygenated blood to mix with deoxygenated blood.

3. Embryological development is orchestrated by multiple genes and gene products (e.g. surface ligands and receptors) which are expressed according to cell type and region. Variable expression of these products governs how an individual cell differentiates. Non-specialised pluripotent ('multiple potential') cells go through several levels of specialisation before finally differentiating into cells which are able to carry out the specific functions of the tissue or organ they are intended for.

4. Unlike in adults, the fetal pulmonary and systemic circuits function in parallel. The supply of oxygenated blood to the systemic circulation relies upon blood mixing (shunting) between the two circuits. The fetal circulation ensures that the head is preferentially supplied with oxygen rich blood, even if this occurs at the expense of the rest of the body.

**Answers** *continued*

5. Normally, shunting of blood through the ductus arteriosus ceases at birth and the duct closes. However, in certain congenital heart diseases the newborn's circulation becomes dependent upon blood shunting across the duct and its closure compromises the circulation. When required, shunting through the ductus arteriosus can be maintained after birth using parenteral prostaglandins (see page 292) until structural correction is undertaken.

6. Coronary anatomy is normally highly variable. Most people have a left and right coronary artery emanating from the corresponding aortic sinus and these arteries usually follow a characteristic path across the myocardium. However, although there are standard methods of naming branches, the manner in which these arteries branch and the amount of myocardium supplied by each branch is highly variable. This can lead to potentially serious clinical problems if the coronary arteries originate from the wrong sinus (i.e. right artery from the left sinus or left artery from the right sinus).

7. Cardiac resynchronisation therapy (CRT) is a common treatment for heart failure (see pages 164 and 248) and relies upon the placement of a LV lead in an epicardial left ventricular vein. Access is gained via the right atrium by passing the lead into the coronary sinus and manoeuvring it within the cardiac veins until a desirable LV location is reached. Coronary venous anatomy is assessed in advance using a CT scan so that an optimal access route and location for the LV lead can be planned.

8. The mitral valve is so-called because the two leaflets resemble a Bishop's mitre (hat).

9. Pieces of blood clots in the deep veins of the leg (deep vein thrombosis (DVT)) can break off (embolise), travel through the blood and lodge in the pulmonary circulation. This occludes arterial blood flow causing a pulmonary embolism (PE). Large emboli occlude large proximal pulmonary arteries causing hypotension and circulatory collapse. Smaller clots occlude smaller, more distal pulmonary arterial branches causing pleuritic chest pain.

10. Pulmonary emboli (PE) are usually a complication of deep vein thrombosis (DVT, see page 316) in the leg or pelvic veins, which occurs due to abnormally reduced blood flow. Risk factors such as immobility, inflammation, surgery, pregnancy, obesity and exogenous oestrogen therapy are over-represented in hospital inpatients putting them at a higher risk of developing a PE. All hospital inpatients in the UK have their DVT risk screened on admission.

11. Access to the heart is required for a variety of procedures such as diagnostic angiography, percutaneous valve insertion and pacemaker implantation. Unless an open surgical approach is used (e.g. midline sternotomy), access is gained via the blood vessels. If followed correctly, all blood vessels eventually lead to the heart. Access to the left heart and coronary circulation is gained via a peripheral artery such as the femoral or radial arteries. Access to the right heart is via a large systemic vein, such as the subclavian or axillary veins. Catheters are used to pass instruments, drugs and devices into the heart and its arteries and veins via these vascular routes.

12. The ability of a tissue to generate an electrical potential spontaneously is called automaticity (see page 40). In a healthy heart the sinoatrial node depolarises more frequently than other areas and therefore controls heart rate. However, almost all regions of the heart demonstrate automaticity. This is advantageous because if the sinoatrial node fails, another region can take over control and the heart continues to beat. If this were not the case sinoatrial node failure or complete heart block would be immediately fatal.

**Answers** *continued*

13. A completely stable potential would never reach threshold and would therefore never trigger a heartbeat. During phase 4, the membrane potential drifts positively until depolarisation (phase 0) is triggered and the threshold potential is reached. This occurs secondary to an inward cation current, i.e. pacemaker potentials. The faster (steeper) the positive drift, the more frequent the threshold is reached and the faster the pacemaker and vice versa.

14. The atria would continue to depolarise as normal and, despite receiving no electrical conduction from the atria, the ventricles would also continue to depolarise but at a different rate. The atria and ventricles would both continue to beat but would not be synchronised. This is know as atrioventricular dissociation. It occurs with complete heart block (see page 218) and ventricular tachycardia (see page 226).

15. Although there are some small differences in cardiac output between the left and right ventricles overall they must balance. The right and left ventricles are arranged in series. Therefore, blood flowing out of the left ventricle must flow into and through the right ventricle. If the cardiac output of either ventricle exceeds the other, blood accumulates in the compartment preceding the affected ventricle. The blood pressure in this compartment rises and eventually fluid leaks out of the capillaries into the tissues causing either pulmonary or systemic oedema (see pages 73 and 96). This explains the clinical features experienced in heart failure (see page 243)

16. Haemodynamic pressure ($P$), flow ($Q$) and resistance ($R$) are similar in their relationships to voltage ($V$), current ($I$) and electrical resistance ($R$), and the relationship between pressure, flow and resistance ($P = QR$) is also identical to Ohm's electrical law ($V = IR$) (see page 54). These relationships can be used to explain the differences in total resistance between parallel and series circulations (see page 54). Electrical components such as batteries, capacitors and resistors can be used to represent components of the cardiovascular system, which allows researchers to model the cardiovascular system using electrical circuits.

17. Stenosed valves do not open well. The corresponding increase in resistance to flow results in a pressure gradient across the valve, the magnitude of which reflects the disease severity. The Bernoulli equation relates pressure gradient to flow velocity, which can be assessed by Doppler echocardiography. The equation is used to calculate the pressure gradient from the flow velocity and thus the severity of the disease.

18. Laminar blood flow is silent, whereas disturbed and turbulent flow creates vibrations which can be heard with a stethoscope as murmurs or bruits. A murmur is caused by abnormal blood flow across a cardiac valve and a bruit is an abnormal sound caused by accelerated blood flow through a narrowed blood vessel. The location, volume, timing and character of a murmur helps diagnose specific valvular heart problems (see page 113). Bruits are used to diagnose peripheral vascular disease (see page 311). Auscultating turbulent blood flow is the basis for measuring blood pressure with a sphygmomanometer (see page 108).

19. At rest, approximately two thirds of the cardiac cycle is spent in diastole with no pressure being generated by the heart. However, diastolic blood pressure normally only falls to 70–80 mmHg. This is because the large elastic arteries distend during systole absorbing energy. They then recoil during diastole, discharging this stored energy and therefore maintaining a diastolic pressure

**Answers** *continued*

20. Breast cancer spreads via the lymphatic circulation. For this reason surgeons remove some, or all, of the axillary lymph nodes during mastectomy, depending upon the nature and spread of the malignancy. Axillary lymph node clearance impairs lymph fluid drainage, resulting in significant arm and chest oedema. This is known as lymphoedema.

21. When there is maximal flow in the arteries downstream autoregulatory mechamisms are able to compensate for upstream blockages, such as those in coronary atherosclerosis, by minimising the resistance of distal small vessels thus maximising flow. Once an occlusion exceeds 50% of the arterial diameter these compensatory mechanisms are exhausted and flow becomes limited by the coronary disease. At this point patients become ischaemic during exertion and experience symptoms such as chest pain. If a blockage exceeds 85% of the arterial diameter, flow becomes limited during resting conditions.

22. In systemic arterioles hypoxia reflects a need for increased blood flow in order to satisfy the metabolic needs of the tissue. It therefore triggers vasodilatation and reduced vascular resistance to increase blood flow. In pulmonary arterioles hypoxia triggers vasoconstriction and reduced blood flow, because the principle role of the pulmonary circulation is to deliver deoxygenated blood to the alveoli for gaseous exchange. In this situation, it is ideal to divert blood towards well-oxygenated areas and away from hypoxic regions to ensure optimal gaseous exchange.

23. Protein synthesis is compromised in advanced liver disease, which results in reduced colloid osmotic pressure. This encourages excess water to exit the vessel into the tissues (i.e. oedema). Hepatic cirrhosis also increases portal circulatory resistance increasing the pressure in the portal venous system. This causes oedema specifically in the the portal venous system which leads to ascites (fluid accumulation in the peritoneal cavity).

24. In heart failure, elevated venous pressures causes a net filtration of fluid into the tissues. The additional effects of gravity mean that the highest venous pressures occur in the most dependent parts of the body. Normally, this is the lower legs but when a patient is bed-bound it is the lower sacral area.

25. Palpating both carotid arteries stimulates baroreceptors. The body interprets the palpation as a rise in blood pressure and responds by acutely reducing blood pressure by reducing heart rate, myocardial contractility and inducing arterial and venous vasodilatation. This can cause hypotension and if blood pressure falls low enough to compromise blood supply to the brain, syncope can occur.

26. Excess dietary salt increases the osmolality of the blood. This is detected in the hypothalamus and stimulates antidiuretic hormone (ADH) secretion from the posterior pituitary. ADH causes peripheral vasoconstriction and water resorption within the kidneys. The net effect is an increase in blood pressure. This is why major public health initiatives have focused on reducing salt consumption.

# Chapter 2
# Clinical essentials

## Introduction

Cardiovascular disease is pathology of the heart and circulation, and includes ischaemic heart disease, heart failure, arrhythmias and other disorders. It accounts for >40% of admissions to hospital and is a leading cause of death. Major risk factors are smoking and high blood pressure.

## Common symptoms and how to take a history

### Starter questions

Answers to the following questions are on page 169.

1. Why might chest pain that lasts for days not have a serious cause?
2. Why might vomiting indicate a cardiac problem?
3. Why does drinking in a pub or eating a meal out no longer increase your risk of cardiovascular disease?
4. What is more serious, a runner collapsing during a marathon or at the end?
5. Why is heart disease so common?

A patient's history comprises their current health problem, previous health problems, medication use, allergies, a family history and a review of all body systems. The history is the foundation of a diagnosis and informs both the examination and subsequent investigations; it should at least produce a shortlist of potential diagnoses.

### General approach

First introduce yourself, initially addressing the patient formally. Then seek their permission to take a history. Choose an area of privacy, such as a side room, for the interview, and ensure that there are no physical barriers (e.g. a desk) between you and the patient.

Next, ask them if you can make notes as you proceed.

History taking requires active listening skills, both verbal (**Table 2.1**) and non-verbal. Non-verbal listening skills include making eye contact throughout the consultation; clinician and patient should be at the same eye level. Adopt an open posture and pay attention to the patient's body language.

The history is organised as follows:

- patient's name, age, sex and date of birth
- the presenting complaint(s)
- history of the presenting complaint(s)
- medical history
- drug history
- allergy history
- family medical history
- social history
- systems review
- summary

## Presenting complaint

The presenting complaint is the 'headline' that summarises the patient's symptoms or presentation in a single phrase or word, such as 'shortness of breath' or 'collapse'. Start with open questions, such as 'What brings you to hospital today?', rather than 'Is it your chest pain again?' This approach allows the patient to tell their story and avoids the use of an inefficient barrage of closed questions (those with only 'yes' or 'no' answers). Also, avoid interrupting the patient's train of thought.

Once an overall picture of the patient's problem has been constructed, discriminating and delineating questions are used to explore each aspect of the history.

## History of the presenting complaint

This part of the history, is the story beneath the headline and comprises details such as when the problem started, its duration and frequency, any exacerbating or relieving factors and associated symptoms. If the symptom has been ongoing for days or weeks, what has changed to make the patient seek medical attention today?

Most patients discuss the presenting complaint and its history in a single, clear narrative. However, some patients, for example those with dementia, may be unable to provide this. In such cases, obtain the information from other sources; paramedics, the referring professional, carers or relatives can give a collateral history.

The art of history taking is in distinguishing the clinically significant from the non-significant. For example, a patient may focus on what their friends think of their ill health, in which case the discussion needs to be tactfully steered back to what the patient, not their friends, think.

A working diagnosis is based on a synthesis of clues, both verbal and non-verbal, gained from interacting with the patient, not the presence or absence of any individual symptom.

> **A diagnosis comprises 75% history, 20% examination and 5% tests.** If the history taking is incorrect, everything that follows will be unhelpful.

## Common symptoms

A symptom, or presenting complaint, is a subjective sensation experienced by a patient that usually indicates the presence of disease. The five key symptoms (**Figure 2.1**) in cardiovascular disease are:

- chest pain
- palpitations
- shortness of breath
- syncope
- ankle swelling

| Active listening skills | | |
|---|---|---|
| Skill | Patient says | Clinician says |
| Acknowledging | 'So I felt like...' | 'Mmm', 'Uh-huh' and 'OK' |
| Encouraging | 'And then...' | 'Please, go on' |
| Repeating | 'I'm in pain!' | 'You're in pain?' |
| Paraphrasing | 'I can never catch my breath' | 'You feel out of breath constantly' |
| Reflecting | 'I'm OK' [Looks sad] | 'Are you sure? You look upset' |

**Table 2.1** Active listening skills

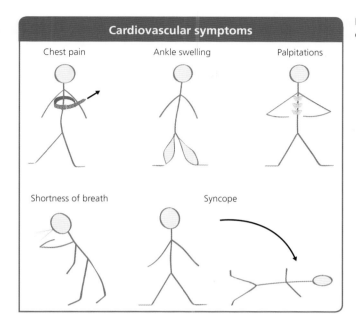

**Figure 2.1** The five common cardiovascular symptoms.

## Pain

Chest pain has many causes and the SOCRATES mnemonic (**Table 2.2**) is used when taking a history of pain. If the patient denies that they are in pain, enquire about chest tightness or discomfort, or use similar descriptions. Its key differentials are shown in **Table 2.3.** A specific form of chest pain is called angina pectoris (Latin for 'strangling of the chest') and refers to a mismatch between myocardial oxygen demand and supply, causing ischaemia.

The ischaemic pain of peripheral vascular disease is experienced in the legs as claudication (Latin: 'limping'). Like angina, this symptom is caused by arterial occlusion from atherosclerosis. Such claudicant pain is brought on by exertion and relieved by rest.

### Site

Angina is felt anywhere on the chest wall, but common sites include behind the sternum, the neck and the epigastrium. Patients use different hand gestures to describe where they have pain, such as a clenched fist, an open palm or touching the opposite arm (**Figure 2.2a–c**). However, use of a single finger means that the pain is localised and therefore usually non-cardiac (**Figure 2.2d**). A non-cardiac cause is also more likely if the same pain is reproduced on palpation.

- Pain behind the sternum (retrosternal pain) is caused by myocardial ischaemia (angina), inflammation of the oesophagus (oesophagitis) or inflammation of the cartilage connecting the ribs and sternum (costochondritis)

| SOCRATES: taking a history of pain | | |
|---|---|---|
| Letter | Meaning | Example question |
| S | Site | 'Where is the pain?' |
| O | Onset | 'When did it start?' |
| C | Character | 'What does it feel like?' |
| R | Radiation | 'Where else is it felt?' |
| A | Associated symptoms | 'What else are you experiencing?' |
| T | Timing | 'How often and for how long?' |
| E | Exacerbating and relieving factors | 'What makes is better or worse?' |
| S | Severity | 'How bad is the pain on a scale of 1 to 10?' |

**Table 2.2** The SOCRATES mnemonic for taking a history of pain

| Features of different causes of chest pain | | | | |
|---|---|---|---|---|
| Type | Gastro-oesophageal reflux disease | Angina | Pericarditis | Pneumonia or pulmonary embolism |
| Site | Epigastric or retrosternal | Retrosternal | Central or left pectoral | Anywhere |
| Character | Burning | Crushing or aching | Sharp | Sharp |
| Radiation | Neck | Arms, neck and jaw | No | No |
| Associated symptoms | Excessive salivation | Nausea, breathlessness and sweating | Fever | Breathlessness, cough and fever |
| Exacerbating factors | Food and lying down | Exertion, cold and stress | Inspiration and lying down | Inspiration and coughing |
| Relieving factors | Milk and antacid | Glyceryl trinitrate and rest | NSAIDs and sitting forwards | Breath holding |

NSAID, non-steroidal anti-inflammatory drug.

*Onset, timing and severity are highly variable so are excluded.

**Table 2.3** Features of the different causes of chest pain*

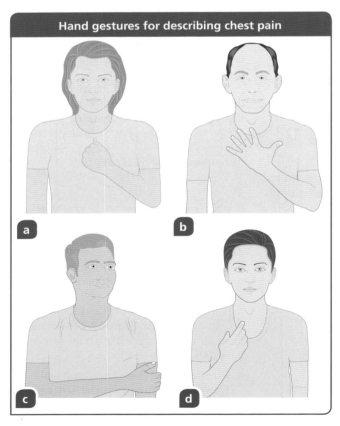

Hand gestures for describing chest pain

**Figure 2.2** The four most commonly used hand gestures for describing chest pain. (a) The clenched fist (Levine's) sign. (b) The palm sign. (c) The arm sign. (d) The pointing finger sign. The ability to localise the pain to a single finger point strongly suggests that the pain is non-cardiac.

- Pain around the left pectoral region is usually the result of inflammation of the heart muscle (myocarditis) or inflammation of the fibroserous sac covering around the heart (pericarditis)
- Pain in the epigastrium usually arises from inflammation of the stomach (gastritis); the stomach is close to the epigastrium

## Onset

Sudden, spontaneous chest pain is usually caused by an ST elevation myocardial infarction, a tear in the aorta (aortic dissection), a collapsed lung (pneumothorax) or a large blood clot blocking the pulmonary artery (massive pulmonary embolism).

Gradual chest pain has several possible causes.

- Gradual chest pain that increases during exertion is due to angina
- Gradual chest pain that increases after exertion is the result of musculoskeletal problems

## Character

Cardiac chest pain feels like a tight band around, or a dull weight on, the chest; it makes breathing difficult. Aortic dissection is usually experienced as a tearing or gripping pain as the intimal lining of the aorta is sheared away.

Non-cardiac chest pain is felt as a local sharpness or diffuse burning. Musculoskeletal chest pain is localised to the structure affected, such as the chest wall muscle, intercostal nerve or costochondral junction. Gastric reflux causes a sensation of diffuse burning of the oesophageal lining along the course of the oesophagus.

## Radiation

Pain that radiates to the neck, the jaw or the shoulders and arms (typically the left) is usually cardiac in origin, and these areas may be the only presenting sites of pain (i.e. no chest pain) indicating angina. Cardiac pain due to myocardial ischaemia radiates here because the area of the spinal cord that receives sensory information from the heart also receives sensory information from the skin over the arms, but the brain is unable to discriminate the two. This phenomenon is called referred pain.

Pain radiating through to the back is usually caused by an aortic dissection. This pattern of radiation occurs because the aorta travels backwards from the heart down through the thorax and abdominal cavity in line with the vertebral column.

Pain radiating through to the left axilla is usually non-cardiac. It has various causes, including anxiety, pleural disease and musculoskeletal disorders.

## Associated symptoms

The pain of a myocardial infarction, pulmonary embolus or aortic dissection is usually associated with a surge in adrenaline (epinephrine). This adrenaline surge causes tachycardia, sweating, nausea and vomiting.

If there is significant left ventricular dysfunction, pain from a myocardial infarction can present with shortness of breath and pulmonary oedema due to acute left ventricular failure.

As well as pain, gastritis and oesophagitis usually also present with an acidic taste in the mouth, increased salivation (water brash) or belching.

## Timing

Information about the timing of pain makes certain diagnoses more or less likely. For example, chest pain that a patient has felt constantly for years is unlikely to be cardiac; it would have already led to serious complications before presentation.

## Exacerbating and relieving factors

Chest pain brought on by exertion and relieved by rest is usually angina. Exertion increases the oxygen requirement of the myocardium. The harder the exercise, the more the heart is deprived of oxygen and the more severe the pain. Oxygen demand is also increased by other exacerbating factors, such as cold weather, consumption of a large meal and stress.

Chest pain that increases during rest and is relieved by exertion is usually non-cardiac; for example, anxiety or a musculoskeletal cause. Musculoskeletal chest pain is also brought on by a specific movement, such as stretching or twisting.

Indigestion usually follows consumption of fatty, spicy or acidic foods. The pain worsens when the patient is lying down, because this position increases reflux through the lower oesophageal sphincter.

Chest pain caused by pericarditis is also worse on lying down, because friction between the two layers of pericardium is increased in this position and therefore pain, and friction, are reduced by sitting forwards.

> The **SPIKES** acronym is a useful framework for breaking any kind of bad news.
>
> **Setting/environment:** Ensure it is private, loved ones are present, sit down, establish rapport with the patient and minimise interruptions.
>
> **Perception:** Determine what the patient understands about their condition and how much they want to know.
>
> **Invitation:** Ask permission from patient to give information. Ask if the patient wants to know the details of the problem.
>
> **Knowledge:** Communicate the medical facts considering the patient's background and level of understanding. Provide information in jargon-free, bite-size chunks, checking understanding at each stage.
>
> **Emotions:** Explore the patient's emotions. Identify and respond in an empathic manner.
>
> **Strategy and summary:** Conclude and outline the plan of action.

## Severity

Patients are asked to rate their pain on a scale of 0–10. Such ratings help clinicians understand the patient's relative concept of their pain. The rating has no bearing on diagnosis but is helpful when monitoring response to treatment. This is because the experience of pain is unique to the individual and relative to their prior experience; for example, one patient may describe the pain of a myocardial infarction as 1/10 and another patient may describe indigestion pain as 9/10.

## Shortness of breath

This is the sensation of being unable to breathe enough to meet the demands of the body.

Shortness of breath is a common symptom occurring with chest pain. However, it has many differential diagnoses (**Table 2.4**), including anxiety, anaphylaxis and panic attacks. The following are common terms for breathlessness.

- Dyspnoea: shortness of breath; a common presenting complaint; the AEROS mnemonic (**Table 2.5**) is used when taking a history of dyspnoea
- Orthopnoea: breathlessness on lying supine, which is common in both heart and lung disease; ask how many pillows the patient sleeps with at night, and whether they are able to lie flat on their back
- Paroxysmal nocturnal dyspnoea: intermittent breathlessness occurring during the night; this usually prompts the patient to sit up or get out of bed
- Tachypnoea: increased respiratory rate (> 20 breaths/min); a clinical sign found on examination

## Associated symptoms

Ask if the patient has any other symptoms during the breathlessness, including pain, wheeze and cough. Chest pain with dyspnoea on exertion suggests myocardial ischaemia. A wheeze in a patient with a history of myocardial infarction or heart failure suggests cardiac asthma. In this condition, pulmonary oedema resulting from left ventricular failure causes narrowing of the airways.

A cough, with or without sputum production, suggests various diagnoses.

- White, frothy sputum suggests pulmonary oedema caused by heart failure
- Pink, blood-stained sputum suggests mitral valve disease causing pulmonary capillary rupture or lung malignancy
- Grey, green, or brown purulent sputum suggests upper or lower respiratory tract infection
- A dry, non-productive, tickly cough is an adverse effect of angiotensin-converting enzyme (ACE) inhibitors; it is experienced by about 30% of patients taking them
- A dry cough with diurnal variation, e.g. worse in the evening, may be the only indication of chronic airways disease

| Features of common causes of shortness of breath | | | | | |
|---|---|---|---|---|---|
| Type | Angina | Asthma or COPD | Heart failure | Pulmonary embolism | Pneumonia |
| Associated symptoms | Chest pain | Wheeze and cough | Fatigue | Pain and cough | Fever and cough |
| Exacerbating factors | Exertion | Allergens and aspirin | Supine | None | None |
| Relieving factors | Rest | β-agonist | Diuretics | None | Oxygen |
| Risk factors | Hypertension and smoking | Occupational exposure to dusts and smoking | Myocardial infarction | Deep vein thrombosis and immobility | Malnutrition and immunosuppression |
| Onset | Gradual | Acute | Gradual | Acute | Gradual |
| COPD, chronic obstructive pulmonary disease. | | | | | |

**Table 2.4** Features of the common causes of shortness of breath

| AEROS: taking a history of shortness of breath | | |
|---|---|---|
| Letter | Meaning | Example question |
| A | Associated symptoms | 'What else are you experiencing?' |
| E | Exacerbating factors | 'What makes it worse?' |
| R | Relieving factors | 'What makes it better?' |
| O | Onset | 'When did it first start and when does it occur?' |
| S | Severity | 'How severe is the breathlessness?' |

**Table 2.5** The AEROS mnemonic for taking a history of shortness of breath

## Exacerbating factors

Most breathlessness is worse on exertion and better at rest. The inverse suggests a psychological cause, such as anxiety.

Breathlessness associated with heart failure is worse when the patient lies flat (orthopnoea). This position removes the effect of gravity on pulmonary oedema, thus increasing fluid blockage of the respiratory membrane.

Patients with airways disease usually find that their symptoms of breathlessness worsen on exposure to common allergens such as animal dander, pollen and air pollutants. It is common to find diurnal variation in asthma; patients usually feel better in the morning and worse in the evening.

Patients who are chronically breathless, such as those with airways or heart disease, can also suffer from anxiety. This can compound the feelings of breathlessness.

## Relieving factors

Other than psychological causes, e.g. anxiety or panic attacks, no cause of breathlessness improves without treatment. If a treatment has been tried (pre-emptively) and the condition has not improved, the diagnosis must be reconsidered.

## Onset

Ascertain when the breathlessness started, how quickly it progressed and whether a precipitant is identified. For example:

- if breathlessness worsens a week after a patient stops taking diuretic medication for heart failure, the medication is the most likely culprit
- rapid onset of breathlessness after a long-haul flight suggest pulmonary embolus
- breathlessness that started some months ago, is intermittent and coincides with palpitations suggests paroxysmal atrial fibrillation

## Severity

This is judged by the level of exertion at which the symptoms become apparent, which can be used to compare against a patient's previous breathlessness. The severity of dyspnoea indicates how advanced the disease process is; it also helps guide and monitor treatment. A commonly used grading system is the New York Heart Association classification.

- I: no limitation of normal activity; patients are breathless only with vigorous activity (e.g. playing competitive sport) and are considered asymptomatic
- II: slight limitation of normal activity; patients are breathless during prolonged or moderate exertion, such as climbing a flight of stairs
- III: marked limitation of normal activity; patients are breathless during minimal exertion, such a walking across one room to another
- IV: inability to perform normal activity; patients are breathless at rest

It is also useful to gauge exercise tolerance by asking the patient how far they can walk before becoming breathless. Onset and progression can also be approximated this way.

# Palpitations

Palpitations are heartbeats that a person becomes aware of. They consist of various unusual sensations in the chest. Common causes are shown in **Table 2.6**. **Table 2.7** shows the FLUTTER mnemonic used when taking a history of palpitations.

## Feeling (character)

Patients describe palpitations in many ways. They call it a 'thump', a fast or slow heartbeat, a 'fluttering' or erratic heartbeat, a general awareness of their heartbeat, discomfort or breathlessness.

A 'thump' is usually an ectopic (extra) heartbeat, also known as a premature ventricular contraction or ventricular extrasystole. It is usually followed by a compensatory pause. Ectopic heartbeats are normal. They originate from the ventricle rather than the sinoatrial node, so there is ventricular but no atrial contraction.

| Features of common causes of palpitations | | | |
|---|---|---|---|
| Arrhythmia | Feeling | Exacerbating factors | Relieving factors |
| Bradyarrhythmias | Tiredness and dizziness | Calcium channel blockers, beta-blockers and ischaemic heart disease | Atropine, permanent pacemaker and stopping medication |
| Ventricular ectopic heartbeats | 'Thump' or missed beats | Electrolyte disturbance and excessive caffeine intake | Correction of electrolytes and reducing caffeine intake |
| Sinus tachycardia | Fast heartbeat | Pain, exercise, anxiety and fever | Treat underlying problem |
| Atrial fibrillation and atrial flutter | Fluttering in chest, dizziness, dyspnoea and transient loss of consciousness | Infection, dehydration, excessive alcohol intake, ischaemia, hyperthyroidism and caffeine | Treat underlying problem, antiarrhythmic medication, direct current cardioversion or ablation of atrial re-entry circuit |
| Atrioventricular re-entry tachycardia and atrioventricular nodal re-entry tachycardia | Fluttering in chest, dizziness, dyspnoea and transient loss of consciousness | Stress, caffeine and alcohol | Anti-arrhythmic medication, direct current cardioversion or ablation of the supra-ventricular re-entry circuit |
| Ventricular tachycardia | Fluttering in chest, dizziness, dyspnoea and transient loss of consciousness | Myocardial ischaemia, heart failure and structural heart disease | Treat underlying problem, anti-arrhythmic medication, direct current cardioversion or ablation of the ventricular re-entry circuit |

*Length, unconsciousness, timing, is the rhythm 'tappable' and related features are highly variable so excluded.

**Table 2.6** Features of the common causes of palpitations*

| FLUTTER: taking a history of palpitations | | |
|---|---|---|
| Letter | Meaning | Example question |
| F | Feeling (character) | 'What does it feel like?' |
| L | Length | 'How long does it last?' |
| U | Unconsciousness | 'Have you ever lost consciousness?' |
| T | Timing | 'How frequently are you having palpitations?' |
| T | 'Tappable' (rhythm) | 'Can you tap out the rhythm?' |
| E | Exacerbating and relieving factors | 'Does anything make it better or worse?' |
| R | Related symptoms | 'What other symptoms are you experiencing?' |

**Table 2.7** The FLUTTER mnemonic for taking a history of palpitations

The normal heart rate is 60–100 beats/min. Faster rates (tachycardia) and slower rates (bradycardia) have various cardiac and non-cardiac causes (see page 105).

'Fluttering' in the chest feels similar to anxiety. The sensation is usually caused by a fast heartbeat, which is regular, as in sinus tachycardia, or irregular, as in atrial fibrillation.

An erratic or irregular heartbeat has one of three causes.

- Atrial fibrillation
- Ectopic heartbeats coupled with normal heartbeats; it is termed bi- or trigeminy depending on whether an abnormal beat is present before one or two normal beats respectively
- Atrioventricular block: this is caused by a disconnect in electrical conduction between the atria and the ventricles

A general awareness of the heart beating is most commonly the result of anxiety or depression.

## Length

The duration of symptoms depends on the cause.

- Seconds: symptoms lasting seconds are usually caused by an ectopic heartbeat rather than serious cardiac pathology

- Minutes: symptoms that last minutes are usually the result of conditions such as atrial fibrillation/flutter, supraventricular tachycardia or sinus tachycardia
- Hours: paroxysmal atrial fibrillation/flutter or supraventricular tachycardia last for several hours but may resolve on their own, without intervention
- Days: long-lasting symptoms are usually caused by anxiety or depression

## Unconsciousness

This is a serious association with palpitations. Following palpitations, loss of consciousness indicates significant cardiac pathology, with reduced cardiac output compromising cerebral hypoperfusion.

## Timing

Ectopic heartbeats are common and benign. They usually occur between once every few minutes and once a week, but they can occur with every other heartbeat.

Atrial arrhythmias such as fibrillation, flutter and supraventricular tachycardia are usually experienced infrequently, only once every few days. Usually, the less frequently an arrhythmia is experienced, the less serious it is.

## 'Tappable' (rhythm)

If the patient can tap the heart rhythm, this can be very informative. Most irregular rhythms are atrial fibrillation. Most regular rhythms are sinus tachycardia, atrial flutter or supraventricular tachycardia.

## Exacerbating and relieving factors

Palpitations caused by ectopic beats feel worse when the patient has fewer distractions or is lying on their left side; this position brings the apex of the heart closer to the chest wall. Palpitations are also exacerbated by caffeine intake.

Patients with atrial fibrillation find that their symptoms worsen with increased alcohol intake. Conversely, their symptoms improve with abstinence from alcohol.

Patients experiencing palpitations resulting from anxiety or depression find that their symptoms reflect their mood.

Patients with postural orthostatic tachycardia syndrome, in which a change of posture from supine to upright causes a rapid increase in heart rate, find that their symptoms are made worse by dehydration, heat, lack of food and stress.

## Related symptoms

Breathlessness, chest pain and presyncope suggest serious cardiac pathology. This is because the tachyarrhythmia prevents adequate cardiac output and the perfusion of coronary arteries and brain.

# Syncope

Syncope, or fainting, is a sudden and transient loss of consciousness with rapid recovery and no long-term sequelae. It is caused by a temporary but global hypoperfusion of the brain as a consequence of hypotension. Syncope can suggest serious cardiac pathology, but other causes include pulmonary embolism, sepsis (severe infection) and significant gastrointestinal blood loss (haemorrhage).

Presyncope is an impending sense of transient loss of consciousness without actual unconsciousness. Symptoms of presyncope include weakness, tunnel vision and dizziness.

Key differential diagnoses are listed in **Table 2.8.** They do not include stroke, in which sustained, focal hypoperfusion of the brain leads to infarction; seizure with a sustained loss of consciousness caused by abnormal electrical activity in the brain; and low blood sugar (hypoglycaemia).

Syncope is described as cardiac or neurocardiogenic in origin.

- Cardiac syncope is uncommon; it is caused by primary disease of the heart, such as an obstructive lesion of the left ventricular outflow tract (e.g. aortic stenosis)
- Neurocardiogenic (vasovagal) syncope is common; it occurs when a stimulus causes an abnormal autonomic reflex that leads to hypotension, tachycardia or both

Stimuli for vasovagal syncope include cough, defecation, micturition, venepuncture (obtaining a blood sample), a strong smell and sudden shock. The condition is exacerbated by heat, dehydration and fasting. The response to the stimulus is cardioinhibitory, with a decrease in heart rate, heart contractility, or both, and consequent insufficient cardiac output. Alternatively there is vasovagal syncope caused by a vasodepressor response (also known as orthostatic hypotension). In this condition, there is a lack of sympathetic response of the peripheral vasculature to standing upright, so gravity causes blood to pool in the extremities. Cerebral hypoperfusion then results from the associated decrease in blood pressure.

The FAINTS mnemonic for taking a history of syncope is shown in **Table 2.9.**

## Frequency

This has no bearing on the diagnosis. However, frequency of syncope does indicate interference in and risk to the patient's life. Response to treatment is more difficult to assess if the episodes of syncope are rare.

## Associated symptoms

Eyewitness testimony and video recordings or both are invaluable. Symptoms before, during and after the attack can suggest the underlying cause.

Symptoms occurring before syncope, such as nausea, reduced hearing, tunnel vision, and dizziness immediately preceding it, usually suggest a neurocardiogenic cause because of the cerebral hypoperfusion. Patients with these symptoms appear pale and sweaty. Palpitations, chest pain and dyspnoea suggest a cardiac cause, such as tachyarrhythmia and cardiac ischaemia. Unusual stereotyped smells or sounds indicate the prodrome of a seizure.

Loss of consciousness suggests global hypoperfusion (syncope) or abnormal electrical activity (seizure). If the patient remains conscious but unresponsive, a non-epileptic attack disorder is likely.

Syncope is usually followed by complete and immediate recovery of consciousness. However, patients have nausea and fatigue shortly afterwards. Seizure is followed by the postictal state of feeling groggy and confused for up to 30 min.

| Features of different causes of syncope | | | | |
|---|---|---|---|---|
| Cause | Speed of onset | Speed of recovery | Initiating event(s) | Associated symptom(s) |
| Carotid sinus hypersensitivity | Sudden | Rapid | Turning head, shaving and wearing a tight shirt collar | Dizziness |
| Hypoglycaemia | Gradual | Gradual | Exercise, hypoglycaemic drugs and missed meals | Sweating and tremulousness |
| Left ventricular outflow obstruction | Sudden | Rapid | Exercise | Chest pain and palpitations |
| Orthostatic hypotension | Sudden | Rapid | Change in posture (from sitting or lying down to standing) and antihypertensive drugs | Tunnel vision and weakness |
| Postural orthostatic tachycardia syndrome | Sudden | Gradual | Increased heart rate on standing | Chronic fatigue syndrome, irritable bowel syndrome and joint hypersensitivity syndrome |
| Pseudoseizure | Gradual | Rapid | Stress and trauma | Psychiatric illness |
| Pulmonary embolus | Sudden | Gradual | Immobility, travel, trauma and surgery | Chest pain and dyspnoea |
| Seizure | Sudden | Gradual | Fatigue, alcohol and flashing lights | Incontinence and tongue biting |
| Stokes–Adams attack | Sudden | Rapid | Prolonged asystole | None |
| Tachycardia | Sudden | Rapid | None | Chest pain and palpitations |
| Vasovagal syncope | Sudden | Rapid | Pain, emotion, coughing and micturition | Dizziness and weakness |

**Table 2.8** Features of the different causes of syncope

| FAINTS: taking a history of syncope | | |
|---|---|---|
| Letter | Meaning | Example question(s) |
| F | Frequency | 'How often do they occur?' |
| A | Associated symptoms | 'What other symptoms are you having?' |
| I | Initiating events | 'What seems to set them off?' |
| N | Nature of recovery | 'How do you recover?' and 'How long does it take?' |
| T | Time | 'How long were you unconscious for?' |
| S | Speed of onset | 'How quickly does it come on?' |

**Table 2.9** The FAINTS mnemonic for taking a history of syncope

## Initiating events

Vasodepressor syncope usually presents with a clear specific trigger, such as sitting or standing upright, from a lying position. Symptoms that occur while sitting or supine are probably cardiac in origin.

■ Symptoms after exercise suggest a loss of postural tone, leading to a vasodepressor response
■ Symptoms occurring during exercise are a red flag for significant cardiac pathology

## Nature of recovery

If recovery from the syncope is prolonged or requires intervention, then the event is unlikely to be a true cardiac syncope.

## Time

The duration of unconsciousness does not inform diagnosis, because syncope of any cause lasts between seconds and minutes.

## Speed of onset

In vasovagal syncope, loss of consciousness occurs up to 2 min after the trigger. Cardiac syncope and seizures usually develop within seconds.

# Ankle swelling

Swelling of the ankles is an abnormal increase in the circumference of the lower limb. The condition usually results from oedema, the collection of excess interstitial fluid. The swelling can extend to the foot, ankle and even the entire leg. Patients usually notice a slow change in shoe or sock size.

Ankle swelling is a sign of serious disease, including heart, liver or renal failure (**Table 2.10**). A thorough history includes ascertaining the location of the swelling, the speed of onset and any associated symptoms (both local, e.g. erythema, and global, e.g. dyspnoea). The PEDAL mnemonic is used when taking a history of ankle swelling (**Table 2.11**).

## Presence

In pitting oedema, the indentation produced by pressure from a finger persists for seconds after the pressure is released (**Figure 2.3**). This effect occurs in heart failure because of an increase in hydrostatic pressure in the venous system, which causes a build-up of fluids in the lungs and legs. In renal and liver failure, pitting oedema is the consequence of a lack of blood protein leading to decreased blood oncotic pressure and leakage of fluid into the subcutaneous tissues; most noticeable in the lower limbs.

Non-pitting oedema occurs with blockage of the lymphatic system (lymphoedema) or hypothyroidism (myxoedema), when protein and fluid leak into subcutaneous tissues. The accumulation of protein leads to proliferation

| Causes of ankle swelling | | |
|---|---|---|
| Type | Category | Cause |
| Non-cardiac | Renal disease | Proteinuria leading to low oncotic pressure |
| | Liver failure | Reduced albumin synthesis leading to low oncotic pressure |
| | Pharmacological | Calcium channel blockers and steroids |
| | Malnutrition | Low dietary protein leading to low oncotic pressure |
| | Travel | Prolonged immobility |
| | Lymphoedema | Lymphatic disease and cancer therapy |
| | Obstetric and gynaecological | Pregnancy, pre-eclampsia and use of the contraceptive pill |
| | Endocrine | Myxoedema caused by hypothyroidism |
| Cardiac | Left-sided | Left ventricular systolic dysfunction (e.g. caused by myocardial infarction) |
| | | Left ventricular diastolic dysfunction (e.g. caused by hypertension) |
| | | Cardiomyopathies |
| | | Mitral and aortic valve disease |
| | Right-sided | Pulmonary embolus |
| | | Posterior myocardial infarction |
| | | Chronic lung disease (cor pulmonale) |
| | | Tricuspid and aortic valve disease |
| | | Pulmonary hypertension |

**Table 2.10** Cardiac and non-cardiac causes of ankle swelling

| Letter | Meaning | Example question(s) |
|---|---|---|
| **PEDAL: taking a history of ankle swelling** | | |
| P | Presence | 'Do you have any swelling in your feet, ankles or legs?' |
| E | Exacerbating and relieving factors | 'Does anything make the swelling better or worse?' |
| D | Development | 'When did the swelling start?' |
| A | Associated symptoms | 'Do you have any other symptoms?' |
| L | Legs: one or both? (Symmetry) | 'Are both legs affected by the swelling? Or just one?' |

**Table 2.11** The PEDAL mnemonic for taking a history of ankle swelling

of fibroblasts and scarring, which results in firm, non-compressible swelling.

## Exacerbating and relieving factors

Pitting oedema usually worsens throughout the day because of the effect of gravity. The condition improves at night, when the lower limbs are elevated.

Oedema improves with treatment of systemic causes, for example the use of diuretics by patients with heart failure, and increased protein intake in malnourished patients.

## Development

If the ankle swelling develops gradually, the cause is a physiological or pathological process.

- In cases of gradual and provoked ankle swelling, patients remember precisely when and why it started, for example during the 2nd trimester of pregnancy or after starting treatment with an antihypertensive agent (e.g. a calcium channel blocker); in such cases, swelling accumulates over days to weeks
- If the swelling developed gradually and spontaneously, patients are unable to recall the onset or trigger; however, in cases of heart, liver and renal failure, other symptoms are present (e.g. dyspnoea, weight loss and fatigue)

Ankle swelling that developed suddenly has a non-cardiac cause; it is the result of localised disease.

- Sudden, provoked swelling is caused by an insect bite or an operation
- Sudden and spontaneous swelling can be caused by cellulitis or deep vein thrombosis

## Associated symptoms

These depend on the cause and include the following.

- Cellulitis: bacterial infection of the lower limb; the patient complains of generalised fever, pain in the limb (from soft tissue swelling) and redness of the limb (from active inflammation)

- Deep vein thrombosis: pain in the limb caused by soft tissue swelling resulting from reduced venous return; if embolism to the lung has occurred, the patient also has shortness of breath
- Heart failure: shortness of breath caused by pulmonary oedema, fatigue as a result

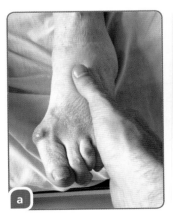
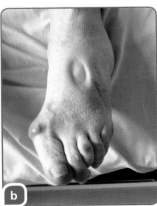

**Figure 2.3** Pitting oedema of the lower limb. (a) The thumb (or a finger) is used to press down over the swelling for 5 seconds.. (b) It is then removed and a pit is left in the swelling.

of reduced cardiac output, and weight loss from loss of muscle mass

■ Renal failure: shortness of breath as a consequence of pulmonary oedema, fatigue caused by anaemia and frothy urine from proteinuria

■ Liver failure: jaundice caused by excessive circulating bilirubin (hyperbilirubinaemia), abdominal swelling resulting from ascites, and easy bruising from impaired blood clotting

■ Myxoedema: weight gain, neck swelling from an enlarged thyroid gland, and fatigue caused by reduced metabolism; all result from hypothyroidism

## Legs: one or both (symmetry)

Unilateral ankle swelling usually has a non-cardiac cause, such as cellulitis, deep vein thrombosis and reduced venous return as a consequence of varicose veins. Bilateral ankle swelling has both cardiac and non-cardiac causes (see **Table 2.10**).

## Medical history

The medical history is a summary of the patient's previous illnesses and their treatment. In cardiology, conditions such as hypercholesterolaemia, diabetes, kidney disease, hypertension and obesity all increase the risk of developing heart disease.

Other chronic diseases cause symptoms that mimic cardiac pathology. For example, breathlessness is caused by chronic airways disease, and weight loss and peripheral oedema by malignancy.

It is useful to speak to the patient's general practitioner. They can provide a printed record of the dates and diagnoses of previous illnesses, as well as information on their treatment.

## Drug history

The drug history comprises the names of current medications and their dosages, routes of administration and frequency. To avoid confusion, generic rather than trade names are recorded. Furthermore, drug names are written in full, not abbreviated, and capital letters

are used. Dosages must be clear as incorrect dosing can significantly harm patients. Spell out units as micrograms or milligrams rather than using the abbreviated form such as mcg or mg respectively.

Record any over-the-counter drugs, including herbal medicines, because they interact with cardiac medications, such as St John's Wort. Drugs that have been stopped, and recent changes in drug therapy, are also noted. Remember that some drugs are cardiotoxic, for example non-steroidal anti-inflammatory drugs (NSAIDs), anabolic steroids and chemotherapeutic agents. Don't forget non-pharmacological treatments such as thoracic radiotherapy, which leads to fibrosis of myocardium and coronary arteries.

## Allergy history

The allergy history includes the name of any drugs to which the patient is allergic, their routes of administration and the nature and severity of the reaction. Allergic reactions vary from a simple skin rash to life-threatening anaphylaxis. Previous adverse effects of drugs are also noted, e.g. dizziness as a result of anti-hypertensives. Reactions to other substances, such as latex, shellfish and peanuts, are equally relevant.

## Family medical history

A number of cardiac conditions, such as cardiomyopathies and arrhythmias, have a genetic element (**Table 2.12**). Therefore a family tree is constructed, documenting any heritable conditions in first-degree relatives (parents, siblings and children). Such conditions include myocardial infarction and sudden cardiac death in those younger than 60 years. Diseases in distant relatives and those over 60 years old are not relevant.

## Social history

The purpose of the social history is to enable understanding of the social context of the patient's health, as well as the effects the presenting complaint or disease has on their life. Ask about the following:

| Inherited cardiac conditions | | |
|---|---|---|
| Disorder | Inheritance | Complications |
| Arrhythmogenic right ventricular dysplasia | Autosomal dominant | Sudden cardiac death |
| | | Arrhythmia |
| Cardiac amyloid | Autosomal dominant | Heart block |
| | | Heart failure |
| Brugada's syndrome | Autosomal dominant | Sudden cardiac death |
| | | Arrhythmia |
| Long QT syndrome | Autosomal dominant or recessive | Sudden cardiac death |
| | | Arrhythmia |
| Hypertrophic cardiomyopathy | Autosomal dominant | Sudden cardiac death |
| | | Arrhythmia |
| Dilated cardiomyopathy | Autosomal dominant or recessive | Heart failure |
| | | Arrhythmia |
| Marfan's syndrome | Autosomal dominant | Mitral valve prolapse |
| | | Aortopathy |
| Atrial myxoma | Autosomal dominant | Stroke |
| | | Syncope |

**Table 2.12** Inherited cardiac conditions

- Occupation: 'What do you do for a living?'
- Smoking: 'Do you smoke or did you used to? If so, how much?'
- Alcohol consumption: 'How much alcohol do you drink per day or per week?'
- Caffeine consumption: 'How many caffeine-containing drinks do you have daily?'
- Use of recreational drugs: 'Do you use illicit substances? If so, how much and how often?'
- Functional capacity: 'How much can you do for yourself when you are well?'
- Exercise: 'How much exercise do you get per day or per week? What kind of exercise do you do?'

## Occupation

A patient's occupation is significant in cardiovascular disease for two reasons. First, certain occupations are associated with risk factors for these conditions. Second, cardiovascular disease limits certain livelihoods or choice of occupation. For example, being the owner of a bar or pub is associated with heavy alcohol consumption, and patients who drive for a living have restrictions placed on their driving licence after a diagnosis, such as cardiac arrest (see page 371).

## Smoking history

Smoking is the most significant risk factor for cardiovascular and peripheral vascular disease. When taking a smoking history, begin by asking the patient if they smoke or if they have ever smoked. If the answer is 'Yes', determine how frequently they smoked and for how long.

Pack-years are units used to compare smoking habits over time: 1 pack-year is the equivalent of someone smoking 20 cigarettes a day for 1 year, and 2 packs daily for 40 years is the equivalent of 80 pack-years.

Patients who smoke are always encouraged to stop, and they should be provided with sufficient information and support to aid cessation.

## Alcohol consumption

Moderate alcohol consumption is beneficial for cardiovascular health, e.g. less than 14 units per week for men and 7 units per week for women. Whilst the relationship is complex, it is believed that alcohol exerts its protective effects by increasing HDL cholesterol, antioxidant properties and inhibiting blood clotting. However, regular and excessive alcohol consumption leads to dilated cardiomyopathy, rhythm disturbances (e.g. atrial fibrillation), or both. Record the patient's weekly consumption in units of alcohol, and pay particular attention to patients who frequently or infrequently drink to excess. If such patients are identified, they should be referred to a local alcohol misuse team and informed of other services available such as alcoholics anonymous.

## Caffeine consumption

Caffeine stimulates the sympathetic nervous system; it is a sympathomimetic. Excessive consumption can lead to sinus tachycardia and ectopic (extra) heartbeats, which patients feel as palpitations or anxiety. Caffeine is contained within coffee, tea, energy drinks, coke and chocolate and is an active ingredient in over the counter pain killers and influenza remedies.

## Recreational drug use

Many recreational drugs have physiological effects with potential short- or long-term cardiovascular consequences. Amphetamines are sympathomimetic and therefore cause palpitations and hypertension. Cocaine, depending on how it is taken and what impurities it contains, can lead to coronary artery spasm, thrombosis, myocarditis and sudden death. Some drugs, such as marijuana, are smoked with tobacco, and tobacco consumption in this form may go unrecognised when taking a smoking history.

## Functional capacity

Functional capacity is a measure of how much activity a patient is capable of in their present state, and significantly influences treatment decisions, the appropriate level of care and the degree of recovery expected. It may fluctuate or differ significantly from what the patient was able to do before they were unwell, i.e. in their premorbid state.

The patient's functional capacity is discussed in terms of activities of daily living: specific tasks of self-care, e.g. mobility, eating, washing, dressing etc. A patient can range from being fully independent to bedbound and doubly incontinent.

Collateral information from third parties, such as family members, carers and nursing staff, can provide a better understanding of the patient's functional capacity. Questions include how they mobilise (e.g. with a stick, frame or wheelchair), their home circumstances (e.g. whether they live in a flat, bungalow or house) and if they have help at home (e.g. from relatives, carers or a warden).

## Exercise

All patients, not just those with cardiovascular disease, are encouraged to exercise.

The recommended minimum is at least 30–60 minutes of moderate exercise (so the patient is short of breath) five times a week. Exercise helps prevent disease, for example by lowering blood pressure. It also helps treat the consequences of disease, for example by increasing exercise tolerance and reducing breathlessness in patients with heart failure.

**Sports cardiology** is the study of how the athlete's heart adapts to exercise. Athletes may have dilated or hypertrophied hearts depending on whether the activity is predominantly resistant, e.g. weight lifting, or endurance, e.g. long distance cycling. The appearance can mimic diseases, such as hypertrophic or dilated cardiomyopathy.

## Systems review

A systems review is an opportunity to ensure that nothing relevant to the presentation has been missed in any of the other major body systems (**Table 2.13**).

## Summary

At the end of the history taking, summarise the history for the patient in a sentence or two. This summary ensures that the facts have been recorded correctly and any areas of doubt clarified. Summarising a history is also good practice when introducing patients to senior colleagues, for example on a ward round.

It is also good practice to ask the patient if they have any questions, or if there is anything that they have not understood, because some are too polite to ask.

**William Osler (died 1919) said, 'Listen to your patient; he is telling you the diagnosis'.** Allow patients to have their say before you interrupt with questions, because the diagnosis is determined through the history.

| Systems review in a cardiology patient | | |
|---|---|---|
| System | Symptom(s) | Cardiac and related causes |
| Respiratory | Cough | Infection, heart failure and angiotensin-converting enzyme inhibitors |
| | Wheeze | Cardiac asthma (a result of heart failure) |
| | Haemoptysis | Pulmonary embolism, pulmonary oedema and mitral stenosis |
| Endocrine | Changes in mood, weight or energy | Thyroid or pituitary disease |
| | Sweating, weakness and headaches | Adrenal disease |
| Musculoskeletal | Myalgia | Statins, exercise to which the patient is unaccustomed and tissue ischaemia |
| Neurological | Dizziness | Postural hypotension |
| | Syncope | Cardiac diseases (e.g. aortic stenosis) and medications (e.g. antihypertensive agents) |
| | Headache | Cardiac medication (e.g. antihypertensive agents) |
| | Stroke | A result of aortic dissection or atrial fibrillation |
| Gastrointestinal | Weight loss | A sign of poor prognosis in heart failure |
| | Gastric reflux | Cardiac medications, e.g. anti-platelet agents causing increased stomach acid |
| | Diarrhoea | Arrhythmia caused by loss of potassium |
| | Nausea and vomiting | Symptom of myocardial infarction |
| Genitourinary | Impotence | Peripheral arterial disease (impotence can be first sign of this) |
| | Haematuria | Glomerulonephritis or endocarditis |
| | Proteinuria | Peripheral oedema with a renal cause (frothy urine) |
| | Frequency | Prostatic disease or diuretic use/abuse |

**Table 2.13** Symptoms to check when taking a systematic history from a cardiology patient

# Common signs and how to examine a patient

## Starter questions

Answers to the following questions are on page 169–170.

6. Can you diagnose patients with cardiovascular disease on sight?
7. What does walking speed tell us about the severity chronic heart disease?
8. Will robots ever replace human doctors?
9. What relevance does the number seven have to presenting patients?

After the history has been taken, a long list of differential diagnoses is formulated. Examination aims to refine this into a short list.

A clinical examination is performed to find clinical signs, the positive and objective findings that demonstrate the presence of disease.

The art is in determining which positive findings are relevant for the particular patient, because multiple signs and therefore pathologies commonly coexist. A stepwise and systematic routine is essential, which is unique to the examiner, but it should be the same for any given system to ensure that nothing is missed. At first, the routine seems formulaic. However, over time it becomes second nature and adaptable to each individual focused examination.

The cardiovascular examination includes the lower limbs and the abdomen. Examination of these areas provides clues as to the presence and severity of other diagnoses.

## Starting the examination

Begin by washing your hands, introducing yourself to the patient and offering to shake their hand. Check the patient's identity and then ask what they would like to be called. Ask if the patient will accept examination of their heart and chest, which requires them to remove their clothing. Inform them why the examination is required and encourage them to ask questions during the process. Ideally perform the examination in a side room or with the curtains closed around the bed if this is not possible. Ensure that women have their modesty preserved at all times; they can use a sheet to cover their breasts while their chest is not being examined and all patient's should be offered a sheet to cover their genitals, in addition to their underwear during examination of the abdomen and lower limbs. The patient should be comfortably positioned at 45°.

> When examining a patient of the opposite sex, it is best practice to have a same-sex chaperone present. This is usually a health professional, such as a fellow medical student, physician or nurse. A relative or friend of the patient is unsuitable as a chaperone, because they are not an impartial observer.

## General inspection

Table 2.14 outlines the cardiovascular examination. The examination starts as soon as you meet the patient. Count from 1 to 10 to ensure that you take the time that this meeting warrants, because a great deal of information is ascertained from first impressions. This encounter also helps set the context for the rest of the examination and helps you relax (especially if in a test situation). While counting, survey both the environment and the patient, looking for clues as to a possible diagnosis or risk factors.

Make an overall assessment of the patient. Do they look well or unwell? For example, are they smiling, well perfused and talkative? Or are they quiet, pale and in pain? Is their face blue suggesting central cyanosis or are the neck veins visible and pulsating, suggesting fluid overload? Are they well nourished, or are they pathologically thin (cachetic) or pathologically overweight (obese)?

Survey the area around the patient, looking for clues to certain diseases. Medications are kept on the cabinet next to the bed, for example a glyceryl trinitrate spray for angina and insulin for diabetes. Look to see if the patient is receiving oxygen for coexisting lung disease or hypoxia, if they are breathless by checking respiratory rate and check for an intravenous infusion, such as antibiotics for an infection or furosemide for heart failure.

After the general inspection, the remainder of the examination proceeds from proximal to distal: hands, wrist, elbow, neck, face and chest.

## Examination of the hands

Start the inspection of both hands by asking the patient to rest them on a pillow. The hands can reveal a plethora of acute and chronic signs.

## Dorsal surface

The dorsal surface is examined for discoloration, clubbing and signs of infective endocarditis.

| Cardiovascular examination | |
|---|---|
| Element | Details |
| General inspection | Appearance: does the patient look systemically well or unwell? |
| | Environment: are there any clues suggesting disease? |
| | Face: is the patient centrally cyanosed? (Look for blue discoloration) |
| | Neck: is there a visible pulsation suggesting fluid overload? |
| | Chest: is the patient breathless at rest, if so what is the respiratory rate? |
| | Is the patient underweight (cachexic), overweight or obese? |
| Hands | Are there any nail abnormalities, e.g. tar staining, clubbing or splinter haemorrhages? |
| | Is there peripheral cyanosis (bluish discoloration)? Is there any evidence of vasculitis, e.g. oslers nodes? |
| Wrist | What is the heart rate and rhythm? |
| Elbow/knee/ankle | Are there any tendon xanthomata? |
| Arm | What is the blood pressure? |
| Neck | Is the jugular venous pressure elevated? What does the carotid pulse feel like? |
| Face | Is there evidence of xanthelasma or corneal arcus? |
| | Is there flushing of the cheeks? |
| | Is there blue discolouration of the lips or tongue? |
| | Is there any dental caries? |
| Chest | Inspection: are there any surgical scars, pacemakers or chest wall deformities? |
| | Palpation: is the apex beat displaced? |
| | Auscultation: are the heart sounds normal, or are there any added sounds? |
| | Lung bases: are there any crepitations? |
| Legs | Examine for swelling (peripheral oedema), venous and arterial disease |
| Abdomen | Examine for fluid in the abdomen (ascites) and vascular disease |
| Fundi | Examine for hypertensive and diabetic eye disease (retinopathy) |

**Table 2.14** The cardiovascular examination

## Splinter haemorrhages

These are short, thin, linear discolorations of the nail (**Figure 7.13a**). Splinter haemorrhages are red at first, before turning brown and finally black within a few days. They are usually caused by trauma, such as that from gardening injuries. However, they are also a sign of arterial vasculitis and infection of the heart valves (infective endocarditis), because these conditions cause microemboli to lodge in the arterioles and cause bleeding (haemorrhage).

## Tar staining

This is often incorrectly referred to as nicotine staining in chronic smokers. The tar contained in tobacco smoke stains the fingers and fingernails yellow-brown (Figure 3.7).

## Finger clubbing

This is an increase in the convexity of the nail and sponginess of the nail bed (Figure 7.13b). Digital clubbing is caused by increased soft tissue and vasodilation, and develops in five stages (**Table 2.15**). Idiopathic clubbing is rare; most cases are secondary to chronic pulmonary, cardiac, liver or gastrointestinal disease, among other conditions. Cardiac causes include:

- benign cardiac tumours (atrial myxoma)
- cyanotic congenital heart disease
- infective endocarditis (see page 277)

| Stages of finger clubbing | |
|---|---|
| Stage | Description |
| 1 | Increased ballotability of the nail bed |
| 2 | Loss of the nail angle (usually < 165°) |
| 3 | Increased convexity of the nail bed |
| 4 | Thickening of the finger (drumstick appearance) |
| 5 | Shiny aspect and striation of finger and nail |

**Table 2.15** The five stages of finger clubbing

The common pathophysiology relates to increased circulating growth factors.

## Capillary refill time

This is the time taken for blood flow to return after occlusion of a capillary bed, for example in the fingernail, by pressure that causes blanching. The patient's fingertip is pressed for 5 s and should return to normal, i.e. the same colour as adjacent fingers, within 2 s. Any delay is caused by reduced peripheral perfusion, which occurs in cardiogenic shock, heart failure, dehydration and acute limb ischaemia.

## Palmar surface

Inspect the palmar surface of the hands for signs of infective endocarditis, peripheral cyanosis and blood disease.

### Osler's nodes and Janeway lesions

These are signs of infective endocarditis.

■ Osler's nodes are tender, raised purple papules in the finger pulps and are the result of deposition of immune complexes
■ Janeway lesions are non-tender, flat purple macules in the palm of the hand (Figure 7.13c), and are caused by septic emboli from endocarditis vegetations.

### Peripheral cyanosis

The blue discoloration associated with low blood oxygen is called cyanosis. Peripheral cyanosis (i.e. in the limbs; **Figure 2.4**) occurs in patients with reduced central circulation, in whom central cyanosis is also present (see page 111). Alternatively, peripheral cyanosis is

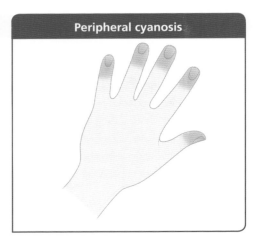

**Peripheral cyanosis**

**Figure 2.4** Peripheral cyanosis.

the result of peripheral factors, such as a cold environment, acute limb ischaemia caused by thromboembolism, or arterial vasospasm.

## Palmar erythema

This is reddening of the thenar and hypothenar eminences of the palm. Palmar erythema occurs in the following conditions:

■ Pregnancy: a third of pregnant women have palmar erythema, which is caused by oestrogen-induced vasodilation
■ Polycythaemia: palmar erythema is a consequence of the excess of red blood cells
■ Syphilis and vasculitis: inflammation causes palmar erythema in these conditions
■ Chronic liver disease: a fifth of patients have palmar erythema, due to increased circulating oestrogens

## Examination of the arterial pulse

Examination of the arterial pulse is a key part of the cardiovascular examination. In emergencies it is used as a proxy for systolic blood pressure measurement and also indicates the presence of arrhythmia, shock or valvular pathology. The pulse can be felt where there is a superficial artery, such as the wrist, neck or groin.

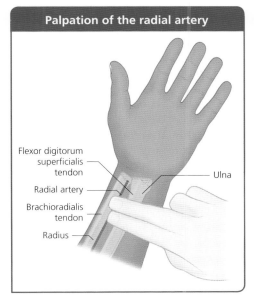

**Palpation of the radial artery**

Flexor digitorum
superficialis
tendon
Ulna
Radial artery
Brachioradialis
tendon
Radius

**Figure 2.5** Palpation of the radial artery in the wrist.

**Causes of abnormal heart rates**

| Rate (beats/min) | Term | Causes |
|---|---|---|
| < 60 | Bradycardia | Sleep, hypothermia, hypothyroidism, athletic training, arrhythmia and certain drugs, e.g. beta-blockers and calcium channel blockers |
| 60–100 | Normal | Not applicable |
| > 100 | Tachycardia | Pain, anxiety, fever, exercise, arrhythmia, shock and hyperthyroidism |

**Table 2.16** Causes of slow and fast heart rates

## Radial pulse

The radial pulse is felt at the base of the thumb, between the radial styloid and the brachioradialis and flexor digitorum superficialis wrist tendons (**Figure 2.5**). It is easily accessible and allows sensitive assessment of pulse rate and rhythm, and detection of a collapsing or delayed pulse.

### Pulse rate

Palpate the radial pulse for 1 min using the index and middle fingers, counting the number of beats throughout, to determine the heart rate in beats/min. To save time, for example in a test setting, palpate for 20 s and multiply by 3 for a less accurate measurement. A heart rate > 100 beats/min is pathologically fast (tachycardia), and one that is <60 beats/min is slow (bradycardia) (**Table 2.16**).

### Pulse rhythm

This refers to the regularity of each pulse wave felt during examination (**Figure 2.6**). The pulse rhythm (heart rhythm) can be one of several patterns (**Table 2.17**).

■ Regularly regular: the period between each pulse wave is the same
■ Regularly irregular: the period varies but has a pattern
■ Irregularly irregular: there is no pattern

### Collapsing (water hammer) pulse

A collapsing pulse is a sign of aortic regurgitation, an incompetent aortic valve. First check

**Figure 2.6** The regularity of the pulse.

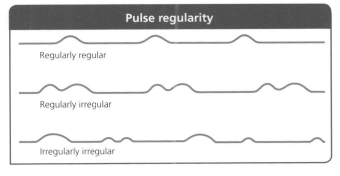

**Pulse regularity**

Regularly regular

Regularly irregular

Irregularly irregular

**Causes of different cardiac rhythms**

| Rhythm | Causes |
| --- | --- |
| Regularly regular | Sinus rhythm |
| | First- or third-degree heart block |
| Regularly irregular | Bigeminy/trigeminy |
| | Second-degree heart block |
| Irregularly irregular | Atrial and ventricular ectopic beats |
| | Atrial fibrillation |
| | Atrial flutter with variable block |
| | Multifocal atrial tachycardia |

**Table 2.17** Causes of different cardiac rhythms

that the patient has no shoulder pain, then place your fingers over the radial pulse and elevate the patient's arm above their head. A collapsing pulse feels as if there is a knocking pulse against your fingertips; it rapidly increases and then collapses. The incompetent valve present in aortic regurgitation remains open during ventricular diastole, allowing the backwards flow of blood into the left ventricle from the aorta and the left atrium, as it relaxes.

## Delayed pulse

Check for any delay between pulses. The radial pulse at one wrist is felt simultaneously with the radial pulse at the opposite (contralateral) wrist to detect any radioradial delay (**Figure 2.7a**). The radial pulse is then felt simultaneously with the femoral pulse on the same (ipsilateral) side of the body to detect any radiofemoral delay (**Figure 2.7b**).

- Radioradial delay suggests an aortic dissection (tear) of the aortic arch proximal to the origin of the left subclavian artery
- Radiofemoral delay suggests coarctation (narrowing) of the aortic arch distal to the origin of the subclavian arteries

## Carotid pulse

This is palpated after the radial pulse. The carotid pulse is found by palpating the common

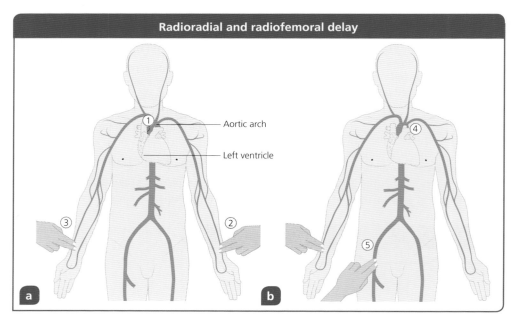

**Radioradial and radiofemoral delay**

— Aortic arch

— Left ventricle

**Figure 2.7** Radioradial and radiofemoral delay. (a) Radioradial delay: a tear in the aortic arch proximal to the left subclavian artery causes a delay between the right and left radial arteries. (b) Radiofemoral delay: a narrowing in the aortic arch distal to the left subclavian artery causes a delay between the right radial and femoral arteries. ①, tear in the aortic arch; ②, left radial artery; ③, right radial artery; ④, narrowing in the aortic arch; ⑤, right femoral artery.

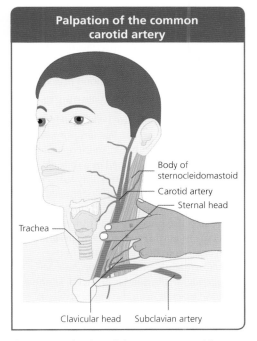

Figure 2.8 Palpation of the common carotid artery.

**Palpation of the common carotid artery**

Body of sternocleidomastoid

Carotid artery

Sternal head

Trachea

Clavicular head    Subclavian artery

carotid artery (see page 13), in the anterior cervical triangle beneath the angle of the jaw, lateral to the trachea but medial to the body of the sternocleidomastoid muscle (**Figure 2.8**).

Like the radial pulse, the carotid pulse is palpated with the index and middle fingers. Unlike the radial pulse, it is a central pulse close to the aorta, and can therefore provide information on pulse character and volume.

## Character

Pulse character is how the pulse feels during palpation, whether it is slow and slight or rapid and pronounced. Assess the carotid pulse for the slow rising pulse of aortic stenosis and the collapsing pulse of aortic regurgitation (**Figure 2.9**). These features are the examination equivalents of a narrow and broad pulse pressure, respectively.

In aortic stenosis, the valve becomes thickened, stiff and narrowed. Therefore it opens for only a short period, which reduces the amount of blood leaving the left ventricle in systole; this results in a slow rising pulse.

## Volume

A low-volume or 'thready' pulse is present in various conditions.

- This type of pulse reflects the reduced stroke volume in cases of shock, heart failure, anxiety and anaemia
- It is also a finding in hyperthermia and hyperthyroidism, because the reduced systemic vascular resistance results in rapid dispersion of the ejected blood.

# Blood pressure

Blood pressure is a measurement of the circulating pressure of blood in the systemic arterial system. It indicates the severity of conditions such as blood loss, heart failure and valvular heart diseases. Furthermore, monitoring of blood pressure is essential in the diagnosis

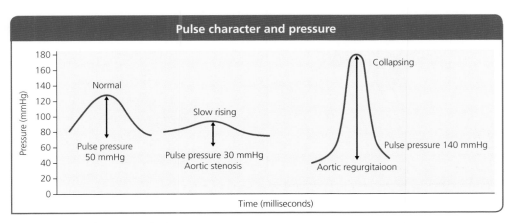

**Pulse character and pressure**

Pressure (mmHg)

Normal

Pulse pressure 50 mmHg

Slow rising

Pulse pressure 30 mmHg
Aortic stenosis

Collapsing

Pulse pressure 140 mmHg

Aortic regurgitaioon

Time (milliseconds)

**Figure 2.9** Pulse character and pulse pressure.

and management of hypertension. Automated blood pressure monitors are available. However, it is good practice to learn how to measure blood pressure manually.

A sphygmomanometer and a stethoscope are required for manual blood pressure measurement. Ask the patient to relax while seated, and request that they remain still and silent, because movement affects blood pressure. The highest and lowest readings are recorded; they are the systolic and diastolic blood pressure, respectively.

Blood pressure is measured as follows (**Figure 2.10**).

1. Place the sphygmomanometer around the patient's upper arm
2. Place the diaphragm of the stethoscope over the brachial artery in the antecubital fossa (the anterior surface of the elbow joint)
3. Inflate the cuff until the radial arterial pulse is no longer palpated; at this point, the pressure in the cuff is suprasystolic
4. Now use the stethoscope to listen to the brachial artery, and deflate the sphymanometer cuff slowly
5. Record the pressure at which Korotkoff sounds are first heard (see **Table 2.18**); this is the systolic pressure
6. Record the pressure at which these sounds disappear; this is the diastolic pressure

# Pulse pressure

The blood pressure measurements are used to check the pulse pressure (**Figure 2.9**).

Pulse pressure = systolic blood pressure – diastolic blood pressure

Pulse pressure is usually 40–80 mmHg.

■ Narrow pulse pressure (< 40 mmHg) occurs in aortic stenosis, cardiac tamponade and cardiogenic shock; an increase in left ventricular afterload or a reduction in left ventricular contractility leads to a reduction in the volume or speed of ejection of blood from the left ventricle
■ Broad pulse pressure (< 80 mmHg) occurs in aortic regurgitation, pregnancy, fever, thyrotoxicosis, arteriovenous malformation and Paget's disease; left ventricular afterload is reduced, so the blood ejected from the left ventricle is equally rapidly distributed

# Mean arterial pressure

The mean arterial pressure is calculated as follows:

mean arterial pressure = diastolic blood pressure + (1/3 pulse pressure)

This is the average blood pressure over the entire cardiac cycle, and is therefore the perfusion pressure supplying organs during

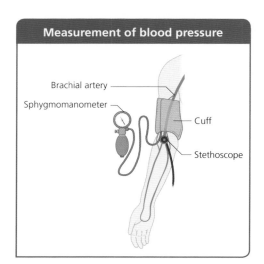

**Measurement of blood pressure**

Brachial artery

Sphygmomanometer

Cuff

Stethoscope

**Figure 2.10** Measurement of blood pressure.

| Significance of Korotokoff sounds | | |
|---|---|---|
| Korotokoff sound | Description | Significance |
| 1 | Crisp, clear tapping | Systolic blood pressure |
| 2 | Softer or longer taps | None |
| 3 | Softer or longer taps | None |
| 4 | Muffled or quiet taps | < 10 mmHg of diastolic blood pressure |
| 5 | Sounds disappear | Diastolic blood pressure |

**Table 2.18** Korotokoff sounds and their significance in the assessment of blood pressure

systole and diastole. Mean arterial pressure is usually 70–110 mmHg. If it decreases to <70 mmHg, tissue ischaemia, infarction and eventually necrosis result.

## Brachiobrachial blood pressure

Systolic blood pressure in both arms is also compared. A difference of >20 mmHg may indicate aortic dissection and is the equivalent of radio-radial pulse delay.

> **Automated sphygmomanometers are not accurate in cases of atrial fibrillation or frequent ventricular ectopy.** The irregularity of the pulse means that blood pressure is overestimated. In such cases, use a manual recording.

## Examination of the elbow, knees and ankles

Inspect the skin on the posterior aspect of the elbow (the triceps tendon), the anterior aspect of the knee (patella tendon) and the posterior aspect of the ankle (Achilles tendon) for yellow xanthomata. These nodular, cholesterol-rich deposits are seen in patients with inherited hyperlipidaemias, a major risk factor for vascular disease.

## The jugular venous pulse

The internal jugular vein (see page 13) is valveless and drains directly via the superior vena cava into the right atrium. Therefore it is used as a barometer of right atrial, and therefore central venous, pressure (**Figure 2.11**). The vein courses from the earlobe to between the sternal and clavicular head of the sternocleidomastoid muscle at the clavicle.

Check the jugular venous pressure as follows.

1. Ask the patient to lay at 45°, turn their head to the left and relax
2. Stand to the left of the patient, and look across the neck for the characteristic double waveform (**Figure 2.12**)
3. The jugular venous pressure is <3 cm vertically above the sternal angle

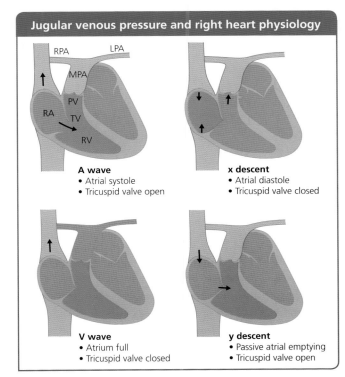

Figure 2.11 The jugular venous pressure and right heart physiology. LPA, left pulmonary artery; MPA, main pulmonary artery; PV, pulmonary valve; RA, right atrium; RPA, right pulmonary artery; RV, right ventricle; TV, tricuspid valve.

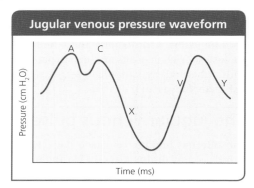

**Figure 2.12** The jugular venous pressure waveform.

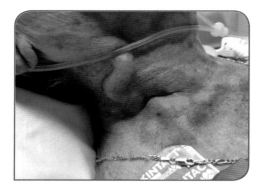

**Figure 2.14** Raised jugular venous pressure (apparent as a visible external jugular vein) caused by heart failure.

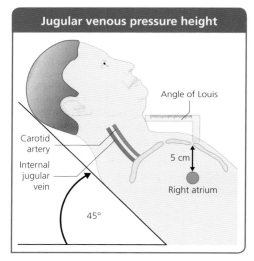

**Figure 2.13** Measuring the height of the jugular venous pressure.

(**Figure 2.13**); 3 cm is equivalent to 3 cm $H_2O$ (2 mmHg)

The jugular venous pressure is usually hidden from view behind the right clavicle, in healthy individuals. It is elevated in:

- biventricular heart failure (**Figure 2.14**)
- right ventricular failure
- right ventricular infarction
- fluid overload

In sinus rhythm, two waves are visible (**Table 2.19**): the A wave before the carotid pulse, and the V wave after it (**Figure 2.16**). Pathologies (**Table 2.20**) include absence of the A wave, which is the result of atrial fibrillation.

> If the jugular venous pressure is difficult to visualise, use the superficial veins of the hand to estimate central venous pressure. With the patient at 45°, lower the arm below the heart to allow the veins to fill, then gradually raise the arm. The height above the clavicle at which they collapse is an estimate of central venous pressure.

## Examination of the face

Gross facial signs noticed on general inspection are inspected more closely.

### Hair

Tar stains hair, like nails, brown.

### Skin

The skin over the cheekbones (malar bones) becomes reddened (erythematous) in conditions such as mitral stenosis (see page 267) or non-cardiac disease such as systemic lupus erythematosus and is called malar flush. A grey malar colour is seen in patients on long-term amiodarone, an antiarrhythmic agent (see page 152).

### Eyes

Xanthalesma are yellow fat deposits in the skin around the eyes (**Figure 2.15**). They are associated with high circulating levels of

| Comparison of jugular venous and carotid arterial pulses | | |
| --- | --- | --- |
| Characteristic | Jugular venous pulse | Carotid pulse |
| Waveform | Double | Single |
| Palpable? | No | Yes |
| Obliterable? | Yes | No |
| Positional? | Yes | No |
| Hepatojugular reflex | Increases | No effect |
| Inspiration | Decreases | No effect |

**Table 2.19** Comparison of jugular venous and carotid arterial pulses

cholesterol, which are caused by both congenital and acquired conditions.

Lipid deposits can also occur in the cornea (corneal arcus). They are visible as a white or grey ring between the white sclera and the coloured iris (**Figure 2.15**). Such deposits are a normal finding in the elderly, when the condition is called arcus senilis.

> A patient cannot have significant anaemia and cyanosis at the same time because cyanosis requires at least 5 g/dL of deoxygenated haemoglobin, which is not compatible with life if there is significant anaemia as well. In fact, many patients with cyanosis have compensatory polycythaemia (increased red blood cell count).

The undersurface of the eyelids has a rich and readily visible blood supply. Therefore this is a good site to judge blood colour. A pale

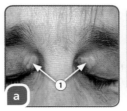 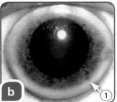

**Figure 2.15** (a) Orbital xanthelasma ①. (b) Corneal arcus ①.

appearance (subconjunctival pallor) is seen in anaemia and is caused by a lack of haemoglobin.

Fundoscopy is performed following examination of the praecordium, abdomen and lower limbs, to examine the retinae.

# Mouth

Inspect the inside of the mouth for dental caries (tooth decay). This is a significant risk factor for bacterial endocarditis, because oral infections or abscesses may spread to the endocardium.

> In a test setting, be sure that the examiner can see what you are doing. Examine the patient in a slower, more pronounced and deliberate way.

Assess the mouth and lips for the blue discoloration of central cyanosis. This is not a sign of anaemia but indicates excessive deoxygenated haemoglobin; it is seen with a concentration of deoxygenated haemoglobin >5.0 g/dL. This occurs in conditions that decrease blood oxygenation, such as chronic lung disease,

| Jugular venous pressure waveform | | | | |
| --- | --- | --- | --- | --- |
| Wave | Descent | Meaning | Physiology | Pathology |
| A | | Right atrial systole | Retrograde venous flow | Big in tricuspid stenosis |
| C | | Right ventricular contraction | Tricuspid valve bulges into right atrium | Not applicable |
| | X | Right atrial diastole | Tricuspid valve pulled down by right ventricle | Not applicable |
| V | | Right atrial diastole | Venous filling of right atrium | Big in tricuspid regurgitation |
| | Y | Tricuspid valve open | Decreased right atrial pressure | Deep in constrictive pericarditis |

**Table 2.20** The jugular venous pressure waveform

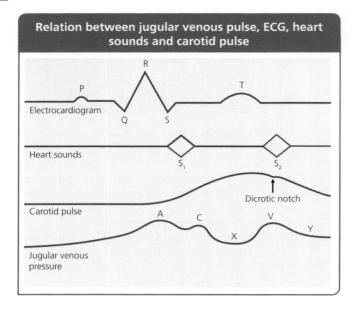

**Figure 2.16** The jugular venous pulse in relation to the electrocardiogram, heart sounds and the carotid pulse.

or in those which decrease blood circulation, such as myocardial infarction, congenital heart disease and cardiogenic shock.

Also assess the colour of the mucous membranes of the gums and lips for the pallor of anaemia. They are a pale pink rather than a deep red.

# Examination of the chest

Examination of the chest wall (praecordium) is the final part of the cardiovascular examination. Listening to heart sounds and making sense of murmurs are difficult skills to master, but structured repetition ensures improvement over time. As with most examinations, the four stages are:

1. inspection
2. palpation
3. percussion (no longer routinely done)
4. auscultation

Key clinical signs discovered at one stage influence subsequent stages. Therefore, although a structured approach is used to ensure that nothing is missed, each examination is tailored to the individual case.

## Inspection

Inspect the chest wall for its shape, any scars or masses, and its movement. Any abnormalities inform subsequent palpation, percussion and auscultation.

## Praecordial scars

Surgical scars may indicate previous cardiac surgery (**Figure 2.17**). For example, a midline sternotomy scar may represent a aortic valve replacement, heart transplant or coronary artery bypass graft operation.

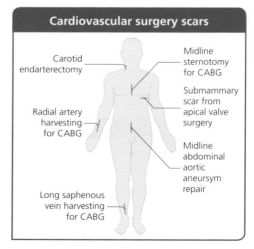

**Figure 2.17** Common scars in cardiovascular surgery. CABG, coronary artery bypass graft.

## Chest shape

Look at the shape of the chest for evidence of congenital abnormality (**Figure 2.18**).

- In pectus carianatum (pigeon chest), the ribs and sternum protrude anteriorly
- In pectus excavatum (hollowed chest), the ribs and sternum are sunken posteriorly

Both abnormalities displace the left ventricular apex.

> **Inspection is done not just with the eyes but also with other senses.** For example, listen for the metallic clicking sound of a metal valve replacement closing.

## Palpation

The praecordium is felt to find any displacement of the apex beat, heaves or thrills, and chest wall tenderness.

### Apex beat

The apex beat of the heart is defined as the most lateral and inferior point on the chest where the cardiac impulse is felt. It is usually in the 5th intercostal space in the mid-clavicular line. Locate it by first palpating the sternal angle; the intercostal space next to this angle is the 2nd intercostal space. Use your right hand to count down to the 5th intercostal space, then across to the midway point along the clavicle. With the index finger parallel to the ribs, feel this area for the forceful impulse of the cardiac apex.

The character and position of the apex beat is altered by cardiac and non-cardiac diseases (**Table 2.21**).

### Heaves

These are strained contractions of the heart. Heaves are felt by the palm of the right hand placed over the left sternal edge. They can indicate right ventricular hypertrophy caused by pulmonary hypertension or pulmonary stenosis.

### Thrills

These are palpable murmurs reflecting turbulent blood flow. Thrills are felt in the four valve areas, in particular those for the aortic and pulmonary valves (**Figure 2.19**). Use your fingertips to feel over each area for any palpable high-frequency vibration.

### Tenderness

The precordium is tender at costochondral junctions in cases of costochondritis.

## Heart auscultation

Use a stethoscope to auscultate the praecordium to detect any altered heart sounds, murmurs or rubs.

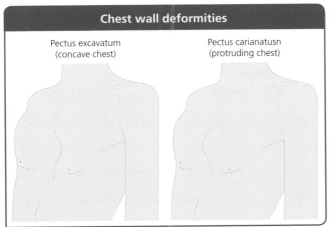

**Chest wall deformities**

Pectus excavatum
(concave chest)

Pectus carianatusn
(protruding chest)

**Figure 2.18** Deformities of the chest wall.

| Apex beat abnormalities | | |
| --- | --- | --- |
| Abnormality | Meaning | Cause(s) |
| Displaced | Left ventricular dilation | Dilated cardiomyopathy |
| | | Left ventricular aneurysm |
| | | Left ventricular systolic dysfunction |
| | | Chest wall deformities |
| | | Chronic lung disease |
| Tapping | Loud $S_1$ | Mitral stenosis |
| Heaving | Left ventricular pressure overload | Aortic stenosis |
| | | Hypertension |
| | | Left ventricular hypertrophy |
| Thrusting | Left ventricular volume overload | Aortic regurgitation |
| | | Iatrogenic fluid overload |
| Absent | Not palpable | Normal in 50% of individuals |
| | | Dextrocardia |
| | | Obesity |
| | | Pericardial effusion |
| Double beat | Forceful left atrial contraction | Hypertrophic cardiomyopathy |

**Table 2.21** Common abnormalities in the apex beat and their causes

## Heart sounds

These are the sounds of the four valves shutting. Two of the heart sounds are usually the most obvious:

- $S_1$, the 'lup' sound of the mitral and tricuspid valves shutting at the start of ventricular systole, when the ventricular pressure exceeds the atrial pressure
- $S_2$, the 'dup' sound of the aortic and pulmonary valves shutting at the end of ventricular systole, when ventricular pressure falls below the pressure in the aorta and pulmonary artery

These sounds are assessed by listening with a stethoscope at the four valve areas (see **Figure 2.19**). These areas are not directly above each valve. Instead, they are the areas of maximal projection of the sound of each valve, and therefore the points at which they are heard most clearly.

Listen to each area in turn with both the bell and the diaphragm. The bell of the stethoscope (the cup shape) is best for low-pitched sounds such as aortic and mitral stenosis. The diaphragm (the cup shape covered with a membrane) is more sensitive for high-pitched sounds, such as aortic and mitral regurgitation.

> The loudness of a murmur is unrelated to the **echocardiographic severity** of the lesion causing it.

On closer listening, $S_2$ is heard to consist of two separate sounds, because the left ventricle typically contracts before the right ventricle:

- $A_2$ when the aortic valve shuts
- $P_2$ when the pulmonary valve shuts

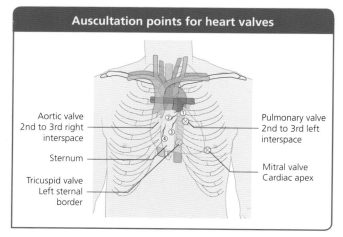

**Auscultation points for heart valves**

Aortic valve 2nd to 3rd right interspace

Sternum

Tricuspid valve Left sternal border

Pulmonary valve 2nd to 3rd left interspace

Mitral valve Cardiac apex

**Figure 2.19** Areas on the praecordium that overlie cardiac valves and are used in auscultation of heart sounds. ①, pulmonary valve; ②, aortic valve; ③, bicuspid (mitral) valve; ④, tricuspid valve; ⊗ aortic valve auscultation point; ⊗ aortic valve auscultation point; ⊗ pulmonary valve auscultation point; ⊗, tricuspid valve auscultation point; ⊗, mitral valve auscultation point.

## Types of heart sound splitting

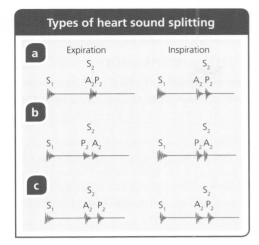

**Figure 2.20** Different types of heart sound splitting. (a) Normal: $S_1$ is usually clearly alone, and $A_2$ and $P_2$ are indistinguishable on expiration but heard individually on inspiration. (b) Reversed: $A_2$ and P2 are split in expiration and indistinguishable in inspiration. (c) Fixed: $A_2$ and $P_2$ are split in both expiration and inspiration.

This splitting of $S_2$ varies with the intrathoracic pressure changes of ventilation in three different ways: normal, reversed and fixed (**Figure 2.20**).

A split of $S_2$ on inspiration is normal. This physiological splitting occurs as chest wall expansion reduces intrathoracic pressure. This effect increases venous return to the right side of the heart, delaying $P_2$, therefore $A_2$ occurs before $P_2$.

A split of $S_2$ on expiration is abnormal. This reversed split is a consequence of prolongation of left ventricular ejection by dysfunction of the heart's conduction system. Examples of such dysfunction are left bundle branch block and structural heart disease, such as aortic stenosis and cardiomyopathy. Prolonged left ventricular ejection causes $P_2$ to occur before $A_2$.

Fixed splitting refers to the presence of splitting of $A_2$ and $P_2$ in both inspiration and expiration. This is abnormal and usually caused by an atrial or a ventricular septal defect. These defects cause shunting of blood down the pressure gradient from the left to the right side of the circulation. This effect delays right ventricular ejection, so $A_2$ occurs before $P_2$.

### Additional heart sounds
Added heart sounds are heard.

- $S_3$ in diastole, between $S_2$ and $S_1$, sounds like 'lup-de-dup'; this sound is normal in children and young adults but can occur because of rapid ventricular filling in cases of heart failure
- $S_4$, which sounds like 'le-lup-dup', is always abnormal; it is caused by a stiff ventricle, usually secondary to left ventricular hypertrophy (**Figure 2.21**).

**Figure 2.21** Cardiac murmurs.

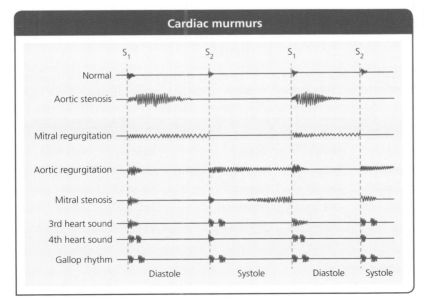

> A 'gallop rhythm' is the simultaneous presence of all four heart sounds, $S_1$ to $S_4$. It sounds like a horse galloping ('le-lup-de-dup') and is typically caused by decompensated chronic or acute heart failure.

## Heart murmurs

These are the sounds of turbulent blood flow through the heart valves (**Table 2.22** and **Figure 2.21**). Forwards blood flow is caused by narrowing, and backwards blood flow by incompetence. Characterise any murmur heard by determining the following.

- Where it is clearest, for example in the aortic or mitral valve area
- When it occurs in the cardiac cycle, for example during systole or diastole
- What it sounds like, for example harsh (high pitched) or blowing (low pitched)
- Where, if at all, it radiates to, for example the carotid artery or left axilla

Not all heart murmurs are pathological. A flow murmur, also described as physiological, innocent or functional, is normal; it is caused by increased flow through a valve in otherwise healthy people. Flow murmurs are typically soft and heard all over the praecordium throughout either systole or both systole and diastole. This type of murmur disappears when the patient stands, because this position decreases venous return to the heart.

## Pericardial rub

This sound is heard in pericarditis when two layers of inflamed pericardium rub against each other. Pericardial rub sounds like the crunching sound of walking on fresh snow.

## Lung auscultation

After auscultating the heart, ask the patient to sit forwards. Then use both palpation and auscultation to examine the lungs.

### Wheeze

Cardiac asthma is when a wheeze is heard in patients with heart failure. Wheeze is a coarse whistling sound heard during expiration, caused by obstruction of the bronchi by pulmonary oedema.

### Crepitations

These crackling sounds are like those made by Velcro. Chest crepitations are heard at the posterior bases of the lungs. They are a sign of pulmonary oedema (fluid in the lungs), which is a result of heart failure.

Crepitations are most pronounced during inspiration. They are produced by the 'popping' open of small airways and alveoli obstructed with fluid.

### Dullness

This is a lack of resonance on percussion. In the lung bases, stony dullness suggests pleural effusion, which is a sign of heart failure. Effusion also presents with reduced chest expansion and quiet breath sounds.

## Examination of the lower limbs

The lower limbs are examined for systemic signs of chronic organ disease. These signs

| Heart murmurs | | | | | |
|---|---|---|---|---|---|
| Cycle | Murmur | Timing | Sound | Location | Radiation |
| Systole | Aortic stenosis | Ejection systolic | Crescendo–decrescendo | 2nd right ICS | Carotid |
| | Mitral regurgitation | Pan systolic | Blowing | 5th left ICS | Axilla |
| Diastole | Aortic regurgitation | Early diastolic | Decrescendo | 2nd left ICS | Carotid |
| | Mitral stenosis | Mid diastolic | Rumbling | 5th left ICS | Axilla |
| ICS, intercostal space. | | | | | |

**Table 2.22** Detection of heart murmurs

include ankle swelling in heart failure, and absent pulses in peripheral vascular disease.

## Ankle swelling

Ankle swelling is seen in kidney, liver and heart failure. Heart failure is a cause of bilateral pitting oedema, when a thumb imprint on the front of the shin (at the anterior tibial border) persists for > 5 s (Figure 6.1).

## Pulses

Assess for the presence of peripheral pulses in both lower limbs. Absence suggests peripheral vascular disease caused by atherosclerosis, indicating associated coronary atherosclerosis. Palpate the four pulses in each limb (Figure 1.1).

- The femoral pulse is in the anterior femoral triangle, medial to the femoral nerve and lateral to the femoral vein
- The popliteal pulse is in the popliteal fossa, between the two heads of the gastrocnemius; it is palpated against the posterior surface of the tibia, with the knee slightly flexed
- The posterior tibial pulse is posteroinferior to the medial malleolus on the medial surface of the ankle
- The dorsalis pedis pulse is palpated on the dorsal surface of foot, medial to the extensor hallucis longus and lateral to the extensor digitorum longus tendons

## Calf tenderness

Squeeze both calves to check for pain caused by deep vein thrombosis.

## Varicose veins

With the patient standing, assess the lower limb anteriorly and posteriorly for varicose veins (saccular venous swelling).

## Lipodermatosclerosis

Look for inflammation of subepidermal skin (lipodermatosclerosis is a form of panniculitis), which is caused by venous disease. The leg resembles an inverted champagne bottle, because it tapers above the ankle; it is also usually reddened and tender.

## Ulcers

Inspect the lower limb for ulcers:

- Arterial ulcers are usually deep, regular and painful, with minimal exudate; they suggest arterial peripheral vascular disease
- Venous ulcers are shallower, irregular and painless, and have heavy exudate; they suggest venous peripheral vascular disease

## Haemosiderin staining

Red or brown deposits in the skin are haemosiderin. Haemosiderin is an iron complex formed as a result of chronic venous congestion and varicose veins; blood that has leaked from the veins is converted in the subcutaneous tissues from haemoglobin to haemosiderin.

## Ankle–brachial pressure index

The ankle–brachial pressure index (ABPI) is the ratio of systolic blood pressure in the arm (brachial artery) to the ankle ( posterior tibial artery). It is measured by inflating a sphygmomanometer until obliteration of the pulse wave being measured by an ultrasound probe, the last recording of which is the systolic blood pressure.

The ABPI is calculated as follows:

$$ABPI = \frac{\text{systolic blood pressure in the ankle}}{\text{systolic blood pressure in the arm}}$$

The ABPI is normally $\geq 1$. A negative ABPI indicates peripheral vascular disease, which causes a relative decrease in leg blood pressure.

## Bedside tests for peripheral vascular disease

Peripheral arterial and venous function is assessed with the Buerger's test and the Brodie–Trendelenburg test, respectively.

### Buerger's test

This is a clinical test to detect arterial insufficiency. Ask the patient to lie flat, and then passively elevate each leg to 45° in turn. If there is significant peripheral arterial disease, the leg turns pale when elevated, and the colour returns only once the leg is hung over the side of the bed.

## Brodie–Trendelenburg test

This clinical test is used to detect and localise venous insufficiency.

1. Ask the patient to lie flat, then tie a tourniquet on one leg, close to the groin, tight enough to prevent superficial (but not deep) venous flow; this stops any reflux from the femoral vein into the long saphenous vein through the saphenofemoral junction
2. Passively elevate the leg to 45°
3. Ask the patient to stand
   - If the distal veins remain collapsed for at least 30 s after standing, release the tourniquet; if the distal veins fill rapidly, then the site of the incompetent venous valve must be above the position of the tourniquet, i.e. the saphenofemoral junction
   - If the caudal veins fill rapidly with the tourniquet in place, perforator incompetence is diagnosed
4. Vary tourniquet position until the incompetent valve is identified, for example:
   - an above-the-knee position suggests mid-thigh perforator incompetence
   - a below-the-knee position suggests calf perforator incompetence

# Examination of the abdomen

The abdomen is examined for signs of ascites, aortic or renal artery disease.

## Ascites

Ascites is an accumulation of fluid in the peritoneal cavity. This is the result of chronic organ failure, such as heart, liver or kidney failure. The abdomen is distended by fluid on palpation; a fluid thrill and shifting dullness can be elicited on percussion. Fluid thrill is where the flanks are dull when the patient is supine, but resonant when they are laid on their side. Shifting dullness is when tapping on one flank creates a wave which is felt on the other.

## Abdominal aortic aneurysm

An abdominal aortic aneurysm is a dilation of the abdominal portion of the aorta. Palpate the abdomen to detect any midline, central and tender expansile mass.

## Renal artery bruit

Listen for any renal artery bruit in both flanks. Renal artery bruits are caused by turbulent blood flow as a consequence of narrowing of the renal arteries, i.e. renal artery stenosis. This condition is a cause of secondary hypertension and sudden pulmonary oedema.

# Examination of the fundi

The last part of the cardiovascular examination is inspection of the fundi (the interior surfaces of the eyes). In fundoscopy, an ophthalmoscope is used to view the retinae. Use of a darkened room is preferable to maximise pupillary dilation and thus facilitate examination. Look for diabetic and hypertensive retinopathy.

## Diabetic retinopathy

Diabetic retinopathy, like neuropathy or nephropathy, is end-organ damage as a result of chronic hyperglycaemia which leads to blindness. It occurs in over 80% of patients who have had diabetes for > 10 years and is the leading cause of blindness in the developed world. Diabetic retinopathy is sub-divided into non-proliferative and proliferative with or without oedema of the macular, which can occur at any stage. Chronic hyperglycaemia leads to damage of the small blood vessels in the eye resulting in ischaemia (cotton-wool spots) and bleeding (dot-blot and flame haemorrhages). This is termed non-proliferative diabetic retinopathy. This leads to a proliferation of new blood vessels, termed proliferative retinopathy.

# Hypertensive retinopathy

Hypertensive retinopathy, like nephropathy or left ventricular hypertrophy, is the end result of hypertension, and as a result is referred to as end-organ damage. There are four stages of increasing severity through which a patient progresses (**Table 2.23**). Up to 10% of healthy adults have grade 1–2 hypertension in the eye; the later stages (3–4) confer a worse prognosis for survival. In a hypertensive emergency, e.g. acute, severe and uncontrolled hypertension, the patient presents with stage IV papilloedema in the presence of hypertension (systolic blood pressure > 180 mmHg and diastolic < 120 mmHg).

| Fundoscopic findings in hypertension | | |
|---|---|---|
| Grade | Finding | Meaning |
| 1 | 'Silver or copper wiring' | Visible atherosclerosis |
| 2 | Arteriovenous nipping | Venous constriction |
| 3 | 'Cotton-wool spots' and flame haemorrhages | Retinal infarcts and bleeds |
| 4 | Papilloedema | Compression of the central retinal vein |

**Table 2.23** Fundoscopic findings in hypertension

# Investigations

## Starter questions

Answers to the following questions are on page 170.

10. When are investigations unnecessary?
11. How can an ECG give insight into a patients diet?
12. When is it normal to have abnormal blood tests of the cardiovascular system?
13. What common errors are made in the care of cardiovascular patients?

The history and examination provide a short-list of working diagnoses, which are then supported or refuted by investigations. Investigation results are generally meaningless without the clinical context provided by the history and examination. The results of investigations determine the nature and severity of a disease, identify any confounding factors and inform a management plan.

The key investigations used in cardiovascular medicine are blood tests, electrocardiogram (ECG), ambulatory blood pressure and electrocardiographic monitoring, exercise tests and imaging studies.

## Blood tests

No investigation should be requested without indication. However, the following 'routine' blood tests are done for nearly all patients.

- Full blood count to detect anaemia, inflammation and infection
- Urea and electrolytes to assess renal function
- Liver function tests to assess hepatic function
- A clotting screen to identify coagulopathy

Additional tests are requested as indicated by the results of the history and examination.

Blood tests whose results are particularly helpful in cardiovascular disease are cardiac biomarkers, which indicate myocardial damage, and lipid profiles, which contribute to the assessment of the risk of vascular disease.

## Cardiac biomarkers

Cardiac biomarkers are specific blood constituents associated with heart disease. They are measured in patients with chest pain and suspected myocardial infarction or with shortness of breath in suspected heart failure.

## Troponin

The troponin complex (**Figure 2.22**; see page 44) is a protein integral to skeletal and cardiac muscle contraction. Its concentration in the blood stream is increased by muscle cell necrosis. Cardiac and skeletal muscle isotypes are assayed separately.

The baseline concentration of troponin is recorded as soon as possible after a suspected cardiac event so that changes are monitored. A second measurement is taken 12 h after the height of the patient's pain, and the result compared with the baseline value to identify any significant increase, for example a doubling, in concentration.

### Creatine kinase

An enzyme in high-energy cells, creatine kinase (**Figure 2.22**) catalyses the following reaction:

$$ATP + creatine = ADP + phosphocreatine + energy$$

Creatine kinase-MB, its myocardial subtype, is released into the bloodstream as a result of myocardial cell death and lysis.

The baseline concentration of creatine kinase-MB is recorded as soon as possible after a suspected cardiac event and then 72 h after the height of the patient's pain, when its concentration peaks. The two values are compared to identify any significant increase.

For example, a doubling in creatine kinase-MB suggests myocardial damage. The creatine kinase-MB test is sensitive, but not specific, for myocardial infarction.

## Myoglobin

This is the muscular form of haemoglobin (**Figure 2.22**). Myoglobin contains an iron-based porpyhrin ring that binds to oxygen in muscle cells. Myocardial damage results in the release of myoglobin into the bloodstream.

Baseline myoglobin is measured as soon as an ischaemic cardiac event is suspected, then at 2 h after the height of the patient's pain, when its concentration peaks. Comparison of the two values identifies any significant increase. However, like the creatine kinase-MB test, the myoglobin test is sensitive but not specific for myocardial infarction.

## Natriuretic peptides

These are short-chain amino acid molecules that cause excretion of sodium in urine (naturesis). Brain natriuretic peptide and its inactive precursor, N-terminal pro–brain natriuretic protein, are released in response to myocardial stretch by the latter inducing sodium excretion and a corresponding decrease in plasma volume and blood pressure (see page 79).

The concentration of natriuretic peptides is increased in heart failure because of salt and water retention which increases plasma volume, myocardial stretch and left ventricular end diastolic pressure. In primary care, blood

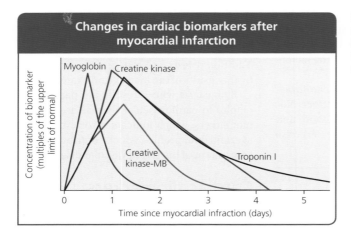

**Changes in cardiac biomarkers after myocardial infarction**

Myoglobin    Creatine kinase

Concentration of biomarker (multiples of the upper limit of normal)

Creative kinase-MB

Troponin I

0    1    2    3    4    5

Time since myocardial infraction (days)

**Figure 2.22** Changes in the concentration of cardiac biomarkers after myocardial infarction. It takes several days for most to return to normal.

tests are used to measure natriuretic peptide concentration to support a diagnosis of heart failure. In secondary care, early echocardiography is the gold standard for heart failure diagnosis.

Natriuretic peptides are also increased in:

- renal failure
- chronic obstructive pulmonary disease
- myocardial infarction
- sepsis
- extreme exercise

## Lipids

Lipids are chemicals with poor water solubility, i.e. they are hydrophobic. Their key functions are as energy stores, hormones and constituents of cell membranes. High circulating levels of lipids, as a result of either inherited or acquired conditions, are a risk factor for vascular disease.

The two main types of lipid in the body are sterols and phospholipids.

- Sterols comprise a hydrocarbon ring attached to one or more glycerides (e.g. triglyceride); this group includes vitamins A, D, E and K, as well as glucocorticoid and oestrogen hormones
- Phospholipids are hydrocarbon chains; they are present in cell membranes

Triglycerides consist of fatty acids and glycerol. They transport and store fatty acids around the body.

Saturated fats, in which all the carbon atoms are saturated with hydrogen, are less healthy. They are usually solid at room temperature and are present in dairy products, red meat and lard. Unsaturated fats are healthier and are present in olive oil, nuts and oily fish such as mackerel.

Lipids are insoluble in water and form emulsion droplets in aqueous solutions such as blood.

### Lipid metabolism

Lipids in food, including triglycerides and cholesterol, combine with bile salts and phospholipids in the gut to form micelles. These are absorbed in the small intestine and combine with apolipoproteins inside intestinal cells to form chylomicrons.

Chylomicrons are released into the blood and metabolised in the liver to form very-low-density lipoproteins. These are converted by peripheral tissues into intermediate-density lipoproteins, with the subsequent release of fatty acids.

Intermediate-density lipoproteins are, in turn, converted by the liver into low-density lipoproteins (LDLs), which release cholesterol into the peripheral tissues. Finally, high-density lipoproteins (HDLs) accept cholesterol from peripheral tissues and transport it back to the liver, where it is metabolised and excreted in bile.

### Measurement of serum lipids

The lipids whose serum concentrations in a venous blood sample taken after overnight fasting are measured include:

- total cholesterol, including LDL, HDL and very low density lipoprotein (estimated); its concentration is normally $< 5$ mmol/L
- triglycerides
- HDL

**Low-density lipoprotein**

This so-called 'bad cholesterol', present in saturated fats, is the major carrier of cholesterol from the liver to the peripheries. LDL is associated with the deposition of cholesterol in arteries to form atheromata leading to atherosclerosis.

The normal concentration of LDL is $< 2.5$ mmol/L. LDL concentration is higher in pregnant women and in patients with conditions such as hypothyroidism and cholestatic liver disease. LDL is also increased in patients receiving corticosteroids.

**High-density lipoprotein**

This 'good cholesterol' is the major carrier of cholesterol from the peripheries to the liver. It reduces cholesterol deposits in arteries.

The concentration of HDL is normally $> 1.5$ mmol/L. HDL is increased by exercise and moderate alcohol consumption, e.g. less than 14 units per week for men and 7 units per week for women, which in turn reduces the risk of vascular disease.

## Triglycerides

A high concentration of triglycerides increases the risk of vascular disease. The normal concentration is < 1.5 mmol/L. However, triglycerides are increased in patients with diabetes, renal failure and obesity, as well as in those using corticosteroids.

> **Cardio-oncology or onco-cardiology** is the study of the adverse effects of both radio- and chemotherapy on the heart. Radiation leads to fibrosis of the arteries, muscle and valves in the heart and anthracycline chemotherapy causes cardiac muscle damage. Patients should be monitored with imaging, e.g. echocardiography, to assess for reduced ventricular function and biomarker, e.g. troponin, to assess for heart damage.

## Electrocardiography

An ECG is a recording of the electrical activity of the heart over a period of time. This investigation is quick, inexpensive, and readily available, and the results provide a wealth of information about cardiac function. Indications for ECG include chest pain, shortness of breath, palpitations, syncope, heart murmur, hypo- and hypertension, and an irregular pulse (**Table 2.24**).

## Principle

All muscle is electrically active: depolarisation occurs just before contraction, and repolarisation precedes relaxation. In an ECG, this electricity is measured by electrodes on the skin; they are placed on the chest and limbs to measure the amount and direction of the electrical activity of the heart muscle. The results are displayed by the ECG machine, which can be printed and placed in the patient's clinical record. Abnormal measurements indicate problems with the heart's blood supply, muscle contraction or electrical circuits.

## Types of electrocardiography

An ECG can be recorded using 3 leads, 12 leads or the paddles of a defibrillator. Confusingly, the term lead refers to both the literal physical electrode and the abstract positional 'view of the electrical heart' that one or more leads represent.

The 12-lead ECG is used to diagnose:

- disturbances of heart rhythm
- myocardial diseases
- focal ischaemia
- drug toxicity

The 3-lead ECG is used to constantly monitor the heart in acute situations, such as after a

| Indications for ambulatory cardiac investigations | |
|---|---|
| **Investigation** | **Indication(s)** |
| ECG | Chest pain, dizziness or syncope, palpitations, breathlessness, heart murmur, hypo- and hypertension, and irregular pulse |
| 1–7 day ECG (Holter monitor) | Daily symptoms, burden of ectopy and conduction defects |
| Up to 2 week ECG (event recorder) | Suspected arrhythmia without daily symptoms (also know as cardio memo) |
| Implantable loop recorder | Very infrequent symptoms (e.g. monthly) |
| Tilt table test | Syncope and suspected orthostatic intolerance |
| 24 hour blood pressure monitor | Diagnosis, and response to treatment for essential hypertension and postural hypotension |
| ECG, electrocardiogram. | |

**Table 2.24** Indications for common cardiac investigations

myocardial infarction. For 24-h ECG recording, three wires are attached to the patient's chest: one on each shoulder, and one on the abdomen.

If a patient is in extremis because of a life-threatening bradycardia or tachycardia, the paddles of a defibrillator machine, which contain electrode sensors, are used to produce a continuous ECG.

# The 12-lead ECG

A 12-lead ECG uses 10 physical leads with 10 electrodes: 4 limb leads and 6 chest leads (**Figure 2.23**). However, the 12-lead signals are from the 6 chest leads and 6 virtual leads created from the 4 limb leads.

## Chest leads

The six chest leads V1–V6 'view' the heart in the horizontal plane (front to back). They are unipolar (as noted by the prefix 'V'), which means they record the difference between the voltage at their location on the chest and zero. They are attached as follows.

- V1: 4th intercostal space (right of sternum)
- V2: 4th intercostal space (left of sternum)
- V3: between V2 and V4

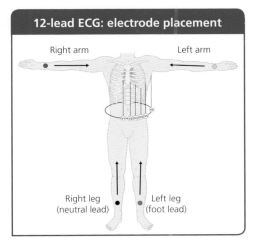

**12-lead ECG: electrode placement**

Right arm    Left arm

Right leg (neutral lead)    Left leg (foot lead)

**Figure 2.23** Placement of the 10 electrocardiogram (ECG) electrodes to create a 12-lead ECG. The six chest leads 'look' at the heart in a coronal plane, and the four limb leads 'look' at it in an axial plane.

- V4: 5th intercostal space (mid-clavicular line)
- V5: between V4 and V6
- V6: 5th intercostal space (mid-axillary line)

## Limb leads

These 'look' at the electrical signal of the heart in the vertical plane (head to toe). The four limb leads are colour-coded (like a traffic light) to aid placement.

- Right arm: red
- Left arm: orange
- Right leg (neutral lead): black
- Left leg (foot): green

## Virtual leads

Limb leads are used to create the six virtual leads displayed on the ECG. They provide a 'view' of the heart's electrical activity from a virtual perspective and are calculated from combinations of lead measurements as follows.

**Unipolar leads**

The first three of these are the unipolar augmented vector leads. They are unipolar because they record the measured electrical signal from one limb at a time using a positive limb lead, which is then referenced against a combination of other limb electrodes (all with a voltage of zero).

- Augmented vector lead of the foot (aVF): left leg – zero
- Augmented vector lead of the right arm (aVR): right arm – zero
- Augmented vector lead of the left arm (aVL): left arm – zero

Zero voltage effectively means that these leads are a 'view' from each limb towards the centre of all three leads.

**Bipolar leads**

Leads I, II and III are bipolar leads, i.e. they record electrical potential differences between two leads. They provide an electrical 'view' from the positive limb lead perspective towards the negative limb lead. Together, the three bipolar leads form Einthoven's triangle (**Figure 2.24**) 'look' at the heart in an axial plane.

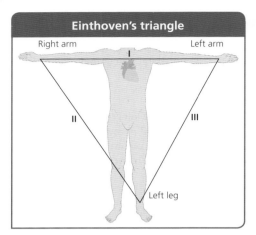

**Einthoven's triangle**

Right arm  Left arm

I

II  III

Left leg

**Figure 2.24** The right arm, left arm, right leg (neutral) and left leg (foot) give three unipolar leads: the augmented vector leads of the right arm, left arm and foot. These unipolar leads create Einthoven's triangle. The bipolar leads I, II and III are the potential difference measured between each.

- Lead I: aVR – aVL views from left arm towards right arm
- Lead II: aVR - aVF views from left leg towards right arm
- Lead III: aVL - aVF views from left leg towards left arm

## Electrocardiographic settings

For consistency of comparison, all ECG machines should be set to record at:

- a speed of 25 mm/s, which means that a large square (5 mm long) represents 0.2 s, and a small square (1 mm long) is 0.04 s (**Figure 2.25**)
- A voltage of 0.1 mV/mm, so that one large square (5 mm long) is 1 mV

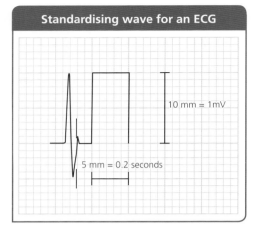

**Standardising wave for an ECG**

10 mm = 1mV

5 mm = 0.2 seconds

**Figure 2.25** Standardising wave for an electrocardiogram, showing the correct paper speed and voltage.

If these standard settings are not used, the results are not comparable with those reported in the literature. However, sometimes very large QRS complexes, such as those caused by left ventricular hypertrophy, make interpretation difficult. Therefore the voltage is halved in such cases.

## The electrocardiogram shape

Each ECG lead displays an electrical signal moving towards it as an upwards voltage deflection, and moving away as a downwards voltage deflection. The bulk of the electrical impulse is during ventricular contraction: the QRS complexes (**Figure 2.26**).

- The Q wave is the first negative deflection; it is not always seen
- The R wave is the first upwards deflection
- An S wave is any negative deflection after the R wave

**Figure 2.26** The different parts of the QRS complex.

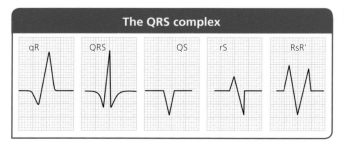

**The QRS complex**

qR  QRS  QS  rS  RsR'

The wave of depolarisation travels across the heart in many directions. However, the shape of the QRS complex shows the average way in which the wave travels through the ventricles. Thus the complex is a summation of the heart's electrical activity. Capitals denote size, e.g. qR indicates that the r wave is larger than the q wave.

## The electrocardiogram axis

The electrical deflection measured by the ECG represents both the amount and the direction of the heart's electrical activity. Therefore the average direction of depolarisation is assessed. This is the cardiac axis, and it is usually between −30° and +90° (11 o'clock to 5 o'clock). Certain diseases deviate the axis (**Table 2.25**).

To calculate the axis, first identify the isoelectric lead which contains the QRS complex with the largest positive deflection, e.g. maximal deflection above the isoelectric line, this is the cardiac axis. Then use the hexaxial reference to find the direction of that lead. For example, if the lead II has the largest positive complex, with R >S, the axis is + 60 degrees

| Causes of right and left axis deviations | |
|---|---|
| Deviation | Example causes |
| Right axis (+90° to +180°) | Often also seen in healthy people, particularly if they are tall and thin |
| | Right bundle branch block |
| | Right ventricular hypertrophy |
| | Pulmonary embolism |
| | Cor pulmonale |
| Left axis (−30° to -90°) | Left bundle branch block |
| | Left ventricular hypertrophy |
| | Cardiac pacemaker |
| | Left anterior hemiblock |

**Table 2.25** Causes of conditions in which right and left axis deviations are present

(**Figure 2.27**). Another method is to imagine the QRS complexes as thumbs pointing up (i.e. R > S) or down (i.e. S > R) (**Figure 2.28**).

- All leads, except III, usually point up
- If lead I is up but the rest are down, there is left axis deviation
- If lead I points down, but the rest are up, this is right axis deviation

**Figure 2.27** The hexaxial reference system is a representation of the 12-lead electrocardiogram to measure the heart's electrical axis.

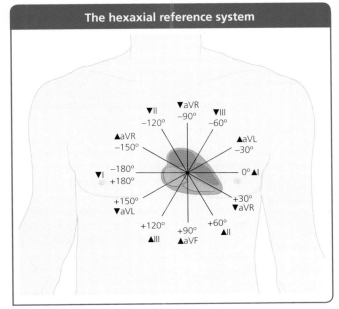

The hexaxial reference system

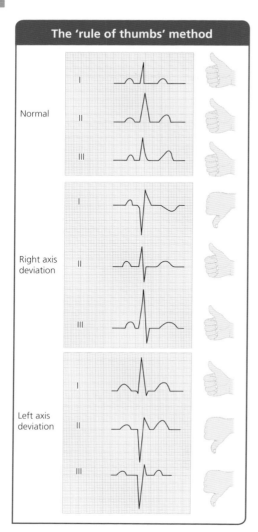

The 'rule of thumbs' method

Normal

I

II

III

Right axis deviation

I

II

III

Left axis deviation

I

II

III

**Figure 2.28** The 'rule of thumbs' method for determining cardiac axis.

## The electrocardiogram elements

An ECG is analysed for heart rate, rhythm abnormalities of conduction and markers of ischaemia. Normal elements of the electrocardiogram are shown in **Figure 2.29**. Non-cardiac causes of ECG abnormalities are listed in **Table 2.26**.

### Rate

The rhythm strip is the long trace (60 large squares; 12 s), usually of lead II, at the bottom of an ECG print-out; it serves as a reference.

The heart rate is best judged on this strip, because it shows the time interval between each R wave: the RR interval. If the heart rate is regular or there is no rhythm strip, count the number of large squares between each QRS complex and divide into 300. Each large square is 0.2 s, so this value is the heart rate in beats/min , e.g. 0.2 s × 300 = 60 s.

If the heart rate is irregular, or if there is a rhythm strip, use a specified length of the ECG, for example 30 large squares (i.e. 30 × 0.2 s = 6 s). Count how many QRS complexes occur during this time, and then multiply by an appropriate factor (in this case, 10) to calculate the heart rate in beats/min (**Figure 2.30**).

### P wave

This represents atrial depolarisation, which originates from the sinoatrial node then travels across the right atrium to the left atrium through specialised conduction tissue. The normal P wave has the following features (**Figure 2.31**):

- a small upwards deflection before the QRS complex
- amplitude <0.2 mV (two small squares)
- duration <0.12 s (three small squares)

Abnormal P wave size or shape indicates atrial pathology. P mitrale is a broad, bifid wave caused by left atrial enlargement and left-sided heart disease. In contrast, P pulmonale is a tall, peaked wave resulting from right atrial enlargement and right-sided heart disease. Atrial repolarisation occurs during, and is hidden by, the much larger ventricular depolarisation (QRS).

### Rhythm

Each QRS complex is usually preceded by a P wave (**Figure 2.29**), representing sinus rhythm, i.e. atrial activity is followed by ventricular activity. If the QRS complex is not preceded by a P wave, this suggests either an atrial arrhythmia causing a tachycardia, or disease of the atrioventricular node causing a bradycardia.

#### Disease of rhythm

Atrial arrhythmias include atrial fibrillation, atrial flutter, wandering atrial pacemaker, atrio-ventricular nodal re-entrant tachycardia and atrio-ventricualr re-entrant tachycardia.

## Electrocardiogram deflections

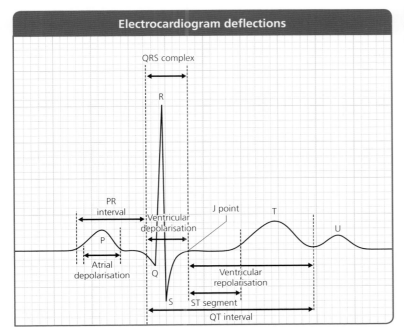

**Figure 2.29** Normal deflections of the electrocardiogram.

## Non-cardiac causes of ECG abnormalities

| Condition | Level | Abnormality |
|---|---|---|
| Hypocalcaemia | < 2.0 mmol/L | Prolonged QT |
| Hypercalcaemia | > 2.5 mmol/L | Shortened QT |
| | > 1 ng/mL | Bradycardia, prolonged PR and junctional escape |
| Hypomagnesemia | < 1 mmol/L | Prolonged PR or QT, wide QRS, ectopic beats and flat T waves |
| Hypermagnesemia | > 3 mmol/L | Heart block and atrial fibrillation |
| Hypothermia | < 35°C | Atrial fibrillation, bradycardia, J waves, ventricular fibrillation and prolonged intervals |
| Hyperthermia | > 38°C | Wide QRS and non-specific ST–T wave changes |
| Hypokalaemia | < 3 mmol/L | Narrow QRS, flat T waves, large P waves and prominent U waves |
| Hyperkalaemia | > 5.5 mmol/L | Wide QRS, tall tented T waves, absent P waves and ventricular fibrillation |

**Table 2.26** Non-cardiac causes of an abnormal electrocardiogram

- In atrial fibrillation, there is no organised electrical activity in the atria and no discernible P wave (**Figure 2.31;** see page 224)
- In atrial flutter, a re-entry circuit in the atria causes a sawtooth baseline comprising flutter (F) waves before each QRS (**Figure 2.32;** see page 224).

In heart block, disease of the atrioventricular node (**Figure 2.33** and page 217) delays the depolarisation wave moving from the atria to the ventricles. As the disease progresses, there is eventually a complete block of conduction between the atria and the ventricles.

- In first-degree atrioventricular block, a P wave is present before each QRS, but the PR interval is prolonged
- In second-degree atrioventricular block, an increasing number of P waves are not

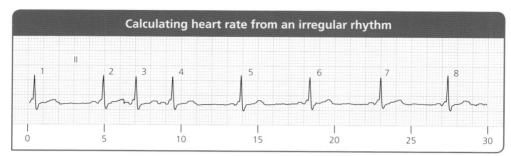

**Calculating heart rate from an irregular rhythm**

**Figure 2.30** Method for calculating heart rate from an irregular rhythm. Eight complexes are counted in 30 large squares, which is equivalent to 6 s. The heart rate is calculated by multiplying the number of complexes in 6 s by 10: 8 × 10 = 80 beats/min.

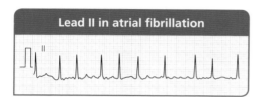

**Lead II in atrial fibrillation**

**Figure 2.31** Lead II in atrial fibrillation.

conducted by the atrioventricular node; the condition has two subtypes
- In Mobitz type 1 heart block, the PR interval is progressively prolonged between each QRS complex until a P wave is 'dropped', i.e. not conducted
- In Mobitz type 2 heart block, two or three P waves are seen before each QRS complex
- In third-degree (complete) atrioventricular block, no P waves are conducted across the atrioventricular node; this leads to a ventricular escape rhythm, with ventricular depolarisation originating in the ventricles, which is evident as bradycardia with broad QRS complexes

## PR interval

This element of the ECG (**Figure 2.29**) is:

- the distance between the start of the P wave and the start of the QRS complex
- the time the P wave takes to pass from the atria to the ventricles through the atrioventricular node and His–Purkinje bundle
- usually three to five small squares (0.12–0.20 s)

A PR interval of <0.12 s suggests ventricular pre-excitation; in contrast, an interval of >0.20 s suggests atrioventricular block (see page 219). The segment of the PR interval is depressed in cases of pericarditis, in which inflammation of the atrial pericardium decreases atrial depolarisation.

## QRS complex

After the PR interval is the QRS complex (**Figure 2.29**). The QRS:

- is the distance from the start of Q to the end of S
- represents the depolarisation of the ventricles, starting in the ventricular septum before moving left to right

**Figure 2.32** Lead II in atrial flutter

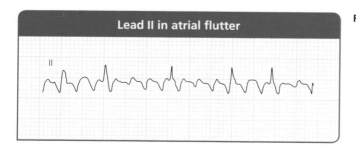

**Lead II in atrial flutter**

## Lead II rhythms in heart block

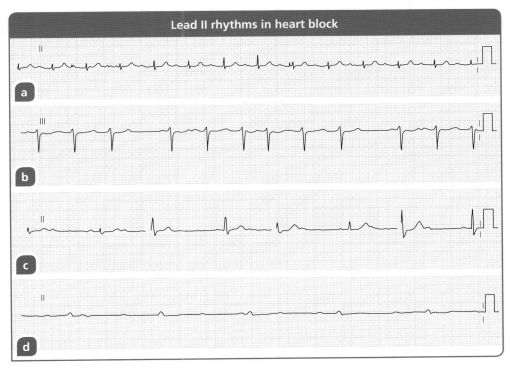

**Figure 2.33** Lead II rhythms. a) First degree AV block. b) Second degree AV block (Mobitz type 1 or Wenckebach). c) Second degree AV block (Mobitz type 2). d) Third degree (complete) heart block.

- is usually less than three small squares (0.12 s)

The left ventricle depolarises before the right, so left ventricular systole occurs before right ventricular systole. The aortic valve (heard as A$_2$) shuts before the pulmonary valve does (P$_2$).

The left ventricle is thicker than the right. Therefore it conducts more electrical current than the right ventricle and makes a greater contribution to the QRS signal and cardiac axis.

A prolonged QRS (> three small squares; 120 ms) duration is seen in bundle branch block (**Figures 2.34** and **2.35**). In this condition, depolarisation travels directly and more slowly through the myocardium, as the fast conduction pathway is not utilised and the ventricles take longer to depolarise, which prolongs the QRS duration. A prolonged QRS duration is also seen in a paced ventricular rhythm, ventricular arrhythmia or an ectopic ventricular beat.

### Right bundle branch block ECG

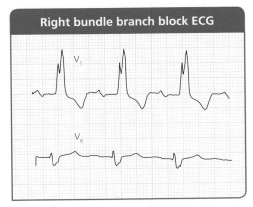

**Figure 2.34** In right bundle branch block, there is a dominant R wave in V1, a QRS complex with an rSR' pattern pronounced rSR prime (the prime denoting a second, e.g. pathological R wave) and slurring of the S wave in V6. Common causes include normal variant, chronic lung disease, pulmonary embolism and Brugada's syndrome.

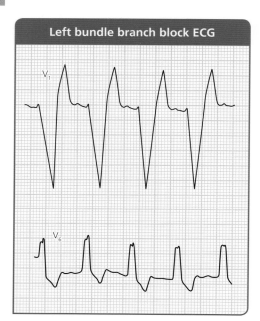

**Left bundle branch block ECG**

V₁

V₆

**Figure 2.35** In left bundle branch block, there is a QS pattern in $V_1$ and an R wave in $V_6$. Common causes include aortic stenosis, myocardial infarction, dilated cardiomyopathy and disease of the conduction system.

---

**Left and right bundle branch block appear different on the 12-lead ECG.**

- Left bundle branch block: WILLIAM (W shape QRS in V1, L for left and M shape in V6)
- Right bundle branch block: MARROW (M shape QRS in V1, R for right and W shape in V6)

---

## Q waves

Q waves are a common normal finding in the septal leads. However, Q waves over one small square (0.04 s) in width or 2 mm (two small squares) in amplitude are pathological. These abnormal Q waves represent a myocardial 'window' of electrically inert myocardium created as a consequence of an ST elevation myocardial infarction. The ST elevation myocardial infarction leads to a focal area death of myocardium, which spans from the endo- to the epicardium which allows detection of the electrical signal from the opposite heart wall.

## ST segment

This part of the ECG (**Figure 2.29**):

- is the region between the S and T waves
- is the period between ventricular depolarisation and repolarisation
- is normally isoelectric, with no deflection from baseline

A depression of the ST region below the iso-electric baseline is called ST depression and is caused by ischaemia. Conversely, ST elevation is due to myocardial infarction, pericarditis or left bundle branch block.

## T waves

These ECG elements (**Figure 2.29**):

- are large positive deflections after the QRS complex
- reflect ventricular repolarisation

Inverted (negative) T waves are normal in the aVR, V1 and V2 leads, as well as any lead in which the QRS is negative. Inverted T waves in other leads suggest ischaemia or structural heart disease. Tall, narrow T waves are seen in hyperkalaemia.

## QT interval

This element of the ECG (**Figure 2.29**):

- lasts from the start of the QRS complex to the end of the T wave
- represents the time taken for depolarisation and subsequent repolarisation of the ventricles action potential cannot be stimulated
- is influenced by heart rate, so needs to be corrected for this

The corrected QT interval (QTc) is calculated thus:

QTc = QT/square root of the RR interval (in seconds)

The QTc is normally <0.45 s in men and <0.40 s in women. A prolonged QT has many causes including ischaemia, drugs and electrolyte dusturbance (**Tables 2.26 and 2.27**) and indicates a risk of arrhythmias (see page 226).

| Drugs that prolong QT interval | | |
|---|---|---|
| Drug class | Name | Example |
| Antianginal | Sodium channel blockers | Ranolazine |
| Antiarrythmic | Class I | Flecainide |
| | Class III | Amiodarone |
| Antibiotic | Macrolides | Erythromycin |
| | Antifolates | Trimethoprim |
| | Quinolone | Ofloxacin |
| | Antifungals | Fluconazole |
| Antidepressant | SSRIs | Citalopram |
| Antiemetic | 5-HT$_3$ antagonists | Ondansetron |
| Antimigraine | Alkaloids | Sumatriptan |
| Antipsychotic | Butyrophenone | Haloperidol |
| | Mood stabilisers | Lithium |
| Chemotherapy | Oestrogen receptor antagonists | Tamoxifen |
| Respiratory stimulant | β-agonist | Salbutamol |

SSRI, selective serotonin reuptake inhibitor.

**Table 2.27** Pharmacological causes of a prolonged QT interval

## U waves

A small positive deflection immediately after the T wave is a U wave (**Figure 2.29**). U waves resemble P waves but are smaller and make the T wave appear bifid. They are usually caused by hypokalaemia.

## J waves

An abnormal positive wave just after the QRS complex is a J wave (**Figure 2.29**). J waves are seen in hypothermia.

## Interpreting a 12-lead electrocardiogram

Use a standardised approach to reading an ECG.

1. Confirm the identity of the patient by checking their name, date of birth and health service or hospital number
2. Check that the time and date of the ECG are correct
3. Ensure that the speed and voltage of the ECG are correct
4. Check the axis: is it normal or deflected to the right or left?
5. Calculate the heart rate (beats/min): is it normal or abnormal?
6. Look at the rhythm: is it a normal sinus (i.e. sinoatrial) rhythm, with each QRS complex preceded by a P wave, or an abnormal rhythm?
7. Think 'PQRST': examine each complex in each lead (e.g. P wave, PR interval, QRS complex, ST segment, Q waves, QT interval and T wave)

## Ambulatory blood pressure and electrocardiographic monitoring

Ambulatory tests, such as an ECG or echocardiogram, are performed on outpatients or on patients who are mobile and performing every day activities. Such monitoring is crucial for the diagnosis of latent and exercise induced arrhythmias, exclusion of white coat induced hypertension syndrome and structural disease of the heart.

**Table 2.24** shows the indications for ambulatory tests.

## Ambulatory blood pressure monitor

The ambulatory blood pressure monitor is a portable sphygmomanometer that measures blood pressure at regular intervals, for example every 20 min over a 24-h period. It is useful to:

- diagnose hypertension
- exclude 'white coat' syndrome (hypertension caused by anxiety in clinical settings)
- assess control of blood pressure with medication
- assess autonomic dysfunction (e.g. a decrease in blood pressure from sitting to standing)

# Short term ECG monitoring: Holter monitor

A three-lead ECG recorder called a Holter monitor is worn for 1–7 days. The more infrequent the symptoms, the longer the period of monitoring required. A cardio memo is a similar device to a Holter monitor, worn for up to 2 weeks. This is activated by the patient during symptoms. Data from the device is sent to the local cardiology department via the telephone.

# Long term ECG monitoring: implantable loop recorder

If the patient's symptoms are very infrequent, a matchbox-sized implantable loop recorder is used for long-term ECG monitoring, for up to 3 years. A local anaesthetic is applied and the device implanted, like a pacemaker, under the skin. It records single-lead ECG data that it transmits directly to a central computer at the local cardiology department.

# Tilt table test

The tilt table test is done to investigate autonomic dysfunction, such as a decrease in blood pressure (postural hypotension) or an increase in heart rate (postural orthostatic tachycardia syndrome) with changes in posture. The patient lies on a platform while ECG and blood pressure monitoring are recorded. The posture of the patient is manipulated, for example from vertical to horizontal, and the effect on the cardiovascular system assessed to determine whether symptoms are provoked. Drugs, such as sub-lingual glyceryl trinitrate, can also be given to induce hypotension and therefore invoke symptoms.

# Exercise testing

The cardiovascular system is dynamic. Therefore cardiac disease usually causes symptoms that occur during exercise, when the heart is under stress. Exercise tests are done, under appropriate supervision, to provoke symptoms and to assess cardiorespiratory function.

# 6-minute walk test

The 6-minute walk test is a useful measure of heart failure. It is used to assess the cardiorespiratory fitness of a patient before treatment, for example a heart transplant.

The patient is asked to walk on a hard, flat surface, such as a corridor, for 6 min, and the distance walked is recorded. The 6-min walk test is a more precise, reproducible and robust measure than the New York Heart Association classification of heart failure. The normal 6-min walk test result is >500 m for healthy adult men and women.

# Exercise tolerance test

In the exercise tolerance test, also known as the cardiac stress test, the patient walks on a treadmill or pedals an exercise bicycle. Their blood pressure and ECG data are recorded before, during and after exercise. The patient is also asked to report any symptoms during the test.

The test continues until a target is met, such as maximal heart rate:

$$\text{maximal heart rate} = 220 - \text{age in years}$$

An exercise tolerance test is considered positive for a diagnosis of ischaemic heart disease if there is horizontal ST depression in more than one lead, as well as provoking the symptoms the patient has been experiencing on exertion.

The exercise tolerance test is used to:

- diagnose ischaemic heart disease, although it has recently been superseded by computerised tomography (CT) coronary angiogram, following new guidelines
- monitor rehabilitation after myocardial infarction
- detect exercise-induced arrhythmias

# Cardiopulmonary exercise testing

This is the gold standard assessment of cardiorespiratory fitness (**Figure 2.36**). Cardiopulmonary exercise testing is used in heart

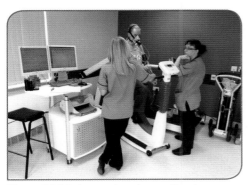

**Figure 2.36** Patient undergoing cardiopulmonary exercise testing on a static pedal cycle, with simultaneous electrocardiographic, blood pressure and gas exchange monitoring.

failure patients to assess the need for transplant. The test is also used for preoperative risk assessment in patients awaiting operations such as abdominal aortic aneurysm repair.

The patient exercises on a static pedal cycle while connected to an ECG machine, a blood pressure monitor and breathing apparatus that record gas exchange and the work done in terms of wattage. The maximum $VO_2$, the maximal uptake of oxygen per kg of body mass per min at peak exertion, is recorded.

The $VO_2$ value provides an objective measure of the ability of the heart, lungs, blood and muscles to uptake, transport and metabolise oxygen.

- $VO_2 > 70$ mL/kg/min is typical in elite athletes
- $VO_2 > 50$ mL/kg/min is normal for healthy active people
- $VO_2 > 30$ mL/kg/min is as expected for healthy sedentary people
- $VO_2 < 20$ mL/kg/min is found in patients with end-stage heart failure.

# Imaging

Cardiac imaging techniques are chest X-ray, ultrasound, echocardiography, nuclear medicine, CT, magnetic resonance imaging (MRI) and invasive angiography. These are used to diagnose ischaemic heart disease,

assess left ventricular and right ventricular function, and detect valve disease.

# Chest X-ray

X-ray radiation is used to provide images of the interior of the thorax. Thus changes in heart size or shape, shadows or silhouettes, and lung fields are visualised.

Chest X-ray enables detection of key features of heart failure, constrictive pericarditis, aortic dissection and pleural effusions. It also shows evidence of interventions and operations, such as sternal wires, artificial valves, left ventricular assist devices and pacemakers.

# Ultrasound

Ultrasound is a diagnostic imaging technique that uses inaudible high-frequency sound waves (>20 mHz) to visualise tissues and organs. The waves are generated by piezoelectric crystals in a transducer. The transducer is housed in a probe held against the body region of interest.

The sound waves pass through certain structures, for example blood and air, but are reflected by denser structures such as muscle and bone. The reflected waves are detected by the transducer and transformed into a digital image.

## Carotid Doppler ultrasound

The Doppler effect of sound waves is used to visualise blood movement; the pitch (frequency) of the sound appears higher as it travels towards the observer, e.g. the probe, and lower as it then moves away.

This technique is used to precisely locate and quantify the degree of arterial narrowing caused by atherosclerosis. Therefore it is used to visualise the carotid arteries, a key site of atheroma. Carotid Doppler ultrasound is also used in patients with suspected carotid atherosclerosis either after a stroke or to assess stroke risk before an operation, such as a coronary artery bypass graft.

## Abdominal ultrasound

This is the first-choice imaging technique to assess for the presence, location and size of an abdominal aortic aneurysm, a focal dilatation of the abdominal aorta. Abdominal ultrasound is inexpensive and quick to carry out, is readily available and involves no radiation. However, it does not visualise the whole abdominal aorta, so other cross-sectional modalities (e.g. CT) are needed to assess its entirety.

## Venous duplex ultrasound

This is used to diagnose deep vein thrombosis, typically in patients with a unilateral painful and swollen leg. An ultrasound probe is used to scan up and down the veins in the lower limb, assessing the anatomy and flow of blood in the veins; deep vein thrombosis renders the vein incompressible and without normal retrograde flow. Venous duplex ultrasound is also used to assess valve competency in patients with varicose veins.

# Echocardiography

Echocardiography, or cardiac ultrasound, uses ultrasound to assess the structure and function of the heart, particularly the muscle and valves. Indications include breathlessness, heart murmur and syncope.

## Transthoracic echocardiography

An ultrasound probe on the thoracic wall is used in transthoracic echocardiography.

### Motion (M) mode

Pulses are emitted in quick succession in a single plane to produce a one-dimensional image. The image represents a single, highly focused section through the heart, with time on the $x$-axis and the depth from the probe on the $y$-axis.

Motion mode can show rapid and small movements well, because the image uses only a single line. This mode is best for fine measurements, such as those of left ventricular wall thickness.

### Brightness (B) mode

This is the most familiar echocardiogram mode. Width is displayed on the $x$-axis and depth on the $y$-axis. The fan-shaped ultrasound beam is projected across the heart to produce a cross-sectional two dimensional tomograph.

Four different viewpoints are typically used (**Figure 2.37**):

- parasternal, next to the left parasternal border
- apical, at the left ventricular apex
- subcostal, from under the diaphragm
- suprasternal, from the neck

The heart is viewed in real time in three planes: sagittal, coronal and transverse. This is done to assess or detect:

- valve structure and function
- chamber size
- function of the ventricles
- cardiac masses
- pericardial disease
- structural heart disease

### Doppler echocardiography

This technique is used to estimate blood velocity, because the frequency of ultrasound waves reflected from moving objects, such as red blood cells, varies according to the speed and direction of movement. Doppler echocardiography is used to quantify the severity of stenotic and regurgitant valve disease (**Figure 2.38**).

## Three-dimensional echocardiography

In this technique, a special ultrasound probe is used to create a three-dimensional cross-sectional image of the heart in any plane. Three-dimensional echocardiography is used to visualise structural heart and valve disease (**Figure 2.39**). However, as with cardiac MRI, image quality is limited because a scan takes several cardiac cycles to generate a single moving three-dimensional image. Therefore several cardiac cycles are required.

Any movement, for example from a patient's failure to hold their breath or irregularity of the heart beat, significantly reduces image quality.

## Transoesophageal echocardiography

In this type of study, an ultrasound probe is inserted orally into the oesophagus while the patient is mildly sedated. Transoesophageal echocardiography produces clearer

## Echocardiographic 'windows'

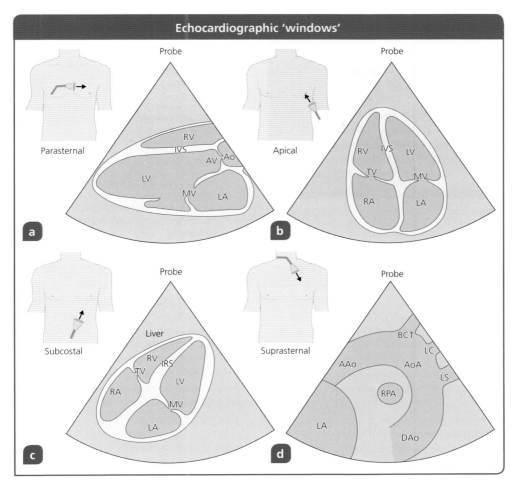

**Figure 2.37** Echocardiography 'windows'. AoA, aortic arch; AAo, ascending aorta; Ao, aorta; AV, aortic valve; BCT, brachiocephalic trunk; DAo, descending aorta; IVS, interventricular septum; LA, left atrium; LC, left carotid artery; LS, left subclavian artery; LV, left ventricle; MV, mitral valve; RA, right atrium; RPA, right pulmonary artery; RV, right ventricle; TV, tricuspid valve.

images of posterior heart structures, including the aortic arch, mitral valve and left atrium.

Transoesophageal echocardiography is used to investigate aortic dissection, endocarditis and left atrial thrombus. It is the key modality for the assessment of mitral valve disease.

### Stress echocardiography

This functional investigation is used to assess ischaemic heart disease. It combines echocardiography of the heart with the use of a cardiac stressor such as exercise or an intravenous sympathomimetic agent (e.g. adenosine or dobutamine).

The test result is positive if areas of ventricle fail to contract adequately in systole in response to stress. Such regional wall motion abnormalities indicate inadequate perfusion as a result of significant ischaemic heart disease in a particular coronary territory.

## Nuclear medicine

In this type of imaging technique, a radio-sensitive camera is used to visualise tissue uptake of a radioactive contrast agent injected

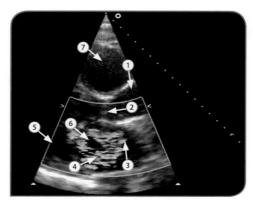

**Figure 2.38** Echocardiogram showing Doppler shift with colour flow mapping. The blue demonstrates severe regurgitating flow through the mitral valve into the left atrium during ventricular systole. ①, Aorta; ②, aortic valve; ③, left atrium; ④, mitral regurgitation; ⑤, left ventricle; ⑥ mitral valve; ⑦, right ventricle.

intravenously. Nuclear medicine studies are done to assess coronary blood flow in patients with ischaemic heart disease for whom exercise testing is contraindicated. For these patients, radiouptake before and after administration of a sympathomimetic drug (e.g. adenosine or dobutamine) are compared. If the images are not the same, this suggests significant ischaemic heart disease with atherosclerosis limiting flow unevenly during stress (**Figure 2.40**).

**Table 2.28** provides a comparison of the radiation dose to the patient from a nuclear medicine study, the doses from other clinical investigations and sources of radiation.

> **Ischaemic heart disease is assessed with anatomical and functional investigations.**
>
> ■ An anatomical study, such as a coronary angiography, locates the atherosclerotic lesion
>
> ■ A functional study, such as stress echocardiography, shows the physiological consequences of the lesion (e.g. chest pain caused by ischaemia)

# Computerised tomography

A CT scan uses ionising X-ray radiation to produce tomographic (i.e. sectional; Greek, *tómos*, 'cut') images of the heart and vessels. The patient lays in a C-shaped CT array that emits radiation. The radiation is absorbed by their tissues to various degrees and is then detected by the same array. Post-processing is then done to create a three-dimensional image from the series of images taken in the axial plane.

Computerised tomography is used to diagnose ischaemic heart disease. It is also used to visualise aberrant vessels and cardiac masses such as tumours.

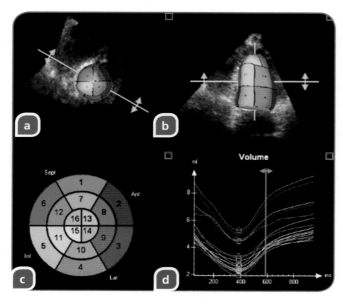

**Figure 2.39** Three-dimensional echocardiogram of the left ventricle. The three-dimensional left ventricle shown in situ in the axial (a) and transverse planes (b). The left ventricle is sub-divided into the 17 standard colour-coded segments (c), with change in volume of each segment over time shown (d).

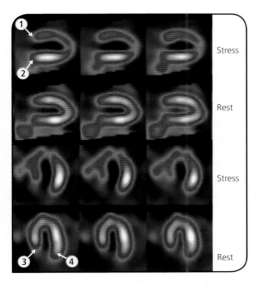

**Figure 2.40** Myocardial perfusion scans taken under stress conditions show a perfusion deficit in the anterior and septal left ventricular walls; the deficit is absent at rest. This finding indicates reversible ischaemia affecting this territory. The probable cause is occlusion of the proximal left anterior descending artery. ①, anterior wall; ②, posterior wall; ③, septal wall; ④, lateral wall.

| Comparison of radiation doses | |
|---|---|
| Radiation | Dose (mSv) |
| Chest X-ray | 0.02 |
| Transatlantic flight | 0.7 |
| Lumbar spine X-ray | 0.7 |
| Annual background radiation (UK) | 2.7 |
| CT calcium scoring | 3.0 |
| Myocardial perfusion scan | 5.6 |
| Coronary CT | 6.6 |
| Invasive angiography | 7.5–15.5 |
| Lethal dose | 5000 |

CT, computerised tomography.

**Table 2.28** Comparison of radiation doses

## CT calcium scoring

Chronic atheroma becomes calcified. Therefore CT calcium scoring is used to provide a low-dose CT assessment of calcium deposition in coronary arterial walls.

The technique is used to assess patients at low risk of ischaemic heart disease (<30% see Table 3.6). The higher the calcium, measured in Hounsfield units, the higher the likelihood of ischaemic heart disease.

- Low calcium (0) suggests no calcium and therefore no ischaemic heart disease
- Moderate calcium (1–400 Hounsfield units) indicates that further imaging is required (e.g. coronary CT angiography)
- High calcium (>400 Hounsfield units) means that invasive angiography should be offered

## Computerised tomography coronary angiography

In this technique, intravenous iodine contrast is used to visualise the coronary arteries. Thus CT coronary angiography allows analysis of blood flow in investigations of coronary artery disease. It is used to locate and assess the severity of atherosclerotic lesions in patients with a moderate likelihood of ischaemic heart disease (30–60%, see Table 3.6), and to assess the patency of coronary artery bypass grafts.

Computerised tomography coronary angiography provides higher tissue resolution than CT calcium scoring and invasive angiography. Furthermore, it can visualise soft, unstable plaques.

## Computerised tomography of the aorta

A CT scan of the aorta and its branches is used in investigations of acute aortic syndromes, aortic root dilatation and thoracic or abdominal aneurysms. The technique may also identify calcification, thrombus, the entry and exit sites of a dissection, and gross pathology of surrounding organs.

**Computerised tomography is used to diagnose acute aortic syndromes.** These include aortic dissection, intramural haemotoma and symptomatic penetrating aortic ulcer.

# Cardiac magnetic resonance

In cardiac MR, a magnetic field at a specific resonance frequency excites hydrogen atoms in the body. The radiofrequency signal emitted by the atoms is then detected and converted into a two-dimensional image.

The patient lies in a doughnut-shaped magnet that oscillates around the body and moves up and down. They are required to lie still in an enclosed and noisy space, and to hold their breath for short periods. Therefore the use of cardiac MR is limited in patients with claustrophobia or lung disease.

Many two-dimensional images are produced and combined to create a three-dimensional representation of the heart (**Figure 2.41**). Cardiac MR is even more specialised than other MR techniques, because the heart moves and its anatomy changes.

Cardiac MR is the best technique for assessing:

- cardiac volumes
- diseases of the right ventricle
- congenital heart disease
- post–myocardial infarction scar tissue

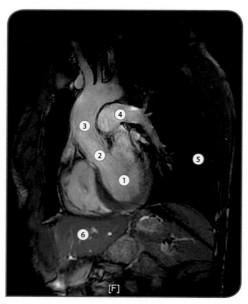

**Figure 2.41** Cardiac magnetic resonance imaging. ① left ventricle; ② aortic value; ③ aorta; ④ pulmonary artery; ⑤ lung; ⑥ liver.

(requires use of intravenous contrast agent)
- coronary perfusion in ischaemic heart disease (requires use of intravenous contrast agent)

> **A normal angiogram in a patient with chest pain, ischaemic ECG changes and significantly increased troponin suggests that there is no ischaemic heart disease.** In such cases, cardiac MRI is invaluable to investigate other causes of the presentation, including acute cardiomyopathies and myocarditis.

# Cardiac catheterisation

This is a contrast-enhanced X-ray imaging technique in which a contrast-injecting and pressure-sensing catheter (a thin, hollow plastic tube) is used to measure blood pressures and visualise blood flow in and around the heart.

Cardiac catheterisation is used to assess the coronary arteries, large vessels, atria and ventricles in investigations of ischaemic heart disease valve diseases and pulmonary hypertension. Catheter studies of the left and right circulations have different indications and procedures.

## Left heart catheterisation

Left heart catheter studies are a combination of coronary angiography, aortography and/or left ventricular ventriculography. They are done to investigate coronary artery disease and aortic valve disease.

### Coronary angiography

In this technique, a contrast agent is injected into an artery to visualise the patency and blood flow of the coronary arteries. Coronary angiography is usually done in patients with a high likelihood of having ischaemic heart disease (>60% see Table 3.6), within <48h of a diagnosis of non–ST elevation myocardial infarction and within 150 min of presentation of an ST elevation myocardial infarction.

The Seldinger, or catheter-over-wire, technique is used.

1. Local anaesthetic is injected around the blood vessel to be accessed, typically the right femoral or radial artery
2. The artery is punctured with the needle, and a short guide wire is passed through the needle and into the blood vessel
3. The needle is removed, and a sheath is placed over the wire into the vessel, keeping the entry site patent. This is the Seldinger technique
4. The short wire is replaced with a long one, which is pushed under X-ray guidance to the coronary ostia and then exchanged for a catheter
5. Radio-opaque iodine-based dye is injected through the catheter, into both coronary ostia, to visualise the vessels

The presence, location and severity of any lesions are assessed, and the results are used to plan treatment. The procedure takes less than 30 min. It carries a 0.1% risk of stroke, myocardial infarction or death, and a 1% risk of pain, bleeding, bruising, pseudoaneurysm or allergic reactions to the contrast media.

### Aortography

To assess the aortic valve, the same Seldinger technique is used to gain access to the aortic root except that a special pigtail catheter is used that can inject contrast in multiple directions.

One example of the use of aortography is to assess patients for whom aortic valve replacement is being considered. Reflux of contrast from the aortic root into the left ventricle indicates aortic regurgitation.

Complications are the same as those for angiography. However, the large amount of dye used in aortography more often results in the patient experiencing a hot flush and feeling as if they want to urinate.

### Ventriculography

To visualise the shape and regional contraction of the left ventricle, the Seldinger technique is used with a pigtail catheter to access the left ventricle, and contrast is injected at high pressure.

Visualisation of the contractile function ventricle helps guide diagnosis, e.g. myocardial infarction, and treatment, e.g. revascularisation. For example, if a regional wall of the left ventricle is not moving (akinetic), there is likely to be no benefit in reopening a blocked coronary artery because the myocardium is dead. Any reflux of contrast from the left ventricle into the left atrium indicates mitral regurgitation. The pressure is recorded in the left ventricle, with the lowest pressure occurring at the end of diastole (left ventricular end-diastolic pressure). If left ventricular end-diastolic pressure is > 30 mmHg, this indicates impaired relaxation of the left ventricle.

After ventriculography, the catheter is pulled back across the aortic valve from the left ventricle to the aortic root to detect any drop in pressure due to aortic stenosis.

## Right heart catheterisation

Right heart catheter studies are used to measure pressures in the right atrium, the right ventricle and blood vessels such as the main pulmonary artery and the pulmonary capillaries. They are used to assess heart transplant recipients, investigate suspected pulmonary hypertension and valve disease (e.g. mitral stenosis). A central venous catheter or line is inserted, using the Seldinger technique, into the femoral or internal jugular vein. Risks include pain, bleeding, infection and pneumothorax (if internal jugular vein is used).

### Pulmonary artery and capillary 'wedge' pressure

The pulmonary capillary wedge pressure is an estimate of pressure in the left atrium. Pressures of the right atrium, right ventricle and pulmonary artery are measured en route.

Following the Seldinger technique, a catheter is passed via the right femoral vein into the right atrium, across the tricuspid valve to the right ventricle and then into the pulmonary artery. A balloon around the catheter is used to 'wedge' it in to a branch of the the pulmonary artery. This gives the pulmonary capillary wedge pressure, which because of the high compliance of the pulmonary circulation reflects the left atrial, and therefore the left ventricular filling, pressure.

- If the wedge pressure is low (< 15 mmHg), the patient is fluid deplete
- If wedge pressure is high (> 15 mmHg), the patient has fluid overload

**Contrast nephropathy is a rare complication in which iodinated contrast agent impairs renal function.** The condition is defined as a 25% increase in serum creatinine within 2–3 days of a procedure. It is treated with intravenous fluids or, in extreme cases, renal replacement therapy. Using < 100 mL of contrast and a 2- to 3-day gap between repeated procedures reduces the risk.

# Management options

## Starter questions

Answers to the following questions are on page 171.

14. How does exercise help treat cardiovascular disease?
15. Can treatments do more harm than good?

The management goals of health professionals are threefold.

- Primary prevention: to prevent disease occurring in the first place
- Secondary prevention: treatment of disease as soon as it occurs
- Tertiary prevention: rehabilitation to reduce the negative impact of established disease

Management depends on the cause, severity and speed of onset of disease. A graded approach starts with conservative management then progresses to the use of medications and finally interventional procedures or surgery if all else fails. The engagement of the patient at every step of management is key to ensure their continuing concordance with treatment, their autonomy is respected and that they understand the nature and likely course of their disease, particularly if they decline treatment.

## Conservative management

Conservative measures are used for primary prevention and for risk reduction in established disease.

## Smoking cessation

Cigarette smoke is the leading preventable cause of vascular disease. Smokers are 5 times more likely than non-smokers to suffer from vascular disease. Therefore, whenever possible, health professionals should attempt a brief intervention with smokers:

- convey the risks
- encourage them to quit
- signpost possible options, including local smoking cessation services

Smoking cessation is supported by nicotine replacement therapy in the form of chewing gum, patches or electronic cigarettes or harm reduction strategies such as hypnotherapy.

The ultimate aim is for the patient to stop smoking entirely.

## Exercise

Regular exercise helps modulate many cardiac risk factors. For example, it reduces weight, blood pressure and LDL cholesterol. Exercise also improves mood, cardiorespiratory fitness, HDL cholesterol and insulin sensitivity. These combined benefits can reduce the risk of vascular disease by up to 50%. For full benefit, the activity needs to be sustained for 30–60 min and done 5 times a week. It also has to be of sufficient intensity to cause shortness of breath. Examples of such moderate intensity exercise are walking, cycling, swimming and dancing.

Exercise is also encouraged in cardiac rehabilitation, because it can help reverse the muscle wasting associated with chronic organ diseases such as heart failure. Furthermore, it reduces symptoms of angina, claudication and dyspnoea because of improved muscle conditioning.

## Alcohol

Alcohol is measured in units (**Figure 2.42**). Guidelines in the UK, for example, advise men to drink no more than 3 or 4 units daily, and women to drink no more than 2 or 3 units daily; furthermore, several alcohol-free days a week are recommended. Alcohol intake above these limits is considered harmful drinking. It can lead to alcohol dependence and the associated increased risks of heart failure, alcoholic liver disease and some cancers, for example. However, a small amount of alcohol reduces the risk of cardiovascular disease.

Health professionals should always assess alcohol intake and inform patients who drink to excess of the associated risks, advise them to reduce their consumption and signpost possible treatments. Treatment options include medications, detoxification regimens, hospital admission and help from organisations such as Alcoholics Anonymous.

## Diet

A healthy, balanced and 'Mediterranean' diet rich in fruit, vegetables, grains, nuts, fish and unsaturated fats and low in red meat, sodium and saturated fat (**Figure 2.43**) helps decrease blood pressure, improve lipid profile and reduce vascular risk by up to 30%.

Dieticians can provide further advice on healthy eating. Referral is appropriate for certain patients, such as those with hypertension who wish to reduce their sodium intake.

## Pharmacological management

Pharmacological management is indicated when a conservative approach to risk factor reduction or disease treatment has failed. At first, drug selection is daunting because of the sheer number of different drug classes, routes, names, dosages, indications, contraindications and adverse effects. With this in mind, never feel pressured to prescribe an unfamiliar medication. View each case as a learning opportunity, and consult a pharmacist, national guidelines, the hospital formulary or a senior colleague.

### Polypharmacy

Increasingly, and unavoidably, patients are taking many medications for comorbidities. However, polypharmacy increases the likelihood of drug interactions. These are potentially harmful and must be taken into account during drug selection, for example a combination of beta-blockers and rate limiting calcium channel blockers can lead

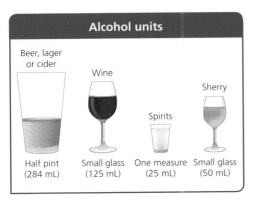

**Figure 2.42** Alcohol units: each item is one unit.

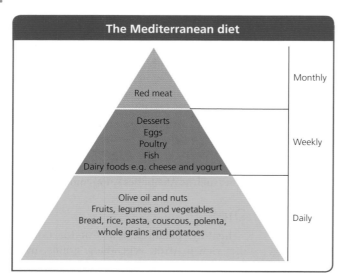

**Figure 2.43** The Mediterranean diet, showing which foods to eat and how frequently.

to bradycardia or heart block.

### Evolving guidelines

Cardiovascular disease is common. Therefore drug treatments for these conditions are the subject of intense research activity, both commercial and clinical. Accordingly, although drug therapies are truly based on evidence rather than anecdote, the accumulation of research findings means that the therapeutic landscape is ever-changing, for example in the past four years, there have been four novel oral anti-coagulants approved for use in atrial fibrillation, with many more in the pipeline. Furthermore, thresholds for the definition and treatment of cardiovascular diseases also change, if they are based not on physiological absolutes but on consensus. When to institute drug therapy for hypertension is one example of this.

### Specialist prescribing

Medications for common conditions, such as angina and hypertension, are initiated equally in primary and secondary care. However, prescribing and funding limitations mean that certain specialist drugs, such as Class I and III anti-arrhythmic agents, are started only by hospital specialists before being continued in primary care.

### Monitoring

Patients must be made aware of why a drug is being initiated, its possible adverse effects and any monitoring requirements. Many cardiac medications require monitoring to ensure that they are not leading to harm (e.g. in the case of amiodarone), or to maintain concentrations in the correct therapeutic range (e.g. in the case of warfarin). Furthermore, consider the impact of starting further medications that augment or inhibit the mechanism of action of the primary drug, for example antibiotics reduce the efficacy of the oral contraceptive pill.

## Lipid-lowering drugs

Hypercholesterolaemia is defined as total cholesterol >5 mmol/L or LDL cholesterol >3 mmol/L. Pharmacological treatment is indicated if the condition is present in isolation in high risk individuals (assessed by smoking, blood pressure and gender) and does not respond to conservative measures, or if it follows a diagnosis of familial hypercholesterolaemia or coronary, carotid and peripheral arterial disease.

The most commonly used agents for hypercholesterolaemia are the statins, i.e. hydroxymethylglutaryl-coenzyme A (HMG-CoA) reductase inhibitors. Statins are also the first-line agents for lowering LDL cholesterol. However, alternative and adjunct drugs are available (**Table 2.29** and **Figure 2.44**): fibrates, the brush border lipase inhibitor ezetimibe, bile acid sequestrants and nicotinic acid.

## Statins

These reduce cardiovascular events and mortality in patients with ischaemic heart disease. They also reduce the likelihood of developing ischaemic heart disease in those at high risk with hypercholesterolemia.

Statins are taken at night, because this is when most endogenous cholesterol synthesis occurs. They improve endothelial function and maintain atherosclerotic plaque stability.

**Drugs in this group** These include simvastatin, atorvastatin and rosuvastatin, and less commonly fluvastatin and pravastatin. The last two are thought to be less hydrophilic, with poorer muscle penetration and as a result less common muscular adverse effects.

**Mode of action** Statins lower LDL by inhibiting hepatic HMG-CoA reductase, the enzyme that synthesises >70% of endogenous cholesterol (**Figure 2.44a**).

**Adverse effects** Between 10 and 20% of patients receiving statins develop adverse effects. These include indigestion, headache, diarrhoea and insomnia. Dose-related and drug-specific adverse effects include liver injury with increased liver enzymes and muscular aches (myalgia), inflammation (myositis) and breakdown (myopathy). If severe, this can lead to kidney injury (rhabdomyolysis).

**Interactions** Other cholesterol-loweringdrugs, such as fibrates, nicotinic acid and inhibitors of the liver enzyme cytochrome P450 (e.g. grapefruit) inhibit the metabolism of statins and as a result lead to increased amounts of the circulating drug, thus increasing the risk of adverse effects.

**Contraindications** These include severe liver and renal disease, and also myopathy, because of the risk of further injury. Statins are contraindicated in pregnant and breast-feeding women where their safety has not been established.

## Fibrates

These are second-line agents for treating hypercholesterolaemia. There is no evidence that fibrates save lives in ischaemic heart disease, but they do reduce the risk of myocardial infarction.

**Drugs in this group** The fibrates include bezafibrate, fenofibrate and gemfibrozil.

| Cholesterol-lowering medications | | | | |
|---|---|---|---|---|
| Type | Mode of action | Effect on cholesterol | Commonly prescribed example(s) | Common adverse effects |
| Statins | Inhibit HMG CoA reductase | Reduce LDL | Simvastatin and atorvastatin | Muscle aches and hepatic impairment |
| Fibrates | Activate PPAR receptors | Reduce LDL and triglycerides | Bezafibrate and gemfibrozil | Indigestion and rash |
| Brush border lipase inhibitor | Inhibits gut absorption of lipids | Reduce LDL | Ezetimibe* | Diarrhoea and headache |
| Bile acid sequestrants | Bind bile in the gut | Reduce LDL | Colestyramine | Diarrhoea and constipation |
| Nicotinic acid | Activates adipocyte receptors | Reduce triglycerides and LDL, and increase HDL | Nicotinic acid† | Flushing and itching |

HDL, high-density lipoprotein; HMG-CoA, hydroxymethylglutaryl-coenzyme A; LDL, low-density lipoprotein; PPAR, peroxisome proliferator-activated receptor.

*The only brush border lipase inhibitor.

†The only drug in this group; it is also known as niacin or vitamin B3.

**Table 2.29** Summary of cholesterol-lowering medications

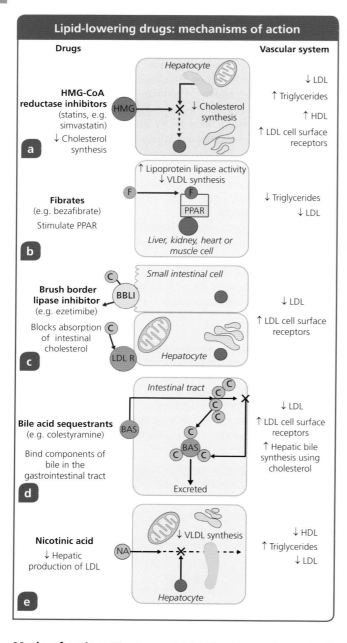

**Figure 2.44** Lipid-lowering medications and their sites and mechanisms of action. (a) Hydroxymethylglutaryl-coenzyme A (HMG-CoA) reductase inhibitors (statins). (b) Fibrates. (c) The brush border lipase inhibitor ezetimibe. (d) Bile acid sequestrants. (e) Nicotinic acid, also known as niacin or vitamin B3. BAS, bile acid sequestrants; BBLI, brush border lipase inhibitor; C, cholesterol; F, fibrates; HDL, high-density lipoprotein; LDL, low-density lipoprotein; LDL R, low-density lipoprotein receptor; NA, nicotinic acid; PPAR, peroxisome proliferator–activated receptor; VLDL, very-low-density lipoprotein.

**Mode of action** Fibrates act by facilitating lipid metabolism. They lower LDL cholesterol and triglycerides by activating intracellular peroxisome proliferator-activated receptor (**Figure 2.44b**).

**Adverse effects** These include indigestion, myositis, rash and anaemia.

**Interactions** Fibrates interact with and potentiate the effect of statins, warfarin, phenytoin and nicotinic acid.

**Contraindications** These include severe liver and renal disease, because of the risk of further injury. Fibrates are contraindicated in pregnant and breastfeeding women because of their safety has not been established. They are also unsuitable for patients with pre-existing gall bladder disease, because these drugs increase the cholesterol content of gallstones.

## Brush border lipase inhibitor

The brush border lipase inhibitor ezetimibe is a second-line agent for treating hypercholesterolaemia. There is no evidence that it reduces cardiovascular mortality or morbidity.

**Drugs in this group** The sole drug in this class is ezetimibe.

**Mode of action** Half of cholesterol absorbed from the gut comes from hepatic secretions, 30% from dietary sources and 10% from the sloughing of epithelial cells. A low-fat diet reduces dietary cholesterol by only 15%; ezetimibe acts on the remaining 85%. This drug inhibits the uptake of dietary cholesterol from the gut at the brush border epithelium, thus reducing plasma LDL cholesterol (**Figure 2.44c**).

**Adverse effects** These include diarrhoea, headache, myalgia and hypersensitivity reactions.

**Interactions** Ezetimibe has no common interactions of note.

**Contraindications** Ezetimibe is contraindicated in patients with liver disease, because of the risk of further hepatic injury. Pregnancy and breasfeeding is a contraindication as safety has not been established.

## Bile acid sequestrants

These are also known as anion exchange resins and are second-line agents for the treatment of hypercholesterolaemia. They reduce the progression of, and mortality in, ischaemic heart disease.

**Drugs in this group** The most commonly used drug in this group is colestyramine.

**Mode of action** Bile acid sequestrants adsorb and combine with bile acids in the intestine, thus preventing their reabsorption; as a result, the bile acids are excreted in the faeces (**Figure 2.44d**). The increased loss of bile acids increases the oxidation of circulating cholesterol to form bile acids. This effect, in turn, increases the activity of HMG-CoA reductase, thus reducing circulating LDL cholesterol.

**Adverse effects** These include constipation, diarrhoea, abdominal pain and itching.

**Interactions** Colestyramine affects the bioavailability of drugs administered concurrently, including warfarin, digoxin, thiazides, propranolol and oral contraceptives. Such drugs should be taken at least 4 h after colestyramine or 1 h before it.

**Contraindications** These include pregnancy and breastfeeding as safety has not been established. Another contraindication is complete biliary obstruction, which reduces the binding of colestyramine to bile acids.

## Nicotinic acid

This is a second-line agent in the treatment of hypercholesterolaemia. It is also known as niacin or vitamin B3. Nicotinic acid reduces the risk of mortality in ischaemic heart disease, but its common adverse effects limit its use.

**Drugs in this group** Nicotinic acid is the only drug in this group.

**Mode of action** Nicotinic acid activates specific G-protein–linked receptors on adipocytes (**Figure 2.44e**). This action inhibits the production of hepatic triglycerides and very-low-density lipoproteins, leading to a reduction in triglycerides and LDL, and an increase in HDL.

**Adverse effects** These include flushing, itching, indigestion, dizziness, peptic ulceration, liver injury, gout and hyperglycaemia.

**Interactions** When administered with antihypertensive medication, nicotinic acid causes postural hypotension. If hot, caffeinated or alcoholic drinks are consumed around the time that nicotinic acid is taken, the likelihood and severity of flushing is increased.

**Contraindications** These include severe liver disease, gout and peptic ulcer disease, because nicotinic acid exarcebates these conditions by increasing levels of uric acid and histamine. It is contraindicated in pregnant and breastfeeding women because their safety has not been established.

# Thrombolytic drugs

Thrombolytic drugs stimulate the breakdown of stable fibrin clots. They are used in the treatment of acute stroke, acute massive pulmonary embolus and in ST elevation myocardial infarctions (not suitable for primary percutaneous coronary intervention).

## Drugs in this group

The main thrombolytic agents are alteplase, tenectoplase and streptokinase.

## Mode of action

They convert plasminogen to plasmin, augmenting the breakdown of stable fibrin clots, e.g. in massive pulmonary embolism with hypotension, collapse and acute right heart failure or acute ischaemic stroke.

## Adverse effects

These include bleeding, allergic reactions, cardiac arrest and arrhythmia.

## Interactions

The risk of bleeding is increased with concomitant use of anti-platelet agents, NSAIDs and anti-coagulants.

## Contraindications

Recent major surgery, bleeding, trauma, hypertension, aortic dissection or pregnancy.

# Anticoagulant drugs

Anticoagulants prevent the coagulation (clotting) of blood. They inhibit clotting factors in the coagulation cascade, thus preventing the formation of a stable fibrin clot (**Figure 2.45**).

The main anticoagulants are coumarins, heparins and novel oral anticoagulants (**Table 2.30**).

## Coumarins

These are present naturally in certain grasses and clover. Coumarins are taken orally to reduce the propagation of venous thrombus, such as those in cases of deep vein thrombosis or pulmonary embolism. They are also taken to prevent formation of arterial thrombus in patients with atrial fibrillation or metallic heart valves. For example, coumarins reduce the risk of embolic stroke by two-thirds in patients with atrial fibrillation.

**Drugs in this group** The drugs in this class include warfarin, and less commonly phenidione.

**Mode of action** The coumarins inhibit the vitamin K-dependent clotting factors II, VII, IX and X, as well as the anticoagulant factors C and S (**Figure 2.46**).

**Adverse effects** These include haemorrhage, easy bruising, hair loss, rash, liver and pancreas injury, and osteoporosis.

**Interactions** Increased consumption of dietary sources of vitamin K, such as green vegetables, antagonise the therapeutic effect of warfarin which acts to inhibit the action of vitamin K. Conversely, cranberry juice, alcohol, some herbal medicines (e.g. arnica, camomile and licorice) and certain drugs (e.g. antibiotics, antiepileptics and immunosuppresants) can enhance its anticoagulant effect.

**Contraindications** These drugs are unsuitable for patients who have frequent falls, because of the risk of intracerebral haemorrhage. Bleeding tendency and recent or planned surgery are contraindications because of the increased risk of bleeding. Coumarins are also contraindicated in pregnancy, because of their teratogenic effects.

## Heparins

These are glycoaminoglycans, naturally occurring molecules in mast cells and basophils that inhibit thrombosis. Synthetic heparins are used to prevent venous thrombosis in high-risk in-patient populations. They also prevent propagation of established thrombus in patients with deep vein thrombosis, pulmonary embolism or myocardial infarction. For example, heparins halve the risk of deep vein thrombosis and pulmonary embolism in orthopaedic patients undergoing total hip or knee replacement.

**Drugs in this group** The most commonly used heparins; are the low-molecular-weight heparins dalteparin, enoxaparin, tinzaparin and fondaparinux, which are administered subcutaneously, and unfractionated heparin, which is given as a continuous intravenous infusion.

**Mode of action** The heparins activate antithrombin III, which inactivates thrombin, and factor Xa, preventing the formation of a stable fibrin clot (see **Figure 2.45**).

**Adverse effects** These include haemorrhage, hyperkalaemia, haematoma, osteoporosis and hypersensitivity reactions.

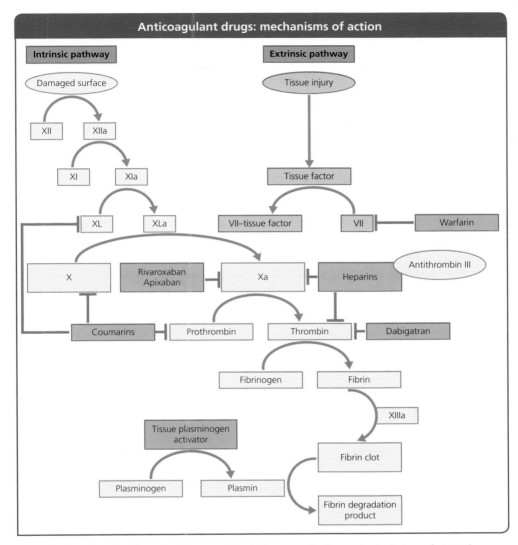

**Figure 2.45** Action of anticoagulant drugs on the clotting cascade. Coumarins include warfarin and phenidione. Dabigatran, rivaroxaban and apixaban are novel oral anticoagulants. Coagulation factors are indicated by their Roman numerals.

**Interactions** Heparins interact with NSAIDs and antiplatelet drugs, increasing the risk of bleeding. They also interact with ACE inhibitors and angiotensin II receptor blockers to increase the risk of high potassium (hyperkalaemia).

**Contraindications** Bleeding tendency, major trauma or cerebral haemorrhage, and severe liver disease are contraindications because of the increased risk of bleeding. Low molecular weight heparins are contraindicated in significant renal impairment.

**Heparin-induced thrombocytopenia (HIT) develops in 3–5% of patients after administration of heparin.** Antibodies to heparin bind to platelets, causing activation, clumping, reduced platelet count and subsequent (paradoxical) thrombosis.

## Novel oral anticoagulants

These drugs were developed to remove the necessity for regular blood tests, required

| Anticoagulant medications | | | | | |
|---|---|---|---|---|---|
| Type | Mode of action | Antidote | Commonly prescribed examples | Common adverse effects | Indications |
| Coumarins | Inhibit clotting factors II, VII, IX and X | Vitamin K | Warfarin and phenindione | Bleeding, bruising, osteoporosis and hair loss | Atrial fibrillation, venous thromboembolism and metallic heart valves |
| Heparins | Activate antithrombin III | Protamine sulfate | Enoxaparin and dalteparin | Bleeding, bruising, hyperkalaemia and thrombocytopenia | Venous thromboembolism and myocardial infarction |
| Novel oral anticoagulants | Inhibit thrombin or factor Xa | Not applicable | Dabigatran and rivaroxaban | Bleeding, bruising, headache and indigestion | Venous thromboembolism and nonvalvular atrial fibrillation |

**Table 2.30** Summary of anticoagulant medications

for warfarin dose optimisation. Novel oral anticoagulants are used as an alternative to heparin or warfarin in patients needing anticoagulation for deep vein thrombosis, pulmonary embolism or atrial fibrillation. However, there is no evidence that these newer drugs are superior to the older agents.

**Drugs in this group** There are several drugs in this class, including dabigatran, rivaroxaban and apixaban.

**Mode of action** Dabigatran is a direct thrombin inhibitor, whereas rivaroxaban and apixaban are factor Xa inhibitors (see **Figure 2.45**). All three prevent formation of a stable fibrin clot.

**Adverse effects** These include bleeding, indigestion, nausea, vomiting and headache.

**Interactions** Concomitant use of antiplatelet drugs or NSAIDs increases the risk of bleeding.

**Contraindications** Bleeding tendency, recent major surgery and intracranial haemorrhage are contraindications because of the increased risk of bleeding. Severe renal disease is another contraindication, because of the impaired excretion of these drugs.

## Antiplatelet drugs

Antiplatelet drugs inhibit platelet adhesion by reducing aggregation and therefore thrombus formation. They are used in the prevention and treatment of coronary, carotid and peripheral arterial disease. Unlike anticoagu-

lants, antiplatelet drugs are effective in the arterial, not venous, circulation.

There are two types of antiplatelet drugs: acetylsalicylic acid and the thienopyridines (**Table 2.31**). They have different mechanisms of action (**Figure 2.46**) and are used together in the treatment of myocardial infarction.

### Acetylsalicylic acid

This was originally derived from willow tree bark and is present in many fruits. It is a minor analgesic and antipyretic, and is also used for lifelong treatment after the diagnosis of peripheral, carotid and coronary artery disease. Acetylsalicylic acid reduces the risk of death and further myocardial infarction by 30% in patients with ischaemic heart disease.

**Drugs in this group** Acetylsalicylic acid is more commonly known as aspirin.

**Mode of action** Aspirin irreversibly inhibits the cyclo-oxygenase enzyme, and thus prevents the conversion of arachidonic acid to thromboxane $A_2$ (**Figure 2.46**). Thromboxane $A_2$, produced in platelets in response to various stimuli, induces platelet aggregation. Therefore inhibition causes dysfunction for the lifetime of the platelet (10 days) and thus prolonged bleeding.

**Adverse effects** These include gout, caused by reduced renal excretion of uric acid; gastric irritation, leading to ulcers and indigestion; bronchospasm; and easy bruising.

**Antiplatelet medications**

| Type | Mode of action | Commonly prescribed example(s) | Common adverse effects | Indications |
|------|----------------|-------------------------------|------------------------|-------------|
| Acetylsalicylic acid | Inhibits platelet cyclo-oxygenase | Aspirin* | Bleeding, bruising, peptic ulceration and gout | Ischaemic heart disease, cerebrovascular disease and peripheral vascular disease |
| Thienopyridines | Inhibit platelet ADP | Clopidogrel, prasugrel and ticagrelor | Bleeding, bruising, thrombocytopenia and dyspnoea | Myocardial infarction, cerebrovascular disease and peripheral vascular disease |

*The only drug in this group.

**Table 2.31** Summary of antiplatelet medications

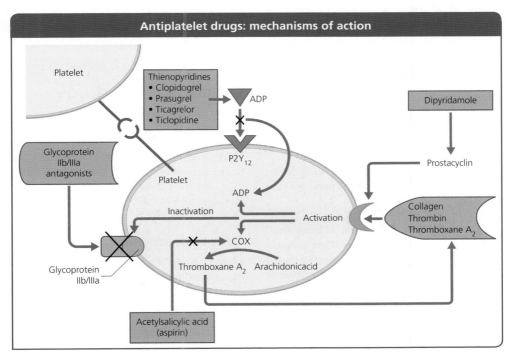

**Figure 2.46** Mechanism of action of antiplatelet drugs. COX, cyclo-oxygenase.

**Interactions** Concomitant use of coumarins, heparins, corticosteroids, alcohol and NSAIDs increases the risk of bleeding.

**Contraindications** These include bleeding tendency and severe renal and liver disease, because of platelet inhibition. In children, there is a risk of Reye's syndrome. Acetylsalicylic acid is contraindicated in patients with aspirin hypersensitivity (e.g. aspirin-induced asthma). Pregnancy and breastfeeding are also contraindications, because of the risk of teratogenesis.

> **Reye's syndrome is potentially fatal.** The condition presents with cerebral oedema, liver failure, hypoglycaemia and coma. It is common in children and is believed to be caused by aspirin.

## Thienopyridines

Members of this class of antiplatelet drugs are used to treat peripheral, carotid and coronary artery disease. They reduce the risk of death and further myocardial infarction by 20% in patients who have had a myocardial infarction.
**Drugs in this group** There are three main drugs in this group: clopidogrel, prasugrel and ticagrelor.
**Mode of action** The thienopyridines irreversibly inhibit the $P2Y_{12}$ ADP receptor on the surface of platelets (see **Figure 2.46**). ADP is a proaggregatory agonist released by these cells. Therefore inhibition prevents platelet aggregation and prolongs bleeding time.
**Adverse effects** These include bleeding, gastric irritation and ulceration (causing indigestion), allergic reaction, rash, thrombocytopenia and dyspnoea. The last of these side effects is caused by ticagrelor only.
**Interactions** Concomitant use of aspirin, NSAIDs and anticoagulants increases the risk of bleeding.
**Contraindications** These include bleeding tendency, because of platelet inhibition. Breastfeeding is a contraindication because of the expression of thienopyridines in breast milk. These drugs are unsuitable for patients with severe liver disease, because of the risk of further injury.

## Glycoprotein IIb/IIIa antagonists

These drugs are used in patients with high risk or unstable acute coronary syndromes who are to undergo percutaneous coronary intervention. Glycoprotein IIb/IIIa antagonists block the final pathway of platelet aggregation.

### Drugs in this group

There are three main drugs in this group: abciximab (a monoclonal antibody), eptifi-batide (a cyclic peptide) and tirofiban (a peptidomimetic inhibitor).

### Mode of action

They block the glycoprotein IIa/IIIb receptor on the surface of platelets (Figure 2.46), stopping the formation of linkages between platelets.

### Adverse effects

Increased risk of bleeding and thrombocytopenia.

### Interactions

Concomitant use of other anti-platelet or anti-coagulants increases risk of bleeding.

### Contraindications

Patients who have pre-existing bleeding disorders or thrombocytopenia are contraindicated.

## Antiarrhythmic drugs

Antiarrhythmic agents are used to suppress abnormal rhythms of the heart, including atrial and ventricular tachycardias. The Vaughn Williams classification divides the drugs into different classes according to their effect on the cardiac myocyte, in particular the action potential (**Figure 2.47**): classes Ia, Ib, Ic, II, III, IV and V (**Table 2.32**).

### Class I antiarrhythmic drugs

Class I agents block the fast $Na^+$ channels of non-nodal cardiac myocytes. The influx of $Na^+$ through these channels is responsible for the rapid depolarisation (phase 0) of the action potential.
**Drugs in this class** These antiarrhythmic drugs include the following.

- Type Ia: quinidine, procainamide and disopyramide
- Type Ib: lidocaine and mexiletine, which suppress ventricular tachycardia
- Type Ic: flecainide and propafenone, which are used to treat paroxysmal atrial fibrillation

**Mode of action** Different class I drugs have different modes of action (**Figure 2.47**).

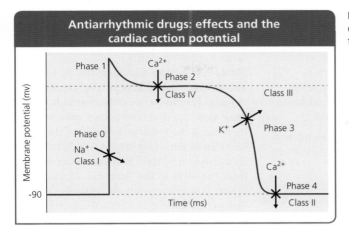

## Antiarrhythmic drugs: effects and the cardiac action potential

**Figure 2.47** Effects of different classes of antiarrhythmic drugs on the cardiac action potential.

### Antiarrhythmic medications

| Class | Mode of action | Effect on cardiac action potential | Commonly prescribed example(s) | Common adverse effects | Indications |
|-------|---------------|-----------------------------------|-------------------------------|----------------------|-------------|
| Ia | Inhibit fast $Na^+$ channels | Lengthen | Procainamide and disopyramide | Dizziness, nausea, arrhythmia, headache and hypotension | Not applicable |
| Ib | Inhibit fast $Na^+$ channels | Shorten | Lidocaine and mexilitine | Dizziness, nausea, arrhythmia, headache and hypotension | Ventricular tachycardia |
| Ic | Inhibit fast $Na^+$ channels | None | Flecainide and propafenone | Dizziness, nausea, arrhythmia, headache and hypotension | Atrial fibrillation |
| II | Block β-adrenergic receptors | None | Bisoprolol, atenolol and propranolol | Bradycardia, depression, bronchospasm and dysglycaemia | Angina, atrial fibrillation, ventricular tachycardia and heart failure |
| III | Inhibit $K^+$ channels | Lengthen | Sotalol and amiodarone | Skin discoloration, thyroid dysfunction, corneal deposits and long QT | Atrial fibrillation and ventricular tachycardia |
| IV | Block $Ca^{2+}$ channels | Shorten | Diltiazem and verapamil | Bradycardia, hypotension and dizziness | Atrial fibrillation/ flutter and angina |
| V | Inhibit $Na^+$–$K^+$ ATPase | None | Digoxin | Anorexia, nausea and bradycardia | Atrial fibrillation or flutter |
| | Transient atrioventricular block | None | Adenosine | Dyspnoea, feelings of apprehension and flushing | Supraventricular tachycardias |

**Table 2.32** Summary of antiarrhythmic medications

- Class Ia drugs lengthen the action potential and refractory period in cardiac myocytes, which reduces the influence of ectopic cardiac pacemakers and increases the fibrillation threshold in both the atria and the ventricles; however, these drugs also lengthen QT interval
- Class Ib drugs reduce the amplitude and duration of the cardiac action potential, the conduction velocity and the refractory

period, which suppresses ventricular re-entry circuits
- Class Ic drugs reduce the amplitude and conduction velocity of the cardiac action potential and lengthen the refractory period, particularly of the His–Purkinje system; these effects decrease conduction speed in the atrioventricular node

**Adverse effects** The range of adverse effects differs between classes. They include the following.

- Class Ia: diarrhoea, nausea, headache and dizziness
- Class Ib: dizziness, bradycardia, hypotension, arrhythmia and cardiac arrest
- Class Ic: dizziness, nausea, dyspnoea and arrhythmia

**Interactions** Be aware of the following interactions.

- Class Ia agents interact with lidocaine and beta-blockers, leading to bradycardia and hypotension
- Class Ib agents have reduced clearance when used with beta-blockers
- Class Ic agents interact with other antiarrhythmic agents, leading to hypotension and bradycardia

**Contraindications** The use of class Ia or class Ib drugs in patients with atrioventricular block can lead to asystole, because of the suppression of escape rhythms.

Class Ic drugs are contraindicated in patients with structural heart disease, for example, those with left ventricular systolic dysfunction and those who have had a myocardial infarction. The use of these drugs in such patients can lead to ventricular arrhythmias.

## Class II antiarrhythmic drugs

These agents are known more commonly as beta-blockers. They suppress atrial and ventricular arrhythmias. They also improve left ventricular function in cases of heart failure, and reduce myocardial oxygen demand in ischaemic heart disease.

**Drugs in this class** Beta-blockers are subdivided according to their selectivity of action on different $\beta$ adrenergic receptors. $\beta_1$ receptors are present in the heart, and $\beta_2$ receptors

in the lung. Atenolol, bisoprolol and metoprolol are selective for $\beta_1$, whereas carvedilol, labetalol and propranolol are non-selective, targeting both $\beta_1$ and $\beta_2$.

**Mode of action** Blocking the $\beta_1$ receptor antagonises the effects of the sympathetic nervous system on the atrioventricular node, thus slowing the conduction velocity and increasing the refractory period of the atrioventricular node (**Figure 2.47**). This slows the transmission of the cardiac action potential from the atria to the ventricle. Blocking the $\beta_2$ receptor leads to smooth muscle contraction in the bronchi and bronchospasm.

**Adverse effects** These include bradycardia, heart block, bronchospasm, hyper- or hypoglycaemia, headache and constipation.

**Interactions** Concomitant use of antiarrhythmic agents may cause hypotension, bradycardia and cardiac arrest.

**Contraindications** Beta-blockers can exacerbate bradycardias, depression, vasospasm and asthma. Their use is avoided in pregnancy, because they can cause intrauterine growth retardation.

## Class III antiarrhythmic drugs

Class III agents are used to manage a wide range of arrhythmias, including atrial fibrillation, ventricular tachycardia and ventricular fibrillation.

**Drugs in this class** There are two drugs in this class: amiodarone and sotalol.

**Mode of action** These agents block the $K^+$ channel in all cardiac tissue; this action lengthens the action potential and refractory period, thus preventing re-entry arrhythmias (**Figure 2.47**). Sotalol also has non-selective class II effects but prolongs the QT interval.

**Adverse effects** These occur in up to 75% of patients taking amiodarone, causing 20% of them to discontinue the drug. The adverse effects of amiodarone include corneal deposits, hypo- or hyperthyroidism, slate grey skin discoloration, pulmonary fibrosis and hepatic injury. The adverse effects of sotalol are those of class II antiarrhythmic drugs.

**Interactions** Amiodarone has synergistic effects with other antiarrhythmic agents, leading to ventricular tachyarrhythmia. It increases the plasma concentration of digoxin and statins, and potentiates the effects of oral anticoagulants. The interactions of sotalol are those of class II antiarrhythmic drugs (see page 152).

**Contraindications** Amiodarone is teratogenic, so pregnancy is a contraindication. Breastfeeding is another, because the drug is excreted in breast milk. Amiodarone is unsuitable for patients with atrioventricular block or cardiogenic shock, because of reduced cardiac contractility.

Sotalol prolongs the QT interval, so it should not be used with other QT-prolonging drugs.

## Class IV antiarrhythmic drugs

Members of this class of antiarrhythmic drugs are more commonly known as rate-limiting calcium channel blockers, as they reduce the heart rate. They are used to treat atrial tachycardias and ischaemic heart disease.

> **Amiodarone is an antiarrhythmic drug with many adverse effects.** Some of these effects occur because of its structural similarity to thyroxine. Each daily dose of amiodarone (200 mg) is equivalent to 20 times the daily requirement of thyroxine (6 mg). The adverse effects of amiodarone, coupled with its long half-life of several months, are reasons why the use of this drug should be considered carefully.

**Drugs in this group** There are two subgroups of calcium channel blocker: the phenylalkylamines (e.g. verapamil) and the benzothiazepines (e.g. diltiazem).

**Mode of action** Calcium channel blockers act on the $Ca^{2+}$ channels of all cardiac tissue; their effects decrease sinus rate and cardiac contractility, prolong the refractory period and slow conduction through the atrioventricular node (**Figure 2.47**). Thus they decrease the ventricular rate in atrial tachycardias and reduce myocardial oxygen demand in ischaemic heart disease. Unlike beta-blockers, calcium channel blockers do not antagonise the action of the sympathetic nervous system, i.e. increasing heart rate and contractility.

**Adverse effects** These include bradycardia, hypotension, dizziness and headache.

**Interactions** Concomitant use of antihyper-

tensive agents can lead to hypotension, and concomitant use of beta-blockers can lead to bradycardia and atrioventricular block.

**Contraindications** Calcium channel blockers cause reduced myocardial contractility. Therefore their use is avoided in patients with cardiogenic shock, heart failure, severe aortic stenosis and hypotension. Pregnancy is a contraindication because of teratogenesis.

## Class V antiarrhythmic drugs

A miscellaneous group of antiarrhythmic drugs, without a common mechanism, are placed in class V. They are used for atrial tachycardias.

**Drugs in this group** Adenosine and digoxin are the main drugs in this class.

**Mode of action** Adenosine is a purine nucleoside present in all cells of the body; it acts on G-protein–linked receptors. In the heart, adenosine acts on the $A_1$ receptor subtype to cause cell hyperpolarisation of both the sinoatrial and atrioventricular nodes, which lengthens the refractory period (**Figure 2.48**). Thus adenosine causes transient heart block in the atrioventricular node and interrupts re-entry pathways through the atrioventricular node, such as supraventricular tachycardias, in particular atrioventricular and atrioventricular node re-entry tachycardias.

Digoxin is a cardiac glycoside derived from the foxglove plant (*Digitalis*). This drug inhibits the $Na^+$–$K^+$ ATP pump in cardiac tissue, leading to an accumulation of intracellular sodium. Consequently, intracellular calcium also increases because of $Na^+$–$Ca^{2+}$ exchange. This increase in intracellular calcium and sodium slows sinoatrial and atrioventricular node conduction velocity, which lengthens the action potential and refractory period. Thus digoxin reduces the rate of ventricular contraction and can cardiovert atrial fibrillation. It also augments cardiac contractility and is used in patients with heart failure, even those with sinus rhythm.

**Adverse effects** Adenosine can cause dyspnoea, facial flushing, asystole, headache and feelings of apprehension.

The adverse effects of digoxin include anorexia, nausea, vomiting and tachy- or bradyarrhythmias.

**Interactions** The effects of adenosine are potentiated by dipyridamole, digoxin and verapamil but antagonised by caffeine.

Digoxin can interact with other antiarrhythmic agents, leading to bradycardia and complete heart block.

**Contraindications** The use of adenosine is avoided in patients with asthma and atrioventricular block, because it can lead to bronchospasm and complete heart block, respectively.

Digoxin is contraindicated in patients with atrioventricular block, because of the risk of complete heart block. Hypokalaemia is a contraindication because it potentiates the action of digoxin. In cardiac accessory pathways, digoxin can accelerate anterograde conduction pathways, leading to ventricular tachycardia or fibrillation.

# Diuretic drugs

Diuretics increase the production of urine. They are used to lower blood pressure in patients with hypertension, as well as to help remove excess salt and water in those with heart failure.

There are four main classes: loop diuretics, thiazide diuretics, mineralocorticoid receptor antagonists and potassium-sparing diuretics (**Table 2.33**). Each class exploits a different mechanism to increase excretion of sodium (natriuresis), and as a consequence, water (diuresis) (**Figure 2.48**).

> **Many patients who need diuretics are elderly.** Be alert to possible electrolyte disturbances; elderly people are more likely to have poor kidney function, and are therefore more susceptible to these adverse effects.

## Loop diuretics

These drugs act on the loop of Henle in the kidney. Loop diuretics are the most powerful diuretics, leading to the excretion of 20% of filtered sodium. They are used to treat pulmonary and peripheral oedema in heart failure. However, although they improve the symptoms of heart failure, they do not reduce mortality.

**Drugs in this group** The main drugs in this group are furosemide, bumetanide and torasemide.

**Mode of action** Loop diuretics act by blocking the $Na^+$–$K^+$–$Cl^-$ cotransporter in the thick ascending limb of the loop of Henle (see **Figure 2.48**). This effect reduces reabsorption of these electrolytes and increases their loss in the urine.

**Adverse effects** These drugs can cause hyponatraemia, hypokalaemia, hypotension,

| Diuretic medications | | | | | |
|---|---|---|---|---|---|
| Type | Mode of action | Site of action | Commonly prescribed examples | Common adverse effects | Indications |
| Loop diuretics | Block $Na^+$–$K^+$–$Cl^-$ cotransporter | Thick ascending limb | Furosemide and bumetanide | Hyponatraemia, hypokalaemia, hyperuricaemia and renal injury | Heart failure |
| Thiazide diuretics | Block $Na^+$–$Cl^-$ cotransporter | Distal convoluted tubule | Bendroflumethiazide and metolazone | Hypotension, dizziness, hyperglycaemia and cholestasis | Heart failure and hypertension |
| Mineralocorticoid receptor antagonists | Block aldosterone receptors | Distal convoluted tubule | Spironolactone and eplerenone | Breast tenderness and hyperkalaemia | Heart failure and hypertension |
| Potassium sparing diuretics | Block epithelial $Na^+$ channels | Collecting duct | Amiloride and triamterene | Hyperkalaemia, dizziness and rash | Hypertension |

**Table 2.33** Summary of diuretic medications

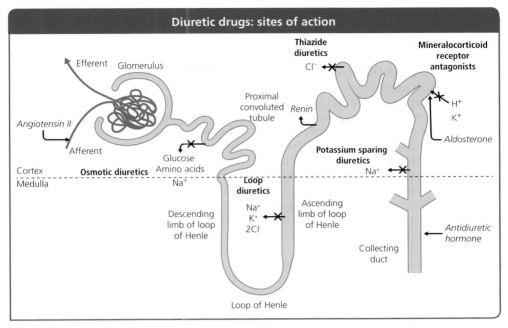

**Figure 2.48** Sites of action in the nephron of different classes of diuretic drug.

cramps, tinnitus, hearing loss, rash and hyperuricaemia.

**Interactions** Concomitant use of other antihypertensive agents can lead to hypotension. Furthermore, the risk of drug toxicity is increased when loop diuretics are used with lithium, NSAIDs, and gentamicin or because of reduced excretion.

**Contraindications** Loop diuretics exacerbate pre-existing renal failure, hypotension, dehydration, hyponatraemia and hypokalaemia.

## Thiazide diuretics

These drugs are used to treat hypertension; they lead to a mean reduction in blood pressure of 10/5 mmHg. Thiazide diuretics are also used in conjunction with loop diuretics in cases of refractory oedema, because of their synergistic effect on natriuresis.

**Drugs in this group** Bendroflumethiazide, chlortalidone, indapamide and metolazone are commonly used thiazides.

**Mode of action** Thiazides bind to and block the $Na^+/Cl^-$ cotransporter in the distal convoluted tubule of the renal nephron (**Figure 2.48**). This effect reduces reabsorption of these electrolytes and increased their loss in the urine.

**Adverse effects** These include indigestion, dehydration, hypotension, dizziness, hyperuricaemia, cholestasis and hyperglycaemia.

**Interactions** Hypokalaemia caused by thiazide diuretics increases the toxicity of antiarrhythmic agents (e.g. amiodarone, flecainide and digoxin) and potentiates the effect of other antihypertensive drugs.

**Contraindications** Thiazides cross the placental barrier and are excreted in breast milk, so their use is avoided in pregnant and breastfeeding women. These drugs exacerbate hyponatraemia and hypokalaemia, so lead to further injury in cases of severe renal or hepatic disease.

## Mineralocorticoid receptor antagonists

These are also known as aldosterone antagonists. They are second-line diuretics used to treat hypertension and heart failure. Mineralocorticoid receptor antagonists reduce blood pressure by up to 17/10 mmHg, and the risk of death by one third, in patients with chronic severe heart failure.

**Drugs in this group** These include spironolactone and eplerenone.

**Mode of action** Mineralocorticoid receptor antagonists competitively bind to the aldosterone receptor in the distal convoluted tubule of the renal nephron (**Figure 2.48**). These drugs block $Na^+/K^+$ exchange, thus reducing the urinary excretion of potassium but increasing that of sodium. They reduce cardiac hypertrophy, fibrosis and arrhythmias, and also improve endothelial function.

**Adverse effects** These include painful breasts (mastalgia), breast swelling (gynaecomastia) and testicular atrophy, which are caused by the antiandrogenic effects of mineralocorticoid receptor antagonists. Other adverse effects are hypotension, hyponatraemia and hyperkalaemia.

**Interactions** Patients receiving mineralocorticoid receptor antagonists have reduced excretion of digoxin and lithium. The effects of other antihypertensive agents are potentiated, and the concomitant use of potassium-sparing diuretics, ACE inhibitors and potassium supplements can precipitate hyperkalaemia.

**Contraindications** Mineralocorticoid receptor antagonists are avoided in patients with severe renal disease and hyperkalaemia, because of the risk of deterioration. Pregnancy and breastfeeding are contraindications, because these drugs are teratogenic and are expressed in breast milk, respectively.

### Potassium-sparing diuretics

These diuretics are 'potassium sparing', because they do not increase the loss of potassium in the urine. They are used in hypertension and heart failure, usually in conjunction with other diuretics, to maintain homeostasis of serum $K^+$.

**Drugs in this group** The most commonly used potassium-sparing diuretics are amiloride and triamterene.

**Mode of action** These diuretics act on the collecting tubules and ducts, blocking epithelial $Na^+$ channels; this effect inhibits sodium reabsorption and decreases potassium excretion (**Figure 2.48**). As a consequence, sodium loss in the urine is increased.

**Adverse effects** The use of diuretics in this group can lead to hyperkalaemia, anorexia, rash, nausea, vomiting, hypotension and dizziness.

**Interactions** Potassium-sparing diuretics interact with drugs such as ACE inhibitors, angiotensin II receptor blockers, mineralocorticoid receptor antagonists and potassium supplements, leading to hyperkalaemia.

**Contraindications** These are concomitant use of potassium-sparing diuretics (e.g. mineralocorticoid receptor antagonists and potassium supplements) and severe renal disease, because of the risk of hyperkalaemia.

# Antihypertensive drugs

Members of this class of drugs lower systemic vascular resistance and consequently blood pressure. They also help prevent the possible consequences of hypertension, including stroke and myocardial infarction. Many antihypertensive drugs also have uses in the treatment of other cardiac diseases , such as heart failure and angina.

Various types of antihypertensive agent are available, which differ in their mode of action: alpha-blockers, calcium channel blockers, hydralazine, angiotensin-converting enzyme inhibitors and angiotensin II receptor blockers (**Table 2.34**).

## Alpha-blockers

These second-line agents in the treatment of hypertension decrease blood pressure by 11/7 mmHg.

**Drugs in this group** Doxazosin, prazosin and terazosin are members of this group.

**Mode of action** Alpha-blockers prevent the binding of noradrenaline (norepinephrine), released by the sympathetic nervous system, to the $\alpha_1$ adrenergic receptors in vascular smooth muscle. This action leads to dilation of arteries and veins, reducing vascular resistance and blood pressure.

**Adverse effects** These include dizziness, hypotension, headache, peripheral oedema, urinary incontinence and nasal congestion.

| Antihypertensive medications | | | | |
|---|---|---|---|---|
| Type | Mode of action | Commonly prescribed example(s) | Common adverse effects | Indications |
| Alpha-blockers | Block $\alpha_1$-adrenergic receptors | Doxazosin | Dizziness, urinary incontinence and hypotension | Hypertension |
| Angiotensin-converting enzyme inhibitors | Block conversion of angiontensin I to angiotensin II | Ramipril, enalapril and lisinopril | Dry cough, hyperkalaemia, renal injury and angio-oedema | Hypertension, heart failure, diabetic nephropathy and myocardial infarction |
| Angiotensin II receptor blockers | Block angiotensin II $AT_1$ receptors | Valsartan, candesartan and losartan | Dizziness, hyperkalaemia, renal injury and angio-oedema | Hypertension, heart failure, diabetic nephropathy and myocardial infarction |
| Hydralazine | Direct peripheral vasodilation | Hydralazine | Allergic reaction, drug-induced lupus and palpitations | Hypertension and heart failure |
| Calcium channel blockers | Block L-type $Ca^{2+}$ channels | Amlodipine, felodipine and nifedipine | Dizziness and flushing ankle or gum swelling | Hypertension and ischaemic heart disease |

**Table 2.34** Summary of antihypertensive medications

**Interactions** Concomitant use with other antihypertensive agents can lead to hypotension.

**Contraindications** Alpha-blockers can increase mortality in patients with heart failure.

## Calcium channel blockers

Unlike class IV antiarrhythmic agents, members of the dihydropyridine group of calcium channel blockers are not rate-limiting. They are used as first-line agents in the treatment of hypertension; they reduce blood pressure by 13/11 mmHg. They are second-line agents in the treatment of ischaemic heart disease, reducing the risk of myocardial infarction by 11%.

**Drugs in this group** Amlodipine, lercanidipine, felodipine and nifedipine are commonly used examples of calcium channel blockers.

**Mode of action** These drugs inhibit the L-type $Ca^{2+}$ channels in vascular smooth muscle. This action causes vasodilation of arteries, thus reducing systemic vascular resistance and blood pressure. Vasodilation of the coronary arteries improves coronary perfusion and reduces angina.

**Adverse effects** These include dizziness, flushing, peripheral oedema, hypotension and enlargement of the gums (gingival hyperplasia).

**Interactions** Concomitant use of other antihypertensive agents augments the effects of calcium channel blockers. Antiepileptic and antifungal drugs affect the metabolism of calcium channel blockers by the liver; antiepileptics increase the level of calcium channel blockers, whereas antifungal drugs reduce it.

**Contraindications** The use of calcium channel blockers in patients with heart failure can exacerbate pulmonary and peripheral oedema.

## Hydralazine

This is a direct peripheral vasodilator used as a second-line agent in the treatment of hypertension and heart failure. In heart failure, hydralazine is used in conjunction with nitrates in patients who are intolerant of ACE inhibitors or angiotensin II receptor blockers.

In hypertension, hydralazine decreases blood pressure by up to 25/17 mmHg. It also reduces mortality in heart failure by 25%.

**Mode of action** Hydralazine targets vascular smooth muscle. It causes the release of $Ca^{2+}$ from the sarcoplasmic reticulum and the opening of $K^+$ channels, leading to hyperpolarisation. Hydralazine also stimulates nitric oxide formation. These effects result in vasodilation and the consequent reduction of systemic vascular resistance and blood pressure.

**Adverse effects** These include tachycardia, palpitations, headache, drug-induced lupus, allergic reaction, rash and dizziness.

**Interactions** Hydralazine interacts with other antihypertensive agents to produce hypotension.

**Contraindications** Hydralazine can exacerbate pre-existing systemic lupus erythematous (an autoimmune condition). It can also lead to acute heart failure in the presence of severe outflow traction obstruction (e.g. severe aortic stenosis).

## Angiotensin-converting enzyme inhibitors

These are used as first-line agents in the treatment of hypertension, heart failure and diabetic nephropathy, as well as after myocardial infarction. ACE inhibitors reduce the risk of myocardial infarction and cerebrovascular accident by 11% in patients with hypertension. In patients who have had a myocardial infarction, they reduce the risk of subsequent death and heart failure by 25%.

**Drugs in this group** The most commonly used examples of ACE inhibitors are ramipril, enalapril, lisinopril and perindopril.

**Mode of action** These drugs block the conversion by ACE of angiotensin I to angiotensin II, thus they inhibit the renin–angiotensin–aldosterone system (**Figure 2.49**). The reduction in angiotensin II leads to arteriolar and venous dilation, which decreases cardiac preload and afterload, improves endothelial function, reduces sympathetic tone and decreases blood pressure. The result is a reduction in cardiac hypertrophy, heart failure progression and proteinuria.

**Adverse effects** These include a dry tickly cough, dizziness, rash, hyperkalaemia, renal injury and angio-oedema.

**Interactions** Concomitant use of mineralocorticoid receptor antagonists, angiotensin II

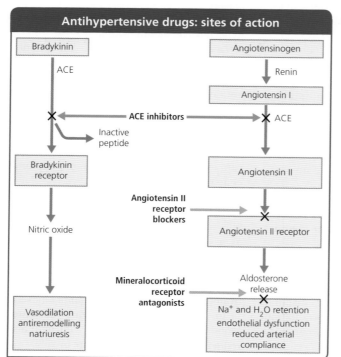

**Figure 2.49** Sites of action of angiotensin-converting enzyme (ACE) inhibitors, angiotensin receptor blockers and mineralocorticoid receptor antagonists.

receptor blockers, NSAIDs, potassium-sparing diuretics and potassium supplements can lead to hyperkalaemia. Use of ACE inhibitors with other antihypertensive agents can lead to hypotension.

**Contraindications** Angiotensin-converting enzyme inhibitors can exacerbate renal artery stenosis, severe renal disease, hyperkalaemia, hypotension and angio-oedema. They also lead to teratogenesis, so their use is avoided in pregnancy.

## Angiotensin II receptor blockers

These are used as second-line agents in the treatment of hypertension and heart failure in cases of intolerance to ACE inhibitors. Angiotensin II receptor blockers reduce the risk of myocardial infarction by 10% in patients with hypertension, and the risk of death by 25% in those with severe heart failure.

**Drugs in this group** Valsartan, irbesartan, candesartan and losartan are the most commonly used examples.

**Mode of action** These drugs inhibit the renin–angiotensin–aldosterone system by blocking the $AT_1$ receptor of angiotensin II (**Figure 2.49**). This action leads to arteriolar and venous dilation, which decreases cardiac preload and afterload, improves endothelial function, reduces sympathetic tone and decreases blood pressure. Consequently, cardiac hypertrophy, progression of heart failure and proteinuria are reduced.

**Adverse effects** These include dizziness, fatigue, hypotension, hyperkalaemia and angio-oedema. However, patients receiving angiotensin II receptor blockers avoid the bradykinin-related adverse effects associated with ACE inhibitors.

**Interactions** Concomitant use of mineralocorticoid receptor antagonists, ACE inhibitors, NSAIDs, potassium-sparing diuretics and potassium supplements can lead to hyperkalaemia. Angiotensin II receptor blockers can lead to hypotension if used with other antihypertensive agents.

**Contraindications** Angiotensin II receptor blockers can exacerbate renal artery stenosis, severe renal disease, hyperkalaemia, hypotension and angio-oedema.

> The most common reason for stopping ACE inhibitors is a chronic, non-productive cough. The cough develops because ACE inhibitors also inhibit the breakdown of bradykinin, a peptide that causes pulmonary irritation and bronchoconstriction.

## Antianginal drugs

This class of drugs is used to treat angina pectoris caused by significant coronary atherosclerosis in patients with ischaemic heart disease (**Table 2.35**). Nitrates are used as first-line agents, together with beta-blockers

| Antianginal medications | | | | |
|---|---|---|---|---|
| Type | Mode of action | Commonly prescribed example(s) | Common adverse effects | Indications |
| First line | Nitric oxide donor | Glyceryl trinitrate and isosorbide mononitrate | Headaches, dizziness and hypotension | Ischaemic heart disease, heart failure and myocardial infarction |
| Second line | Sodium channel blocker | Ranolazine | Palpitations, long QT and indigestion | Ischaemic heart disease |
| | 'Funny' Na+ channel agonist | Ivabradine | Flashing lights, bradycardia and dizziness | Ischaemic heart disease |
| | Nitric oxide donor and K+ channel agonist | Nicorandil | Palpitations, flushing and gastric ulcers | Ischaemic heart disease |

**Table 2.35** Summary of antianginal medications

and calcium channel blockers (see page 157). However, if patients are intolerant to these, or if their symptoms are inadequately controlled, the second-line agents ranolazine, ivabradine and nicorandil are indicated.

## Nitrates

These are first-line agents in the treatment of angina, hypertensive crises, acute coronary syndromes and acute heart failure. In cases of intolerance to ACE inhibitors, they are used in conjunction with hydralazine in patients with chronic heart failure, leading to a 34% reduction in mortality.

**Drugs in this group** The most common drugs in this class are glyceryl trinitrate and isosorbide mononitrate.

**Mode of action** These drugs are organic nitrates that, after enzymatic reduction, donate nitric oxide. This leads to the relaxation of vascular smooth muscle, which causes veins and coronary arteries to dilate. This vasodilation reduces cardiac preload, afterload, myocardial oxygen demand and blood pressure.

**Adverse effects** These include headaches, dizziness, nausea, vomiting and hypotension.

**Interactions** Concomitant use of antihypertensive agents can lead to hypotension. Life-threatening hypotension can result from the use of nitrates with phosphodiesterase type 5 inhibitors such as sildenafil, which is used to treat for erectile dysfunction.

**Contraindications** Nitrates are contraindicated in patients with hypotension, infarction of the right ventricle and aortic stenosis, because the reduction in preload can exacerbate these conditions.

## Ranolazine

This is a second-line agent used to treat symptomatic chronic refractory angina. Its mechanism of action is not fully understood. Unlike the other antianginal agents, it has minimal effect on blood pressure and heart rate. Ranolazine reduces episodes of angina by one or two episodes per week, but it has no impact on the risk of myocardial infarction or mortality.

**Mode of action** Ranolazine is believed to inhibit the late inward $Na^+$ current in myocardial cells by blocking $Na^+$-dependent $Ca^{2+}$ channels. This effect reduces intracellular $Ca^{2+}$ and consequently myocardial ischaemia.

**Adverse effects** These include constipation, diarrhoea, indigestion, palpitations and prolonged QT interval.

**Interactions** The plasma concentration of ranolazine is increased by concomitant use of antifungal agents, calcium channel blockers and macrolide antibiotics, but decreased by antiepileptic agents.

**Contraindications** Ranolazine is contraindicated in patients with pre-existing long QT syndrome and those using drugs that prolong the QT interval. Severe renal or hepatic impairment is a contraindication because of the reduced excretion of the drug.

> **A long QT interval, either inherited or acquired, increases the risk of sudden cardiac death**. This is because the long QT leads to abnormal repolarisation in an effect called the R-on-T phenomenon. The result is an increased risk of re-entry ventricular arrhythmias, such as torsades de pointe ventricular tachycardia..

## Ivabradine

This is a second-line agent used to treat symptomatic chronic refractory angina in patients with normal sinus rhythm and heart rate >70 beats/min. Ivabradine does not reduce mortality, but it does decrease the risk of myocardial infarction by a third. Its use is generally reserved for patients who are intolerant to beta-blockers.

**Mode of action** Ivabradine blocks the 'funny' $Na^+$ channel (see page 37) in the cells of the sinoatrial node. Thus it reduces heart rate and therefore cardiac work, myocardial oxygen demand and the symptoms of angina.

**Adverse effects** These include flashing lights, atrioventricular block, bradycardia, dizziness and blurred vision.

**Interactions** The plasma concentration of ivabradine is increased by antifungal agents, macrolide antibiotics and calcium channel blockers. Antiepileptic agents reduce it.

**Contraindications** Bradycardia, atrioventricular block, heart failure and cardiogenic shock are exacerbated by ivabradine.

## Nicorandil

This is a second-line agent used to treat symptomatic chronic refractory angina. It is a nitrate derivative of nicotinamide, which itself originates from vitamin B3 (niacin). The use of nicorandil results in a 15% reduction in myocardial infarction risk and the number of admission to hospital with chest pain.

**Mode of action** As an organic nitrate, nicorandil is a nitric oxide donor. As such, it causes the relaxation of vascular smooth muscle, thus dilating the veins and coronary arteries. Nicorandil also activates K+ channels, leading to further arterial and arteriolar dilation.

**Adverse effects** These include palpitations, flushing, weakness, headaches and gastrointestinal ulceration.

**Interactions** There are no interactions of note.

**Contraindications** Concomitant administration of phosphodiesterase type 5 inhibitors such as sildenafil can produce profound hypotension. Nicorandil exacerbates cardiogenic shock, acute pulmonary oedema, hypotension and hypovolavemia.

# Interventional management

If conservative and pharmacological management fail, the next step is to try an interventional approach. Interventional approaches use minimally invasive transcutaneous techniques. These procedures are not operations; however, the patient's skin is broken. The patient is conscious during the procedure, and only local anaesthesia is required.

The minimally invasive approach is often favoured by patients, because it means a smaller scar, shorter recovery time and earlier discharge. A multidisciplinary team compromising cardiologists, radiologists, surgeons and other paramedical staff discuss the pros and cons of each strategy and agree on a common approach.

## Angioplasty and stenting

Angioplasty is the technique of mechanically opening an artery that has been narrowed or blocked by atherosclerosis. Once the artery is open, a metal scaffold called a stent is inserted to maintain patency.

### Indications

This procedure is indicated for significant atherosclerosis, typically lesions more than 70% stenosed. It is used in the carotid artery to treat transient ischaemic attack, the coronary artery to treat angina (ischaemic heart disease) and the lower limb arteries to treat claudication (peripheral arterial disease).

### Procedure

The Seldinger technique (see page 138) is used to access the diseased artery. Radiopaque dye is then injected into the artery to identify any flow-limiting lesions.

Once a lesion is identified, a wire with a deflated balloon at its tip is inserted to cross the narrowing. Next, the balloon is inflated to reopen the narrowing. This process is then repeated but with a collapsed stent, which is expanded in the lesion to restore distal arterial flow.

The only exception to this technique is for the aorta, which in cases of abdominal aortic aneurysm is repaired by using a covered stent. The stent seals the aorta proximal and distal to the aneurysm. In this way, normal blood flow is maintained and the risk of rupture reduced, but the aneurysm remains in situ.

### Complications

Angioplasty and stenting carries a 1% risk of significant bleeding and arterial damage, and a 0.1% risk of stroke, death and myocardial infarction during the procedure. There is also the risk of the stent becoming blocked by thrombus. Furthermore, the patient may need a repeat procedure or a bypass operation should angioplasty and stenting fail.

# Structural intervention

Structural intervention is the term for the treatment of non-coronary cardiac disease by a percutaneous approach.

## Septal ablation

This procedure is used for patients with hypertrophic cardiomyopathy and symptomatic obstruction of the left ventricular outflow tract (see page 328).

## Indications
In some cases of hypertrophic cardiomyopathy, there is interventricular asymmetrical septal hypertrophy of the myocardium. This causes narrowing and subsequent dynamic obstruction of the left ventricular outflow tract.

## Procedure
The Seldinger technique is used to gain access to the left coronary arteries. A septal branch supplying the thickened myocardium is chosen and injected with pure ethanol, which leads to a localised infarction of the hypertrophied septum.

## Complications
The procedure fails in 30% of cases, and complete heart block (see page 219) occurs in 5–10% of cases.

## Transcatheter valve implantation
This technique was developed to treat aortic stenosis (see page 258) without the need for open heart surgery.

## Indications
Transcatheter valve implantation is indicated for patients with severe symptomatic aortic stenosis (mean valvular gradient > 40 mmHg) who have > 50% risk of death if they undergo conventional aortic valve replacement, and whose life expectancy is > 1 year.

## Procedure
The Seldinger technique (see page 138) is used to reach the aortic root. The aortic valve is crossed with a deflated balloon on a wire. Next, the balloon is inflated to crush the native aortic valve against the aortic root. Another wire, with the valve collapsed around a deflated balloon, is then passed immediately into the same position; the balloon inflated and the prosthetic valve expanded into place at the left ventricular outflow tract.

## Complications
There is a risk of death, stroke, aortic dissection (see page 308), aortic regurgitation (see page 265), complete heart block (see page 219), embolisation of the valve and failure of the procedure.

## Closure devices
These are used to close holes, repair leaking valves and occlude potentially thrombogenic orifices by using a minimally invasive technique.

## Indications
The procedure is indicated for the closure of holes between the left and right atrium (see page 288) in patients with a patent foramen ovale or atrial septal defect and who have had paradoxical emboli, for example a venous clot leading to an arterial embolism because of a right-to-left shunt.

Percutaneous mitral valve repair can be performed to improve the function of a failing valve in patients with primary severe mitral regurgitation (see page 270) and who are too unwell to undergo open heart surgery. The mitraclip is such a device.

For patients with atrial fibrillation (see page 224) and for whom anticoagulation is unsuitable, a left atrial appendage occlusion device can be used to prevent thrombus formation.

## Procedure
The Seldinger technique (see page 138) is used to reach the right atrium for closure of a patent foramen ovale or an atrial septal defect, the septum of which is then punctured to access the left atrium for percutaneous mitral valve repair or left atrial appendage occlusion.

For patent foramen ovale or atrial septal defect closure, a self-expanding umbrella device is deployed in the defect to plug the gap.

For the left atrial appendage occlusion device, a self-expanding plug is deployed into the narrow blind-ending tube of the appendage. It plugs the hole and prevents clot formation.

For percutaneous mitral valve repair the $A_2$ and $P_2$ leaflets are gripped with the clip. The clip is then left in place to improve mitral regurgitation.

## Complications
These include the standard risks of the Seldinger technique, such as vascular injury and bleeding.

For the left atrial appendage occlusion device, the complication rate is 5%. Complications include failure of the device, dislodgement, embolisation and clot formation.

For the MitraClip, the rate is 3% and includes failure of the device and embolisation.

For closure of a patent foramen ovale or an atrial septal defect, the rate is 5% and includes pericardial tamponade, failure of the device, dislodgement, embolisation and clot formation.

# Pacing and devices

This term refers to the use of internal and external pacemakers and defibrillators to speed up or slow down abnormally slow or fast hearts rates, respectively.

## Defibrillation

This is an electric shock used to restart the heart of a patient in extremis with atrial or ventricular tachycardias.

### Indications

Defibrillation is used to restore normal sinus rhythm in patients with dangerous ventricular rhythms, such as tachycardia or fibrillation (see page 228). The same technique is used for electrical cardioversion in patients in extremis with atrial tachycardias. Synchronisation of the shock, in ventricular tachycardia or atrial fibrillation, ensures that the energy is delivered during the R wave (depolarisation) and not the T wave (repolarisation), and thus prevents the R-on-T phenomenon (see page 357).

### Procedure

The shock of external cardiac defibrillation is painful. Therefore general anaesthesia is first administered to render the patient unconscious. Shocks of increasing intensity are delivered by paddles applied to the chest to cardiovert the heart back into normal sinus rhythm.

To insert an implantable cardioverter defibrillator, a local anaesthetic is first injected subcutaneously in the left pectoral region. Next, a small incision is made and a pocket created to contain the device's battery and circuitry, called the pulse generator. The pulse generator is then inserted under the skin and the Seldinger technique is used to place a pacing wire via a large central vein, e.g. axillary, cephalic or subclavian, into the right ventricle.

The defibrillator senses when the heart develops a malignant ventricular rhythm, such as tachycardia or fibrillation and delivers an electric shock in response. The device can also use antitachycardia pacing to break the ventricular tachycardia cycle, before a shock is deployed.

### Complications

For external cardiac defibrillation or cardioversion, there are risks from the anaesthetic, failure, stroke and skin burns.

For implantable cardioverter defibrillator, there are the risks of the Seldinger technique, pacemaker implantation , e.g. failure, lead displacement, infection, pnemothorax, and inappropriate shocks.

## Ablation

This refers to the destruction of faulty neural or electric pathways using local heating or freezing.

### Indications

Failure of pharmacological treatment for cardiac arrhythmias such as atrial fibrillation, atrial flutter, supraventricular tachycardias, ventricular tachycardias and abberant pathways is an indication for cardiac ablation. Patients with hypertension that is not controlled by pharmacological management are suitable candidates for renal sympathetic denervation, but the efficacy of this procedure is currently controversial.

### Procedure

The Seldinger technique (see page 138) is used to gain access to the cardiac chambers. The chamber in which the arrhythmia is believed to be located is stimulated to trigger the arrhythmia, map the conduction tissue and localise the abnormal pathway. The abnormal pathway is then destroyed.

### Complications

These include the complications of the Seldinger technique (see page 138), pericardial effusion and the need for a permanent pacemaker.

## Pacing

If the sinoatrial node (the heart's pacemaker; see page 219) or any of the conduction tissue becomes diseased and causes symptomatic bradycardia or heart block, pacing is required. Pacing can include the use of transcutaneous pads, a temporary pacing wire or a permanent pacemaker.

### Indications

Patients with symptomatic bradycardia (heart rate, <60 beats/min), daytime pauses (>3 s) or high-degree atrioventricular block (e.g. second- or third-degree or sick sinus syndrome; see page 219) require a permanent pacemaker. Heart failure, breathlessness on mild exertion, optimal pharmacological therapy and bundle branch block are indications for cardiac resynchronisation therapy.

### Procedure

Acute symptomatic bradycardia requires transcutaneous pacing provided by energy delivered by a defibrillator through pads attached to the chest. This is uncomfortable and requires sedation. Transcutaneous pacing is a bridging measure to a more definitive therapy.

The Seldinger technique (page 138) is used to gain access to the femoral or internal jugular vein. A temporary pacing wire is then passed into the right ventricle. The right ventricle is then paced using an external pulse generator, and the ECG will develop left bundle branch block.

To insert a permanent pacemaker, local anaesthetic is injected subcutaneously into the left pectoral region. A small incision is then made and a pocket created to contain the pacemaker's pulse generator. Next, the pacemaker is inserted and the Seldinger technique used to place a pacing wire through a large central vein into the right heart. Depending on the conduction disease, the right atrium, right ventricle or both chambers are then paced. Next, the wires are connected to the pacemaker in the left pectoral region, which is then programmed to sense the heart's intrinsic rhythm and provide pacing when appropriate.

Cardiac resynchronisation therapy is provided by a three-lead pacemaker, which paces the right atrium and both ventricles (**Figure 2.50**). The right heart is paced endocardially, but the left ventricle is paced epicardially, by accessing the coronary sinus in the right atrium. This resynchronises the heart, improving left ventricular function, functional capacity and reducing mortality. The pacemaker may also be combined with a defibrillator as a cardiac resynchronisation therapy efibrillator.

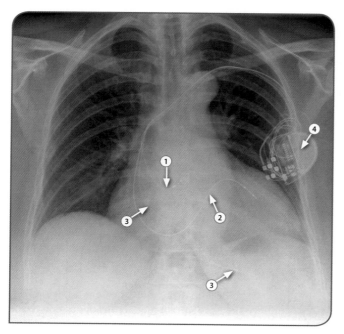

**Figure 2.50** Chest radiograph showing a cardiac resynchronisation device in-situ. ①, right atrial lead; ②, left ventricular lead; ③, right ventricular lead; ④, pulse generator.

## Complications

These include those arising from the Seld-inger technique (see page 138), failure, lead dislodgement, pneumothorax, infection and venous thrombosis.

## Endovenous therapy

These techniques were developed as an alternative to venous stripping (see page 168).

### Indications

Endovenous therapy is used for symptomatic varicose veins causing pain, swelling and fatigue.

### Procedure

In sclerotherapy, a sclerosant (a substance which damages tissue causing sclerosis and thrombosis) such as polidocanol is intravenously injected into the varicose veins. The resulting inflammatory response leads to irreversible fibrotic occlusion. The vein remnants remain in situ.

In endovenous thermal ablation, or laser therapy, an ablation catheter is inserted into the varicose veins. The veins are then heated to cause irreversible occlusion, and the remnants are left in situ.

### Complications

These include bleeding, failure, the need for a repeat procedure, pain, venous thrombosis and scarring.

# Surgical management

The final echelon in the management of cardiovascular disease is surgery. Cardiac and vascular surgeons perform both invasive and open procedures. Other approaches attempt to optimise the patients native diseased tissue, but the surgical approach to treatment is to resect, transplant, bypass or replace.

Surgery is indicated if both the following criteria are met.

- The patient remains symptomatic or at risk despite a combination of conservative risk reduction and optimal pharmacological management
- An interventional approach is not possible, is not indicated or has failed

Cardiac surgery is only carried out by cardiac surgeons in tertiary centres after referral by cardiologists, radiologists and other specialists. In contrast, vascular surgery is done at most hospitals; although there is now a move towards centralisation in a fewer number of large centres. This is because the evidence suggests that outcomes are improved and complications are reduced in centres with a higher volume of such operations and procedures.

# Risk

The risk of death from cardiac and vascular surgery is very real. For this reason, cardiac surgeons were one of the first groups in the UK to make public their mortality rates. Risks are associated with all stages: preoperative (e.g. from complications of anaesthesia), perioperative (e.g. from blood loss) and postoperative (e.g. from infections). Close liaison between the surgeon and the anaesthetist is required, and they combine anaesthesia with work in an intensive care or high-dependency setting.

Risk management includes ensuring that preoperative assessment of cardiovascular patients is robust and based not only on subjective measures (e.g. a surgeon's intuition) but also on objective measures such as risk score, comorbidity, functional status and cardiovascular fitness.

> **Informed consent for cardiac or vascular surgery requires a frank discussion with the patient, covering the common and serious risks of surgery, and its benefits, as well as other treatment options.**
> A clinician with relevant experience, preferably the person doing the operation, should talk to the patient; this task should not delegated to a junior member of the team.

# Arterial bypass

In arterial bypass, a synthetic or transplanted vessel is used to bypass a section of artery that is significantly occluded by atherosclerosis. The patient requires general anaesthesia.

## Indications

Patients with significant atherosclerotic lesions in either the coronary or the lower limb arteries are considered for arterial bypass surgery.

Left main stem and triple-vessel ischaemic heart disease are best suited to bypass graft surgery. Internal mammary, radial artery or long saphenous vein grafts are used to bypass blockages. Patients with peripheral arterial disease may have significant aortic, femoral, tibial or peroneal artery stenoses.

## Procedure

The process for coronary artery bypass surgery is as follows.

1. The chest is opened with an incision through the sternum.
2. The circulation is connected to a bypass machine, which does the job of the heart and lungs
3. The heart is cooled by a process termed cardioplegia. Injecting cold, potassium rich fluid (5C) stops and protects the heart
4. The grafts are harvested, washed and sewn proximal to the blockage, typically in the aorta, and distally past the blockage
5. The patient is taken off the bypass machine, then the chest is closed and the anaesthesia reversed

Peripheral artery bypass surgery is done as follows.

1. The patient's native vessels are bypassed using conduits made of polytetrafluoroethylene (Teflon)
2. An incision is made at the point of the blockage, then the artificial conduit is sewn to points proximal and distal to the blockage (e.g. femoral–popliteal, tibioperoneal, aortofemoral and even axillofemoral)
3. The incision is closed and the anaesthesia reversed

## Complications

These include death, bleeding, thromboembolism, graft failure, infection, myocardial infarction and cardiac arrhythmia.

# Arterial repair

Abnormal dilations, acute dissections and focal atherosclerosis of large arteries, such as an abdominal aortic aneurysm, are repaired with the patient under general anaesthesia.

## Indications

Large abdominal aortic aneurysm (>5.5 cm; normal width, <3.0 cm), acute dissection of the ascending aorta and symptomatic, moderate to severe (50–99%) blockage of one or both carotid arteries are indications for arterial repair.

## Procedure

The process for abdominal aortic aneurysm repair is as follows.

1. An incision is made in the abdomen
2. The aneurysm is located and clamped above and below
3. The aneurysmal segment is removed and a Teflon conduit sewn in place
   - The iliac arteries are also repaired, if necessary
4. The abdomen is then closed and the anaesthesia reversed

An aortic dissection requires the following.

1. The chest is opened
2. The dissection is located and clamped above and below
3. The dissected segment is removed and a Teflon conduit sewn in place

   - Depending on the site of the dissection, the three branches of the aortic arch, the aortic valve and even the coronary arteries may also need to be repairedor bypassed.
4. The clamps are removed and the chest closed

For an endarectomy, the following process is required.

1. An incision is made over the carotid artery and a clamp placed above and below the blockage
2. The artery is cut open and the atherosclerotic lesion removed
3. The skin is then closed and the anaesthesia reversed

## Complications

These include death, stroke, bleeding, thromboembolism, graft failure, infection, myocardial infarction and cardiac arrhythmia.

# Heart transplantation

Heart transplantation is a life-saving treatment for end-stage heart disease. The diseased heart is replaced by a healthy one from a recently deceased donor.

## Indications

Cardiac transplantation is indicated in patients with acute or chronic severe heart failure that is refractory to pharmacological and device therapy.

## Procedure

After induction of general anaesthesia, the process is as follows.

1. The chest is opened through a midline sternal incision
2. The patient is attached to a bypass machine
3. The diseased heart is isolated from the major vessels and then removed
4. The donor heart is put in place and sewn to the major vessels
5. The patient is taken off the bypass machine, the chest is closed and the anaesthesia is reversed

## Complications

These include death, stroke, bleeding, thromboembolism, transplant failure, rejection of organ, infection, myocardial infarction and cardiac arrhythmia.

# Valve repair or replacement

Severe heart valve disease causing significant symptoms or heart failure requires valve repair or replacement.

## Indications

This option is used for patients with symptomatic and severe disease of any four of the heart valves which is not suitable for minimally invasive repair, such as those requiring additional surgery to correct co-existing ischaemic valve disease, arrhythmia, aneurysms or infection.

## Procedure

After induction of general anaesthesia, the process is as follows.

1. The chest is opened through an incision in the sternum
2. The patient is attached to a bypass machine, then the heart is cooled by a process called cardioplegia
3. The diseased valve is located and either repaired or removed
4. The patient is taken off the bypass machine, the chest is closed and the anaesthesia is reversed

## Complications

These include death, stroke, bleeding, thromboembolism, valve dehiscence, infection, myocardial infarction and cardiac arrhythmia.

# Myocardial repair or support

Certain myocardial defects are suitable for repair, the use of an artificial pump to support the failing myocardium, or both.

## Indications

Patients can have a left ventricular assist device inserted while awaiting heart transplantation (in 'bridge-to-transplantation therapy') or to support myocardial recov-ery in cases of reversible acute heart failure, such as fulminant myocarditis or post-partum cardiomyopathy. Newer technologies to fulfil the function of the entire heart, such as the artificial heart, may provide a permanent but totally artificial solution (Figure 2.51).

Left ventricular restoration therapy is used to improve left ventricular function in patients with a left ventricular aneurysm after a myocardial infarction resulting in significant left ventricular systolic dysfunction.

Patients with functionally significant septal defects, such as atrial septal defect and ventricular septal defect, which cannot be closed using a device, may require surgical closure.

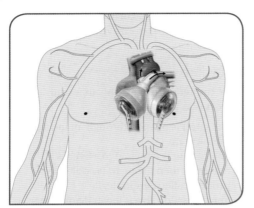

**Figure 2.51** A total artificial heart in-situ, demonstrating turbines driving blood through both the pulmonary artery and aorta.

## Procedure

After induction of general anaesthesia, the procedure is as follows.

1. The chest is opened through an incision in the sternum
2. The patient is attached to a bypass machine, then their heart is cooled
3. Next is one of three options
   - For left ventricular restoration therapy, the diseased myocardium is located and removed, then the heart is closed
   - For insertion of a left ventricular assist device, the pump inlet is sewn to the left ventricular apex and the pump outlet to the ascending aorta
   - For repair of an atrial or a ventricular septal defect, the defect is exposed and a patch sewn into place using native pericardium, bovine pericardium or Teflon
4. The patient is taken off the bypass machine, the chest is closed and anaesthesia is reversed

## Complications

These include death, stroke, bleeding, thromboembolism, infection, myocardial infarction and cardiac arrhythmia.

# Venous repair

Varicose veins are removed by venous stripping.

## Indications

Venous stripping is indicated in patients with symptomatic varicose veins in the lower limbs. The vains cause pain, swelling and fatigue.

## Procedure

The following is done after induction of general or local anaesthesia.

1. An incision is made over the origin and termination of the varicose vein
2. A wire is passed into the vein distally, tied and advanced proximally to a point
3. The wire is pulled, which strips the vein from the body
4. The skin is closed and the anaesthesia reversed

## Complications

These are bleeding, venous thromboembolism and infection.

**Reversible causes of heart failure may require only temporary placement of a left ventricular assist device.** This may suffice to allow the heart to recover before resuming its normal function. Examples of cases in which this approach is appropriate include post-partum cardiomyopathy and fulminant myocarditis.

# Answers to starter questions

1.  Chest pain that is neither brought on by exertion, relieved by rest, localised to a finger-point, is palpable or lasts either for seconds or continues for days, is unlikely to have a serious cause. This is because it is unlikely to be cardiac in origin; the pain is atypical and not brought on by stressing the cardiovascular system. Pain that has been present for days, which hasn't caused serious harm to the patient, e.g. collapse, loss of consciousness or admission to hospital, cannot be due to cardiac disease; if it was, it would have manifested itself as a myocardial infarction, heart failure or cardiac arrest.

2.  Systemic symptoms such as nausea, vomiting, dyspnoea and diaphoresis increase the likelihood that pain is cardiac in origin, because cardiac ischaemia causes an increase in sympathetic drive, e.g. fight/flight response. Palpitations and dizziness suggest a symptomatic tachycardia or bradycardia, which lead to haemodynamic compromise e.g. hypotension and cerebral insufficiency, e.g. loss of consciousness.

3.  The musician Roy Castle's death from lung cancer was attributed to years of playing and singing in smoke filled clubs. Since 2007, in the UK, smoking cigarettes in enclosed work places has been banned. This is arguably one of the greatest public health interventions in the 21st century as it has reduced the passive exposure to the harmful effects of cigarette smoke, which is as harmful as active smoking.

4.  Collapse at the end of the race (exercise associated collapse) occurs due to a buildup of lactate, dehydration, vasovagal syncope, hypoglycaemia and fatigue. It is common and harmless, as ultimately the cardiovascular system has coped with the physical test of running a marathon. However, a collapse during a marathon is a different issue because the stressor (the marathon) has unearthed an underlying problem. For those under 35, the cause is most likely structural heart disease and for those over 35 ischaemic heart disease is most likely.

5.  The move from manual to sedentary jobs, increased car use, reduced recreational physical activity and diets richer in highly processed foods have increased the incidence of diabetes and obesity, which greatly increase the incidence of coronary atherosclerosis. Despite advances in health, such as smoking reduction, improved housing and increased immunisation, more people are living long enough (with increased risk) to develop atherosclerosis, increasing the incidence of heart disease.

6.  Patients suffering from acute heart failure or ST elevation myocardial infarction have a characteristic appearance that can often be identified on sight: typically they look grey, clammy and breathless. In contrast, patients with arrhythmias often have nothing outward to differentiate them from a healthy person.

7.  Assessment start with a patient's physical condition: is their walk quick or slow? Aided or unaided? Demonstrating pain or breathlessness? Essentially, does the patient look well or unwell? Is their current state new or chronic? A well patient will have a quick, purposeful and unaided stride, which means, regardless of the nature or severity of their underlying disease, they are minimally symptomatic. Stratifying criteria such as the New York Heart Association (NYHA) for heart failure, the Canadian Cardiovascular Society (CCS) for angina and the European Heart Rhythm Association (EHRA) for atrial fibrillation help to grade symptom severity and facilitate communication with other clinicians.

**Answers** *continued*

8.   While a large part of reaching a diagnosis is following specific steps in the history and examination, there are subtle aspects in assessing a patient that can hint at a diagnosis. Clinicians with years of experience can often have their suspicions aroused by patient who just 'don't look right'and can look at the finer details as well as the bigger picture. Robots would be able to follow diagnostic algorithms but the personal aspects of a clinician's experience would be lost. This is a problem for modern medicine with its increasing use of guidelines, which are often evidence-based for a population but can sometimes inadequately guide management decisions for an individual.

9.   The working memory of the human brain has the ability to store 7 (+/–2) pieces of information. When presenting patients to senior doctors, the key is to convey the pertinent points without being verbose or digressing. The patient's notes may be several pages long but should be summarised in a couple of sentences otherwise the relevant information will be lost, e.g. 'Mr Smith is a 54-year-old train driver with a 1-week history of cardiac-sounding chest pain and without past, drug or family history. The examination was unremarkable and the working diagnosis is angina'. Only include relevant positives, e.g. smoking, and negatives, e.g. no family history.

10.  Investigations are unnecessary when their results will not affect the management given to the patient. For example, whilst the finding of a new murmur in asymptomatic patient may seem interesting, if that patient is > 80, bed bound, doubly incontinent and suffering from dementia, then it is irrelevant. This is because the patient is asymptomatic, they would not be considered fit for any intervention and subjecting them to echocardiography is cruel and a waste of limited resources. Think through investigations before they are ordered as nothing is routine and may have unforeseen consequences, such as an incidental finding requiring regular follow-up.

11.  The limitation of the ECG is that it is a 2D electrical study of a 3D moving muscle with blood, wiring and valves. However, it is not just the heart that has an impact on the ECG. For example, in patients with eating disorders, e.g. bulimia, the repeated vomiting can lead to depletion of potassium (hypokalaemia) putting them at risk of life threatening arrhythmias. The ECG can be the first suggestion of this, as it is not seen on an echocardiogram or cardiac MR scan.

12.  Blood tests require clinical context to have meaning in cardiovascular disease. For example, after an iron man triathlon (3.8 km swim, 180 km bike, 42 km run) a healthy athlete will have raised troponin and BNP as a result, both of which are also signs of cardiac damage. In a normal patient this would be considered abnormal (symptoms of heart disease) and would be cause for further investigation. However, iron man athletes have endured 8–17 hours of vigorous exercise, inducing a high-output cardiac state, not unlike high-output heart failure; a small elevation in cardiac biomarkers is therefore expected.

13.  There are different types of error in the management of patients with disease, including biases of attribution, e.g. a patient of a particular type is presumed to have a diagnosis of a certain type; confirmation, e.g. overemphasising evidence to support not refute the diagnosis; framing, e.g. diagnosis unduly influenced by how the problem is described; overconfidence, e.g. overestimate ones diagnostic acumen and anchoring, e.g. locked into a pertinent part of narrative too early in diagnosis. Being mindful of such pitfalls in the diagnosis and management of patients helps prevent harm from wrong, delayed or missed diagnoses.

**Answers** *continued*

14. The heart depends on well-functioning musculoskeletal, circulatory and respiratory systems to deliver oxygen to tissues. If a patient becomes physically deconditioned from lack of exercise, then symptoms such as chest pain and breathlessness can get worse. Exercise improves symptoms in all types of heart disease, and reduces the risk of developing cardiovascular disease and the risk of mortality following a cardiac insult.

15. Treatment of a patient's disease serves many purposes: reduce their symptoms, improve their quality of life, prevent deterioration in the condition and prolong life. It may also serve to reassure the clinician, the patient or their relatives that something is being done, especially in the absence of a firm diagnosis. However in individuals with asymptomatic disease, such as hypertension, there is considerable risk to the individual from the harms of being labelled as unwell and from the side-effects of medications. In such patients, more harm than good may be served by initiating treatment as it may negatively impact on their autonomy. Ultimately, it is the patient's decision whether they feel the risks of treatment are greater than the benefits and this must be respected, even if it is the 'wrong' decision.

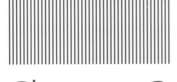

# Chapter 3
# Ischaemic heart disease

## Starter questions

Answers to the following questions are on page 193.

1. Do all patients with heart attack experience chest pain?
2. Why is thrombolysis no longer first line treatment for myocardial infarction?
3. Can ischaemic heart disease be prevented?
4. Why do stents inserted into arteries not promote clotting?
5. Are heart attacks more common on Monday mornings?

## Introduction

Ischaemic heart disease is caused by coronary arterial blood flow becoming restricted secondary to an accumulation of atherosclerotic plaque. Ischaemia occurs when myocardial oxygen demand exceeds supply, often presenting as chest pain. The terms ischaemic heart disease, coronary artery disease and coronary heart disease are all used to describe the same condition. Chest pain is one of the most frequent presenting complaints to the accident and emergency department and to primary care clinics.

Ischaemic heart disease has been considered primarily a disease of western populations. However, its global burden is growing rapidly with the adoption of the western-style diet by other populations, as well as the increasing prevalence of non-dietary risk factors (e.g. smoking, hypertension, hypercholester-

olaemia and diabetes). According to the World Health Organization, ischaemic heart disease is now the single leading cause of death and disease burden in the world. In 2013 it was responsible for 7 million deaths per year which represents just over 11% of all deaths worldwide. However, in the past 10 years, death rates have halved. This is largely the result of efforts to reduce risk factors, such as the ban on smoking in enclosed public places.

Patients with ischaemic heart disease are at risk of acute coronary syndromes: unstable angina, non–ST elevation myocardial infarction (NSTEMI) and ST elevation myocardial infarction (STEMI). Acute coronary syndromes occur when an atherosclerotic plaque ruptures. The subsequent platelet activation and blood clotting result in occlusion of the coronary artery. Blood flow becomes blocked which results in ischaemia. Unless blood flow is restored rapidly this leads to necrosis of the myocardium and a myocardial infarction (commonly known as a heart attack).

The broad aims of treatment are to:

- control risk factors
- reduce myocardial oxygen demand
- reopen blocked arteries
- reduce the coagulability of blood

Myocardial ischaemia is less frequently caused by disease processes other than atherosclerosis, which reduce coronary blood flow via other mechanisms, for example coronary arterial spasm, embolisation of a blood clot or infective vegetation, or a vasculitic process such as Wegener's granulomatosis with polyangiitis. Myocardial ischaemia also occurs secondary to dissection of a coronary artery.

## Case 1 Pain radiating across the chest and down the left arm

### Presentation

Mr Baylis, who is 58 years old, presents to his local accident and emergency department complaining of central chest pain radiating down his left arm. He had been suffering with the pain, on and off, for a week, but it had suddenly become worse that morning.

### Initial interpretation

Mr Baylis's presenting complaint is chest pain. There are many causes of chest pain, several of which are very serious. Mr Baylis's symptoms need to be explored further, for example by using the SOCRATES mnemonic.

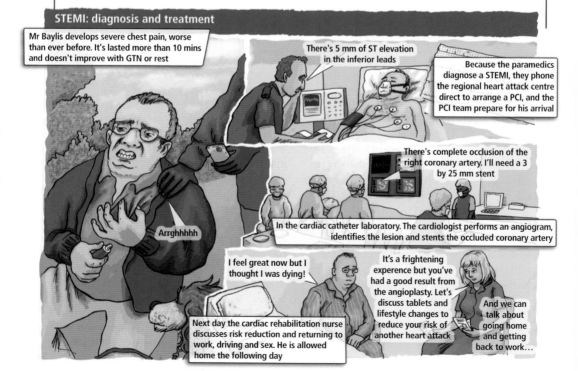

**STEMI: diagnosis and treatment**

Mr Baylis develops severe chest pain, worse than ever before. It's lasted more than 10 mins and doesn't improve with GTN or rest

There's 5 mm of ST elevation in the inferior leads

Because the paramedics diagnose a STEMI, they phone the regional heart attack centre direct to arrange a PCI, and the PCI team prepare for his arrival

Arrghhhhh

There's complete occlusion of the right coronary artery. I'll need a 3 by 25 mm stent

In the cardiac catheter laboratory. The cardiologist performs an angiogram, identifies the lesion and stents the occluded coronary artery

I feel great now but I thought I was dying!

It's a frightening experience but you've had a good result from the angioplasty. Let's discuss tablets and lifestyle changes to reduce your risk of another heart attack

And we can talk about going home and getting back to work...

Next day the cardiac rehabilitation nurse discusses risk reduction and returning to work, driving and sex. He is allowed home the following day

**Case 1** *continued*

> SOCRATES is a mnemonic used in the assessment of pain.
>
> **S**ite: central, unilateral, diffuse or focal?
>
> **O**nset: over minutes, hours, days or weeks?
>
> **C**haracter: sharp, dull, stabbing, heavy or constricting?
>
> **R**adiation: neck, jaw, back or arm?
>
> **A**ssociated symptoms: nausea, vomiting, dizziness, dyspnoea or collapse?
>
> **T**iming: when did the pain start and is it constant or intermittent?
>
> **E**xacerbating and relieving factors
>
> **S**everity: graded out of 10

## History

Mr Baylis's medical history includes ischaemic heart disease, hypertension and hypercholesterolaemia, but not diabetes. He suffers from angina infrequently, always on exertion and typically resolving with rest or a single use of his glyceryl trinitrate spray. However, over the past week he has been experiencing pain on and off, at a much lower exercise threshold than usual. Unusually, the most recent episode did not resolve with rest or glyceryl trinitrate.

Not wanting to ruin his holiday, he had dismissed the symptoms as indigestion and took an over-the-counter indigestion remedy from the local pharmacy. On further questioning, it becomes apparent that Mr Baylis is not nauseous or dizzy, nor is he experiencing palpitations. The pain is not related to meals, and the medication for indigestion has had no effect.

## Interpretation of history

Episodic pain over a week suggests unstable angina, and the sudden deterioration may have been caused by a myocardial infarction. Other diagnoses are possible,

such as stable angina, a pulmonary embolus or pneumonia (see **Table 3.1** for help with diagnosing chest pain).

It is important to determine whether the patient has had this pain before. If so, what was the cause, and was it similar in severity? The heart is not the only structure in the chest that causes chest pain. Therefore it is useful to think about the possible sources of pain according to their anatomy (see **Table 3.1** and text box).

> In the differential diagnosis of chest pain, consider the possible sources of pain in terms of their anatomy.
>
> - Skin: herpes zoster infection (shingles)
> - Musculoskeletal system: costochondritis, fibromyalgia or delayed-onset muscle soreness
> - Lungs: disease affecting the parietal pleura, e.g. pulmonary embolus or pneumonia
> - Heart (non-atherosclerotic causes): pericarditis, coronary spasm or coronary dissection
> - Oesophagus: spasm, gastro-oesophageal reflux disease or rupture
> - Others: aortic dissection, panic attack or anxiety

Patients with angina often become very familiar with their own pain and know what is 'normal' for them. Consequently, they usually know when the pain becomes more persistent or more severe, or when it is experienced at a lower-than-normal threshold. These changes suggest an acute coronary syndrome. In any of these situations, patients are advised to seek immediate medical advice.

Patients, and their physicians, often mistake the pain of indigestion for that of myocardial ischaemia – and vice versa. Furthermore, up to a third of myocardial infarctions are silent (i.e. without significant chest pain). However, worsening central chest pain in a middle-aged man with known ischaemic heart disease is serious and should be treated as an acute coronary syndrome until proven otherwise.

**Case 1** *continued*

| The characteristics of pleuritic, ischaemic and musculoskeletal chest pain | | | |
|---|---|---|---|
| Characteristic | Pleuritic | Ischaemic | Musculoskeletal |
| Site | Focal (single finger point) | Central and retrosternal | Variable |
| Character | Sharp or 'stabbing' | Heavy or tight, with sensation of pressure | Tender |
| Precipitating factors | Deep inspiration and coughing | Any factor that increases physical demand on the heart:<br>■ exercise<br>■ cold<br>■ heavy meals<br>■ stress | Movement, postural change or palpation |
| Relieving factors | Shallow breathing | Rest and nitrates (in cases of stable angina) | Staying still |
| Radiation | Rare | Into jaw and into arms and back | Rare |
| Other | Caused by friction between inflamed visceral and parietal pleural or pericardial layers | Stable angina eases with rest and nitrates, but pain in acute coronary syndromes is resistant to these relieving factors | Tenderness to palpation (common) |
| Causes | Respiratory disease and pericarditis, for example:<br>■ pneumonia<br>■ pericarditis<br>■ pulmonary embolism | Ischaemic heart disease | Trauma, costochondritis, arthritis and post-exercise muscle tenderness |

**Table 3.1** Characteristics of the three main diagnostic categories of chest pain

**Several groups of patients are at increased risk of a silent myocardial infarction.**

■ The elderly: because of late onset, atypical or absent symptoms
■ Heart transplant recipients: because of destruction of nervous pain afferents during surgery
■ Patients with diabetes: because of neuropathy

## Further history

Regarding Mr Baylis's family history, his brother and father died in their fifties of heart attack. Enquiries about his drug history reveal that, along with the glyceryl trinitrate spray, he is taking atenolol and atorvastatin; he has no known drug allergies. He drinks 10–14 units of alcohol per week and has never smoked. He works as a taxi driver and is married, with no children. The systems review is unremarkable.

## Examination

Mr Baylis is dyspnoeic, pale and clammy. His heart rate is 90 beats/min, and his blood pressure is 110/60 mmHg. His jugular venous pulse is not raised. Capillary refill time is about 2 s. Respiratory rate is 18 breaths/min, and oxygen saturation is 95% on room air.

Auscultation of Mr Baylis's precordium reveals that his chest is clear and his heart sounds are normal, with no added

**Case 1** *continued*

sounds. No peripheral oedema is present. He is apyrexial, his chest pain is not reproducible with palpation and his abdominal examination is unremarkable.

## Interpretation of findings

Mr Baylis's history of more persistent, more severe pain occurring at a lower threshold suggests that his 'usual' angina progressed into unstable angina which is an acute coronary syndrome. His pain is now constant and severe which suggests he is now experiencing a myocardial infarction (**Table 3.2**).

Unless ischaemia or myocardial infarction has caused heart failure or arrhythmia, examination findings are sometimes normal, even during a myocardial infarction. However, pallor, nausea and clamminess (secondary to vagal activation) are common in patients experiencing severe ischaemia and myocardial infarction.

> A standard 12-lead ECG (e.g. Figure 3.1) does not 'look at' the posterior aspect of the heart. Therefore, in a posterior territory STEMI, ST segment elevation is seen as ST depression in the anterior leads. Posterior leads can be positioned across the patient's back if a posterior myocardial infarction is suspected.

## Investigations

Chest X-ray using a portable machine in the accident and emergency department shows clear lung fields. However, Mr Baylis's electrocardiogram (ECG) shows convex ST elevation > 5 mm in leads II, III and aVF (**Figure 3.1**). The results of baseline blood tests, including full blood count, renal function test, liver function test and troponin, are all normal.

> **Patients with ischaemia often deny being in any pain.** They may instead describe 'pressure', 'tightness' or 'heaviness' in the chest. Therefore it is important to ask about any discomfort in the chest, as well as any pain.

## Diagnosis

An ST elevation myocardial infarction (STEMI) is diagnosed. The ECG suggests that this is affecting the inferior myocardial territory; it is therefore likely to be secondary to obstruction of the right coronary artery.

Mr Baylis is transferred to the closest primary percutaneous coronary intervention (PPCI) centre to reopen the blocked coronary artery. **Figure 3.2** shows PPCI of his obstructed right coronary artery.

| Diagnosis of acute coronary syndromes | | | | | | |
|---|---|---|---|---|---|---|
| Diagnosis | Exertional central chest pain relieved by glyceryl trinitrate | | Electrocardiogram | | Troponin concentration | |
| | Yes | No | Normal | Abnormal | Normal | Increased |
| Stable angina* | ✓ | | ✓ † | | ✓ | |
| Unstable angina | ✓ | | ✓ † | | ✓ | |
| NSTEMI | | ✓ | | ✓ | | ✓ |
| STEMI | | ✓ | | ✓ | | ✓ |

NSTEMI, non–ST elevation myocardial infarction; STEMI, ST elevation myocardial infarction.
*Stable angina is not an acute coronary syndrome, but is included for comparison. †In angina the ECG looks non-ischaemic between episodes (which is most of the time) but develops changes during ischaemia.

**Table 3.2** Diagnosis of acute coronary syndrome based on symptoms, electrocardiogram and troponin concentration.

**Case 1** *continued*

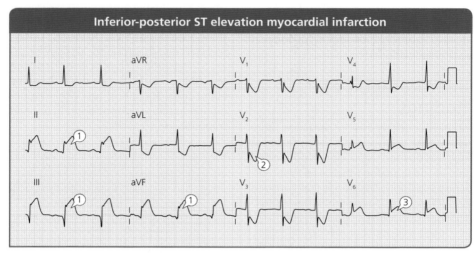

## Inferior-posterior ST elevation myocardial infarction

**Figure 3.1** Mr Baylis's ECG demonstrates inferior-posterior ST elevation. There are no posterior leads in a standard 12-lead ECG. In posterior STEMI ST depression is seen in the anterior leads instead. Inferior STEMIs normally occur secondary to right coronary artery occlusion but may involve the left circumflex artery if the circulation is left dominant (i.e. the posterior descending artery is a branch of the circumflex artery). ① ST elevation in the inferior lead; ② ST depression in the anterior leads; ③ ST elevation in the lateral leads

### Infarct territory, ECG changes and culprit vessel

| Site of infarct | | ST elevation | Culprit vessel |
|---|---|---|---|
| Left ventricle | Anterior | V1–V4 | Left anterior descending artery |
| | Septal | V3–V4 | Left anterior descending artery |
| | Lateral | I, aVL and V5–V6 | Left circumflex artery |
| | Inferior | II, III and avF | Right coronary artery or left circumflex artery |
| | Posterior | V7–V9 | Diagonal or left circumflex artery |
| Right ventricle | | V1 | Right coronary artery (proximal to right ventricular branch origin) |

**Table 3.3** Site of infarct, corresponding electrocardiographic changes and culprit vessel. Note the significant crossover between these patterns. For example, a large anterior infarct may extend across the septal and lateral regions. Similarly, a large inferior infarct (right coronary artery) may extend into the lateral regions of the left ventricle.

**Case 1** *continued*

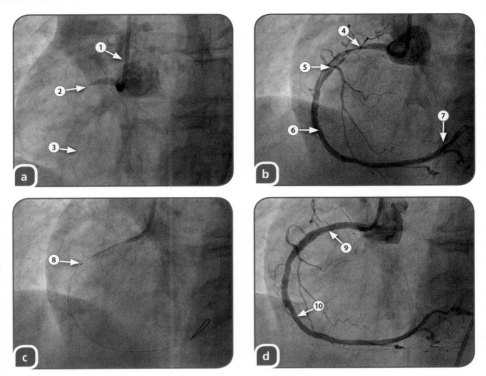

**Figure 3.2** Primary percutaneous coronary intervention to reopen the right coronary artery. Four stages of a primary PCI procedure. (a) Blocked RCA. ① Catheter in RCA. ② RCA is completely occluded by atherosclerotic plaque and clot at this point. ③ Absence of distal RCA flow. (b) After balloon inflation. ④ Deflated balloon in the RCA. ⑤ Clot (pale area) in the RCA. ⑥ Flow restored in the distal RCA. ⑦ Intracoronary wire seen in the RCA (only the distal tip is radiopaque). (c) Clot aspiration. ⑧ Aspiration catheter sucking the clot out of the RCA. (d) Final result after stenting. ⑨ Stented segment (stent not visible). ⑩ Excellent distal flow.

# Angina

Angina is the clinical manifestation of myocardial ischaemia. It is typically characterised by 'heavy' or 'crushing' central chest pain on exertion, which is relieved by rest.

Angina is classified according to the Canadian Cardiovascular Society Angina Grading Scale (**Table 3.4**), which is similar to the New York Heart Association system for the classification of heart failure (see page 244).

| Class | Definition |
|---|---|
| 1 | Angina only during strenuous or prolonged physical activity |
| 2 | Slight limitation, with angina only during vigorous physical activity |
| 3 | Symptoms with everyday living activities (i.e. moderate limitation) |
| 4 | Inability to perform any activity without angina or angina at rest (i.e. severe limitation) |

**CCS Angina Grading Scale**

**Table 3.4** The Canadian Cardiovascular Society Angina Grading Scale

## Epidemiology

In the UK, the incidence of ischaemic heart disease is 21,000 cases/year; stable angina accounts for a significant proportion of this. Its prevalence in people older than 55 years is 12% in men and 5% in women.

## Aetiology

Risk factors for the development of ischaemic heart disease are divided into those that can be modified and those that cannot, as well as probable risk factors that increase risk through an unknown mechanism (**Table 3.5**).

## Prevention

Primary prevention of ischaemic heart disease focuses on controlling or reversing modifiable risk factors. Key interventions include:

- smoking cessation
- strict control of hypertension and diabetes (if present)
- regular exercise
- a Mediterranean-style diet, which is rich in fresh fruit and vegetables

## Pathogenesis

Ischaemia occurs when myocardial oxygen demand is greater than supply. Ischaemia is a consequence of luminal atherosclerosis which restricts coronary arterial blood flow. In stable angina, blood flow across the diseased section is sufficient at rest but becomes limited during times of increased flow demand.

Ischaemic heart disease arises from the development of atherosclerotic plaques in the coronary arterial lumen (**Figure 3.3** and **Figure 3.4**). The major risk factors are smoking, hypercholesterolaemia, hypertension, diabetes and a positive family history (a first-degree relative with premature coronary artery disease, i.e. diagnosed before the age of 65 years) (**Table 3.5**).

## Clinical features

### Symptoms

The key symptoms of ischaemic heart disease are chest pain and dyspnoea.

- Chest pain is typically central or retrosternal. Its character is crushing or tight; it is often described as 'like a band across the chest' (**Figure 3.5**). The pain often radiates to the arms (often the left arm), neck or jaw (**Figure 3.6**). The discomfort is sometimes sensed primarily in these sites, without any overt chest pain. Exacerbating factors include the cold, exertion, large meals and stress. Relieving factors include use of glyceryl trinitrate and rest.

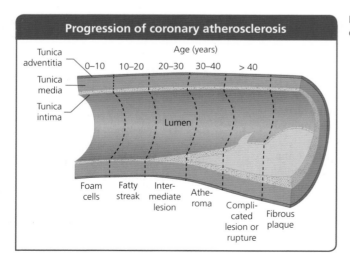

**Figure 3.3** Progression of coronary atherosclerosis.

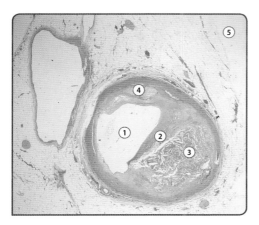

**Figure 3.4** Haematoxylin and eosin staining of coronary artery (right) and vein (left). The artery shows a markedly diminished lumen ① due to encroachment of the atherosclerotic plaque. There is a fibrous cap ② overlying necrotic core matrix and cholesterol crystals ③. Some calcification is also present ④. Supporting fibrofatty tissue ⑤.

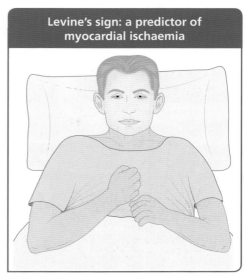

**Levine's sign: a predictor of myocardial ischaemia**

**Figure 3.5** Patients may use a clenched fist in the centre of the chest when describing their chest pain; this gesture (Levine's sign) predicts myocardial ischaemia. Pointing with a single finger does not; it suggests non-ischaemic chest pain instead.

### Risk factors for ischaemic heart disease

| Non-modifiable | Modifiable | Probable |
| --- | --- | --- |
| Advanced age | High blood pressure | Obesity |
| Male gender | Diabetes | Poor diet |
| Personal history of ischaemic heart disease | Smoking | Chronic kidney disease |
| Family history of ischaemic heart disease | Hypercholesterolaemia | |

**Table 3.5** Modifiable, non-modifiable and probable risk factors for the development of ischaemic heart disease

- Dyspnoea is sometimes experienced, particularly when ischaemia causes left ventricular systolic impairment. The impairment leads to increased pressure in the pulmonary vasculature. Breathlessness may be the patient's primary complaint.

## Clinical signs

Between attacks, patients usually have no obvious signs of cardiac ischaemia on clinical

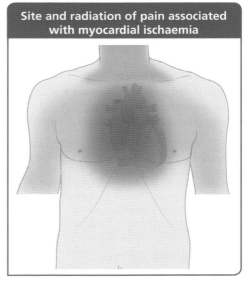

**Site and radiation of pain associated with myocardial ischaemia**

**Figure 3.6** Pain associated with myocardial ischaemia is typically experienced across the centre of the chest and often radiates into the arms, neck and jaw.

examination. However, clinical evidence of risk factors may be found (**Figure 3.7**), for example:

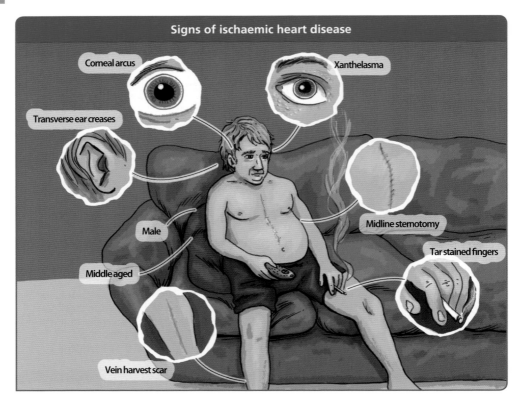

**Figure 3.7** Signs of ischaemic heart disease.

- glycosuria (diabetes)
- high blood pressure (hypertension)
- tar-stained fingers (smoking)
- xanthelasma (hypercholesterolaemia)

**Angina pain is similar in nature to that of an acute coronary syndrome.** However, stable angina results in stable symptoms. Pain precipitated by exertion or stress which quickly resolves (within 10 min) with either rest or use of a glyceryl trinitrate spray is more likely to be angina.

Worrying signs are:

- an increase in the severity or duration of symptoms, or in the patient's feeling of fear
- a reduction in the threshold for symptoms (a sudden change in classification)

These signs suggest that the patient's condition has become unstable and may have developed into an acute coronary syndrome.

## Diagnostic approach

Patients with suspected angina typically undergo electrocardiography at rest. If the clinical index of suspicion is significant, a functional test is done to identify inducible ischaemia. The test is often done in the emergency department or a chest pain clinic at the local cardiology department.

If the patient has inducible ischaemia, they may then undergo invasive coronary angiography to investigate the burden of disease. **Table 3.6** helps assess the pretest likelihood of ischaemic heart disease based on the patient's symptoms and risk factors.

## Investigations

### Electrocardiography

The ECG is typically normal in patients with ischaemic heart disease, unless they have had a prior myocardial infarction or there are signs of risk factors such as hypertension. Signs of current ischaemia include ST segment depression

| Pretest likelihood of ischaemic heart disease | | | | | | | | | | | |
|---|---|---|---|---|---|---|---|---|---|---|---|
| Type of chest pain | Non-anginal | | | | Atypical angina§ | | | | Typical angina | | | |
| Gender | Male | | Female | | Male‡ | | Female§ | | Male‡ | | Female§ | |
| Degree of risk*,† | Low | High | Low | High | Low | High | Low | High | Low | High | Low | High |
| Age (years) 35 | 3 | 35 | 1 | 19 | 8 | 59 | 2 | 39 | 30 | 88 | 10 | 78 |
| 45 | 9 | 47 | 2 | 22 | 21 | 70 | 5 | 43 | 51 | 92 | 20 | 79 |
| 55 | 23 | 59 | 4 | 25 | 45 | 79 | 10 | 47 | 80 | 95 | 38 | 82 |
| 65 | 49 | 69 | 9 | 29 | 71 | 86 | 20 | 51 | 93 | 97 | 56 | 84 |

*Low risk: no diabetes, smoking or hypercholesterolaemia.

†High risk: diabetes, smoking or hypercholesterolaemia.

‡ Men > 70 years with typical or atypical symptoms are assumed to have >90% likelihood of ischaemic heart disease.

§ Women > 70 years are assumed to have 61–90% likelihood of ischaemic heart disease (women at high risk with typical symptoms are assumed > 90% likelihood).

Presence of ischaemic ECG changes automatically increases risk above cited values.

Adapted from National Institute for Health and Care Excellence (NICE). Chest pain of recent onset: assessment and diagnosis of recent onset chest pain or discomfort of suspected cardiac origin. London: NICE; 2013.

**Table 3.6** Percentage pretest likelihood of ischaemic heart disease, based on symptoms and risk factors

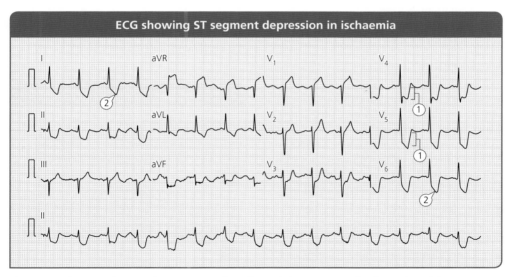

**Figure 3.8** Electrocardiogram showing signs of significant ischaemia. Note the depression of the ST segments in leads I, II, aVF and V3–V6 ① and the inverted T-waves also seen ②.

**(Figure 3.8)**, T-wave flattening or inversion, and sometimes left bundle branch block.

## Functional testing

Investigations done to look for evidence of ischaemia when the heart is stressed are known as functional tests. Stress, and subsequently ischaemia, may be induced by exercise or by the use of pharmacological agents. Functional tests include:

- exercise electrocardiography
- single-photon emission computed tomography scanning (also known as perfusion scanning)
- stress echocardiography
- perfusion magnetic resonance imaging

As well as provoking and detecting ischaemia, functional tests may also differentiate between scarred myocardium and ischaemic myocardium. They can also indicate the site of the ischaemia.

## Anatomical testing

Coronary anatomy is assessed using coronary computed tomographic angiography (CCTA) and invasive angiography (see page 137). CCTA is good at detecting atherosclerotic plaques and calcium in the coronary tree. However, invasive angiography is better for assessing the severity of disease and therefore guiding therapy because there is less distortion of the images and a more accurate assessment of the impingement on the lumen by the atherosclerotic plaque can be made.

# Management

## Medication

The management of ischaemic heart disease is divided into symptomatic therapies, which reduce symptoms, and prognostic therapies, which improve outcome.

Symptomatic therapies reduce cardiac preload and afterload, and encourage coronary dilation, by vasodilating systemic (and coronary) arteries and veins. These therapies include:

- nitrates such as glyceryl trinitrate (short acting) or isosorbide mononitrate (long acting)
- calcium channel antagonists such as amlodipine
- potassium channel blockers such as nicorandil

Prognostic therapies include:

- cardioselective beta-blockers (e.g. atenolol), which reduce sympathetic stimulation of the myocardium and reduce myocardial work
- aspirin, which reduces platelet function and the progression of atherosclerotic plaques

- statins (3-hydroxy-3-methylglutaryl coenzyme A reductase inhibitors; e.g. simvastatin), which stabilise existing plaques by reducing blood cholesterol

## Surgery

Patients with uncontrolled anginal pain despite medical therapy are considered for percutaneous coronary intervention (PCI). In this procedure, also called an angioplasty, a balloon is used to force the narrowed coronary lumen open and squeeze the fatty plaque to either side. A scaffold called a stent is then inserted in the arterial lumen to keep the plaque in position and the lumen open (**Figure 3.9**).

A coronary artery bypass graft (CABG) is considered for patients with:

- severe disease (e.g. affecting all three vessels or with very tight stenosis of the proximal left coronary artery)
- triple vessel or proximal main stem disease
- disease that is unsuitable for PCI

This procedure typically uses the long saphenous veins from the legs or the internal mammary arteries from the thorax to bridge the blocked vessel (see page 165).

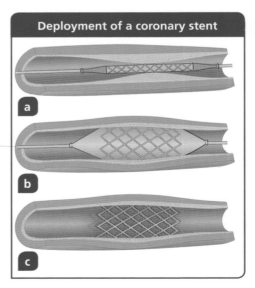

**Figure 3.9** Deployment of a coronary stent. (a) The stent crimped over the balloon and guide wire. (b) The balloon inflated, thus expanding the stent. (c) The stent in situ after removal of the deflated balloon and guide wire.

# Acute coronary syndromes

Like stable angina, acute coronary syndromes (ACS) are caused by ischaemic heart disease arising from atherosclerosis in the lumen of a coronary artery. However, acute coronary syndromes have a different underlying pathological process and are much more serious, acute and life-threatening than angina.

Acute coronary syndrome is an umbrella term for the following conditions.

■ Unstable angina: best thought of as a potentially 'pre–myocardial infarction' condition
■ Non–ST elevation myocardial infarction (NSTEMI): a type of myocardial infarction
■ ST elevation myocardial infarction (STEMI): a type of myocardial infarction caused by an acute and complete obstruction in one of the main coronary arteries

> Be careful when differentiating between stable and unstable angina. Stable angina is very different from unstable angina in terms of pathology, risk and treatment. Unstable angina can quickly progress to NSTEMI or STEMI.

## Epidemiology

Acute coronary syndromes are rare in people younger than 35 years. Their prevalence is estimated to be about 0.6% in people aged 35–74 years and about 2.3% in people aged ≥ 75 years. In England, about 233,600 new cases of acute coronary syndrome are diagnosed annually, an estimated three quarters of which are unstable angina or NSTEMI. STEMI affects 5 people in 1000 per year in the UK.

The prevalence of NSTEMI is rising year on year relative to the number of STEMIs.

## Prevention

The following interventions are used to prevent acute coronary syndrome. They focus on management of risk factors, with the aim of stabilising coronary plaques and reducing progression.

■ Smoking cessation
■ Cholesterol reduction through drug therapy as well as dietary improvement
■ Optimisation of hypertension and diabetes mellitus control
■ Reduction of the likelihood of platelet aggregation through antiplatelet therapies (e.g. aspirin or clopidogrel) or $P2Y_{12}$ inhibitors (e.g. prasugrel or ticagrelor)

## Pathogenesis

The pathological changes underlying stable angina and acute coronary syndromes are shown in **Figure 3.9**. Stable angina is caused by a stable atherosclerotic plaque inside the coronary artery. If the plaque becomes unstable, it may fissure and expose the underlying plaque to the flowing blood. This is a stimulus for platelet aggregation and the coagulation cascade. The resulting clot acutely obstructs the artery, causing a sudden reduction in blood flow to the myocardium. This is an acute coronary syndrome.

If the ischaemia is not reversed quickly (within about 10 min), it results in myocardial necrosis. This is known as myocardial infarction.

## Clinical features

The clinical features of unstable angina, NSTEMI and STEMI are similar. However, the pattern, nature and severity of the pain and other symptoms differentiates these syndromes from stable angina and provide clues as to which syndrome the patient has.

### Chest pain

Pain associated with acute coronary syndromes is typically central and retrosternal, and crushing or tight in character. The feeling is often described as 'like a band across the chest'. The pain sometimes radiates from the chest to the left arm, neck or jaw, or is sensed primarily in these areas rather than in the chest.

## Dyspnoea

The patient may feel breathless, particularly if ischaemia causes left ventricular systolic impairment.

## Signs

Patients often have no obvious signs on clinical examination. However, evidence of risk factors may be present, including complications of diabetes, increased blood pressure, tar staining on the fingers and xanthelasma. During severe cardiac ischaemia, the patient may look clammy and pale because of reduced cardiac output and subsequent sympathetic activation. If ischaemia has induced an arrhythmia or acute heart failure, signs of these conditions may be detected during the examination.

**Myocardial infarction leads to sympathetic activation.** The sympathetic nervous system is activated in response to the patient's pain, anxiety and reduced cardiac output. The resulting phenotype is similar to that seen in the fight-or-flight response.

**Table 3.1** outlines how unstable angina, NSTEMI and STEMI are differentiated clinically. However, acute coronary syndromes are a spectrum (**Figure 3.10**):

- the milder the symptoms and signs, the more likely the diagnosis is unstable angina
- the more severe and acute the symptoms and signs, the more likely the diagnosis is NSTEMI or STEMI

Unstable angina is not associated with infarction of the myocardium itself. However, it is considered a serious diagnosis, potentially 'pre-myocardial infarction', requiring admission to hospital for in-patient care.

## Diagnostic approach

The clinical history gives the diagnosis in most cases of acute coronary syndromes; it usually includes chest pain that seems to originate from the heart.

Diagnosis of an acute coronary syndrome also requires a finding of the ECG abnormalities with which these conditions are typically associated. Therefore patients who present with chest pain always require an ECG on arrival to hospital.

Myocardial infarction is detected biochemically as an increase in serum cardiac-specific biomarkers such as troponin I or T, which leak from dead myocytes. Evidence of cardiac myocyte death is required for a diagnosis of myocardial infarction.

# Investigations

## Chest X-ray

Patients require chest X-ray to exclude pulmonary oedema and aortic dissection (see pages 133 and 308).

## Electrocardiography

Electrical evidence of arrhythmia is sometimes present.

- Unstable angina or NSTEMI: the ECG usually shows signs of ischaemia (Figure 3.8) without ST segment elevation
- STEMI: by definition, this presents with ST segment elevation in a pattern that reflects the myocardial territory affected

Electrocardiographic changes associated with myocardial infarction of all subtypes are shown in **Figure 3.11**. Examples of inferior and anterior territory STEMIs are shown in **Figures 3.1** and **3.12**.

## Blood tests

A full blood count, urea and electrolytes test and lipid profile are needed. Cardiac markers (e.g. troponin I or T, and creatine kinase) are increased in cases of myocardial infarction but normal in unstable angina.

Cardiac markers are measured 12 h after the onset of pain, because results are not conclusive if done earlier; however, a 6 h result will give a good indication as to whether the troponin is increased or not. Increases in the concentration of cardiac biomarkers are the only essential criterion for a diagnosis of myocardial infarction.

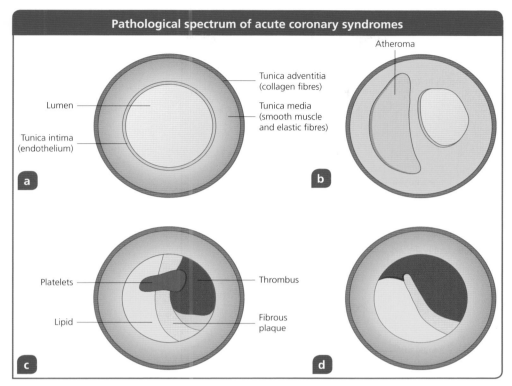

**Pathological spectrum of acute coronary syndromes**

**Figure 3.10** The pathological spectrum of acute coronary syndromes. (a) Normal artery. (b) Artery in a patient with stable angina. (c) Artery in a patient with unstable angina. (d) Artery in a patient with myocardial infarction.

## Coronary angiography

This procedure shows the nature and extent of the narrowing (or narrowings) within the coronary arteries. It also allows the anatomy of the coronary arteries and the nature and extent of the coronary disease to be understood, so that an appropriate revascularisation strategy can be planned.

## Management

A main aim of angina therapy and care for patients who have had a heart attack is to keep coronary plaques as stable as possible. Acute clot occlusion of a coronary artery is partial or full. Therefore the clinical sequelae vary from those of unstable angina to those of STEMI.

■ Unstable angina: a significant worsening of angina symptoms but no evidence of myocardial death (i.e. myocardial infarction)

■ STEMI: acute, complete obstruction of a main coronary artery, with myocardial death in the territory it supplies, severe pain and risk of sudden death

## Management of unstable angina

Unstable angina typically presents as sudden worsening of angina combined with normal cardiac biomarkers measured 12 h after onset of pain.

### Medication

Patients with unstable angina require the following medication.

■ Antiplatelet or antithrombotic therapy: dual antiplatelet therapy with aspirin and another agent (clopidogrel, ticagrelor or prasugrel) are given. Patients are started on an anticoagulant such as

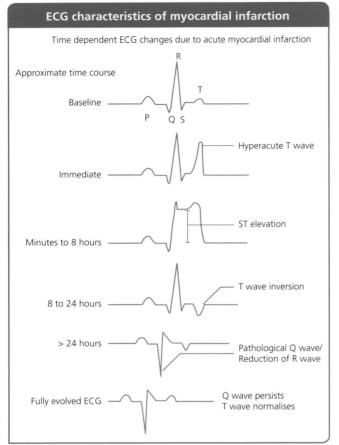

**Figure 3.11** Electrocardiographic characteristics of myocardial infarction.

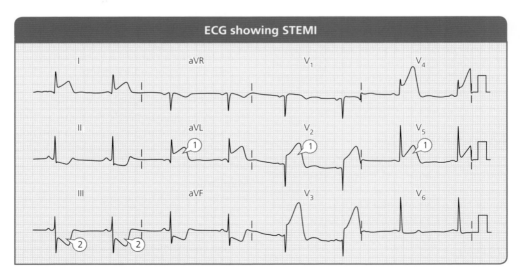

**Figure 3.12** Electrocardiogram showing an anterior ST elevation myocardial infarction: (1) ST elevation in V2–V5 and (2) reciprocal changes in leads II, III and aVF.

a low-molecular weight heparin or a factor Xa inhibitor (e.g. fondaparinux), unless cardiac catheterisation is planned for the same day. For patients with renal impairment, unfractionated heparin is used (with close monitoring) for anticoagulation.

■ Analgesics: intravenous nitrates are often required to control pain. Opiates are often also required (always give with an appropriate antiemetic).
■ Secondary prevention: this includes treatment with a statin, an angiotensin-converting enzyme (ACE) inhibitor and a beta-blocker.

### Percutaneous coronary intervention and surgery

Patients in whom unstable angina is confirmed usually undergo coronary angiography once their condition has been stabilised. At this point, significant coronary lesions are assessed and treated either medically, with stent insertion (PCI) or surgically (with CABG), depending on the severity and pattern of disease.

## Management of NSTEMI

Non–ST elevation myocardial infarction presents with persistent pain or discomfort combined with increased cardiac biomarkers. Its presentation is usually more severe than that of unstable angina but less severe than that of a STEMI.

### Medication

The following are given to patients with NSTEMI.

■ Antiplatelet and antithrombotic therapy: the same medications are prescribed as for unstable angina. Patients who have ongoing pain with dynamic ECG changes also have a glycoprotein IIb or IIIa inhibitor (e.g. tirofiban) started as a bridge to transfer to invasive assessment and management.
■ Analgesics: the same medications are prescribed as for unstable angina.

### Percutaneous coronary intervention and surgery

Patients with NSTEMI usually undergo coronary angiography within 72 h of admission. Significant coronary lesions are assessed.

Once the severity and pattern of disease have been determined, the decision is made to treat the lesions medically, with stent insertion (PCI) or with surgery (CABG).

## Management of STEMI

**ST elevation myocardial infarction** is the most severe and acute of the presentations of acute coronary syndromes.

If the ECG shows ST elevation, the patient is referred to the local heart attack centre for PPCI. It is crucial to transfer the patient to the nearest PPCI centre as soon as possible.

Because of the severity of a STEMI (a large proportion of the myocardium is affected), patients are more likely to present with acute complications such as arrhythmia or cardiogenic shock and acute heart failure.

> **Criteria for referral for PPCI vary by locality.** They usually include a combination of chest pain <12 h in duration (from the most severe pain) and ST segment elevation of ≥1 mm in the limb leads and ≥2 mm in the chest leads, in two contiguous leads.

### Medication

The following are used for patients with a STEMI.

■ Thrombolysis: this is now used much less frequently and is reserved for patients who cannot undergo PPCI in a timely fashion (door-to-balloon time > 120 min). Recombinant human tissue plasminogen activator is given intravenously as soon as possible (< 12 h from onset of pain). Patients need monitoring on a coronary care unit or equivalent ward. Contraindications to thrombolysis must be assessed before the drug is given.
■ Antiplatelet therapy: patients are given aspirin 300 mg and another antiplatelet agent (e.g. clopidogrel, ticagrelor or prasugrel according to local protocol) as soon as the diagnosis is made.

Following a STEMI, all patients, assuming no contraindications, receive the following medications.

- Aspirin 75 mg once a day: required lifelong
- An additional antiplatelet agent: usually a P2Y$_{12}$ inhibitor (e.g. clopidogrel, ticagrelor or prasugrel) for ≥ 1 year
- Statins: to achieve target cholesterol concentrations
- Angiotensin-converting enzyme inhibitors and beta-blockers: to aid myocardial recovery

### Percutaneous coronary intervention and surgery

Primary percutaneous coronary intervention (**Figure 3.2**) is the treatment of choice. A tiny wire is passed down the occluded artery and a balloon used to open the vessel and implant a stent (or stents). The stent acts as a scaffold and keeps the artery open.

Some patients undergo CABG instead of PPCI, although this is rare in the acute setting. Patients are typically considered suitable for CABG if their disease is not amenable to PCI or if they have myocardial infarction despite previous PCI therapy.

The 'hub and spoke' approach to the management of myocardial ischaemia is outlined in **Figure 3.13**.

> **Door-to-balloon time is crucial for treatment of STEMI.** PPCI should be done within 120 min of chest pain to achieve maximum benefit.

### Prognosis

The mortality of STEMI is 4.4% for patients who reach hospital. However, 30% of patients die before reaching hospital.

Patients occasionally need further coronary angiography to deal with any other significant coronary lesions after the PPCI procedure, because PPCI deals only with the 'acute' lesion.

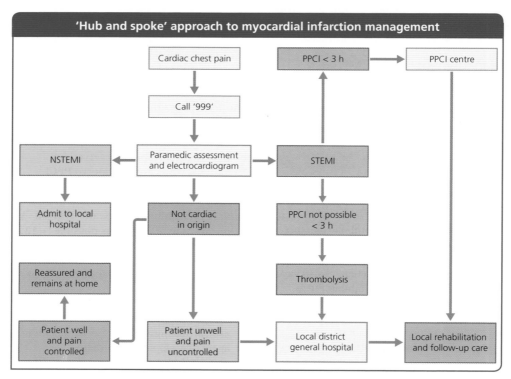

**Figure 3.13** The 'hub and spoke' approach to management of myocardial infarction. NSTEMI, non–ST elevation myocardial infarction; PPCI, primary percutaneous coronary intervention; STEMI, ST elevation myocardial infarction. Adapted from Boyle R. Mending hearts and brains – clinical case for change. London: Department of Health; 2006.

# Complications of myocardial infarction

Scarred myocardium does not contract, so heart failure (discussed in Chapter 6) remains the most prevalent complication after myocardial infarction. This section covers the other complications of myocardial infarction that need to be considered in the period after a myocardial infarction.

## Arrhythmia

Arrhythmias such as paroxysms of non-sustained ventricular tachycardia (<30 s), supraventricular tachycardia, accelerated idioventricular rhythm and ventricular ectopic beats are common after a myocardial infarction and usually resolve spontaneously. Cardiac arrest is also more common after a myocardial infarction.

Atrioventricular heart block is common in inferior territory infarcts, because the artery supplying the atriventricular node originates from the posterior descending artery. However, atrioventricular block in the context of an anterior infarct indicates extensive infarct territory and poor prognosis, and therefore requires early pacing.

### Clinical features

Patients are often asymptomatic or may experience syncope, palpitations or light-headedness. Signs include tachycardia, bradycardia and hypotension. Arrhythmia is diagnosed from a cardiac monitoring system or ECG.

### Management

To detect and diagnose arrhythmia promptly, patients are best treated in a coronary care unit. Such units provide continuous monitoring of cardiac rhythm.

Arrhythmias usually resolve spontaneously within 48 h. If they remain asymptomatic and the patient is not compromised, they are simply monitored.

Cardiac arrest requires cardiopulmonary resuscitation and defibrillation (discussed in Chapter 11). The frequency of ventricular fibrillation or ventricular tachycardia can be reduced by administration of beta-blockers. If either recurs after 48 h, or if the patient is considered at high risk of future cardiac arrest (left ventricular ejection fraction <40%), they are considered for an implantable defibrillator. Otherwise, arrhythmia is managed according to the same principles discussed in Chapter 5. Cardiac arrest is a very serious event, but long-term prognosis is unaffected if it is limited to the first 48 h.

In inferior infarcts, asymptomatic, uncompromised atrioventricular block is just monitored, because it usually resolves spontaneously within 10 days. Temporary and then permanent pacing are considered more urgently in the context of an anterior infarct, because of the poor prognosis.

## Rupture of myocardial structures

Myocardial necrosis rarely results in rupture of an individual cardiac structure. This is more common with extensive, 'full thickness' infarcts and is less common when patients receive prompt and successful revascularisation.

### Clinical features

Rupture of the left ventricular free wall causes collapse, shock and cardiac arrest (pulseless electrical activity). The condition is usually rapidly fatal. An echocardiogram sometimes shows a pericardial collection of blood. Immediate surgical referral is warranted, but few patients survive.

In rare cases, a ventricular septal defect develops post infarct as a result of a ruptured interventricular septum. Rupture of a sub-mitral valve papillary muscle can also occur causing mitral regurgitation. These complications present with symptoms and signs of acute heart failure and a new pansystolic murmur.

## Management

Suspicion of rupture requires immediate echocardiography and referral for urgent surgical repair.

> **Post–myocardial infarction mitral regurgitation** may also, and more commonly, occur secondary to papillary muscle dysfunction (without rupture). After a myocardial infarction, be alert for signs and symptoms of heart failure and for new murmurs.

## Ongoing ischaemia or recurrent myocardial infarction

Patients occasionally experience ongoing ischaemia (angina), a recurrent infarction in the same territory or in a new territory. Those who have received PPCI rarely suffer acute stent thrombosis if a clot forms inside the newly deployed stent.

> **There are two types of stent. These are used in different situations** depending upon the diameter of the vessel being treated and the length of the affected vessel to be stented.
>
> - Bare metal stents are made from a cobalt–chromium alloy without a coating
> - Drug-eluting stents are similar to bare metal stents but coated with chemotherapy agents, such as sirolimus or paclitaxcel, to inhibit cell proliferation and prevent restenosis

## Clinical features

Patients often complain of chest discomfort. Daily ECG recordings are taken until discharge and must also be performed when patients complain or chest pain or ischaemia is suspected. Acute stent thrombosis usually presents with severe pain and ST segment elevation on the ECG, in the same territory as the stented artery.

## Management

Urgent coronary angiography is warranted for patients with repeat infarction or with ongoing ischaemia. Antianginal therapy is discussed on pages 184 and 368. Definitive therapy is usually repeat PCI to remove the acute thrombus.

## Left ventricular thrombus

Clots sometimes form on the endocardial surface where blood flow is reduced over akinetic and scarred myocardium.

## Clinical features

Left ventricular thrombus is more common after an anterior territory myocardial infarction and is usually identified by echocardiography. Sadly, the first sign of thrombus formation is a stroke if the thrombus embolises.

## Management

Patients with post infarct left ventricular thrombus receive long-term anticoagulation to reduce the risk of stroke, because the precipitating cause (scarred myocardium) is permanent.

## Pericarditis

If the infarct related inflammation involves the pericardial membrane then pericarditis will occur. In this condition, patients complain of a chest pain that is different to the pain they experienced when they had a heart attack (see page 343 for more details).

## Clinical features

Chest discomfort is the main symptom. Pericarditic pain is pleuritic in nature, and a pericardial rub may be heard on cardiac auscultation.

> **The sound of a pericardial rub** is said to resemble the sound of snow crunching underfoot.

## Management

Patients with pericarditis are treated with anti-inflammatory medications such as high-dose aspirin or colchicine. Interval echocardiography is required (at diagnosis and at about 7 days) to identify and track any pericardial effusion that develops.

## Answers to starter questions

1. Patients experiencing a heart attack do not necessarily suffer from chest pain. They may describe their symptoms using other words, have predominantly arm or neck pain or experience a silent heart attack with no pain at all. This may be because they genuinely don't feel the pain due to neuropathy or transplant surgery, deny the feeling because they are afraid of what the pain signifies or mistake the pain for something else, e.g. indigestion.

2. Thrombolysis is no longer used as first line treatment for STEMI. Primary PCI (PPCI) is used instead because it is safer and provides the definitive investigation (allowing direct visualisation of the coronary disease and clot), diagnosis and treatment at the earliest possible opportunity. Patient outcomes are also improved. Thrombolysis is still used for heart attacks where PPCI would be delayed for >120 minutes, some cerebrovascular strokes and severe pulmonary emboli.

3. There are no direct causes of ischaemic heart disease but there are multiple risk factors. Common modifiable risk factors are smoking, diabetes, hypertension and hypercholesterolemia, therefore the risk of developing ischaemic heart disease can be reduced by treating high blood pressure, high cholesterol and stopping smoking, but it still cannot be prevented completely.

4. The incidence of stent thrombosis (clotting) is approximately 1%. Stents are made of metal (e.g. cobalt, chromium) and as foreign bodies can induce a response from the body in the form of thrombosis. However, over time the body of the stent is incorporated into the wall of the artery and the chance of stent thrombosis is reduced greatly.

5. There is no direct evidence that heart attacks are more common in the mornings. Stress is a recognised contributor to myocardial infarction, although the mechanism for this is unclear.

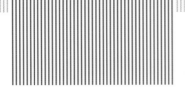

# Chapter 4
# Hypertension

## Starter questions

Answers to the following questions are on page 210.

1. Why do many hypertensive patients fail to take their prescribed medication?
2. Why are an estimated 500 million people worldwide unaware of their hypertension?
3. Why is reducing blood pressure alone not good enough when treating hypertension?
4. What key strategies are used to treat hypertension?
5. When is urgent secondary care required for hypertension?

## Introduction

Hypertension is a state of chronically and abnormally high arterial blood pressure. The condition is common, and one that physicians encounter daily. Globally, hypertension affects nearly 1 billion people, a figure that is likely to increase to more than 1.5 billion by 2025.

Hypertension is the major risk factor for cardiovascular disease, which is the commonest cause of death in the world. However, the condition is largely asymptomatic, so diagnosis depends on clinician awareness and the opportunistic measurement of blood pressure. It is vital for all clinicians, regardless of seniority, speciality or locality, to have a good understanding of how to diagnose, assess and manage hypertension.

This chapter focuses purely on systemic arterial hypertension, as opposed to pulmonary arterial hypertension, which is a quite distinct condition.

## Case 2 Opportunistic blood pressure measurement

### Presentation

Mrs Johnson, aged 57 years, visits her general practitioner (GP) for an annual review of her type 2 diabetes mellitus. Her GP measures her blood pressure as 167/98 mmHg. Measurement is repeated later in the consultation; the second reading is 170/95 mmHg.

### Initial interpretation

Two blood pressure readings > 140/90 mmHg indicate that Mrs Johnson may have hypertension, the pathological effects of which will be compounded by her diabetes. Both conditions are key risk factors for cardiovascular disease (ischaemic heart disease), peripheral vascular disease and stroke.

### Further history

Mrs Johnson is an office worker with a sedentary lifestyle. She eats processed foods but little fresh fruit and vegetables. She smokes 20 cigarettes daily and drinks about 35 units of alcohol most weekends.

She has a family history of heart disease. Her uncle and father both died from heart attacks in their late fifties.

### Examination

Her GP assesses her heart, eyes and kidneys because these are the main systems affected by hypertension. Cardiovascular examination is normal except for the high blood pressure and high body mass index (33 kg/m$^2$). Dipstick urinalysis shows glycosuria and proteinuria. Fundoscopic examination excludes optic disc oedema, retinal infarcts ('cotton-wool spots') and retinal haemorrhage **(Table 4.1 and Figure 4.1).**

| Grades of hypertensive retinopathy | | |
|---|---|---|
| Grade | Feature(s) | Description |
| 0 | Normal | |
| 1 | 'Silver wiring' and arterial attenuation | Increased arterial tortuosity and light reflex |
| | | Arteries attenuated and look shiny, like copper or silver wire |
| 2 | Grade 1 changes + | |
| | Arteriovenous nipping | Areas where the veins are constricted by crossing arteries |
| 3* | Grade 2 changes + | |
| | 'Cotton-wool spots' | Retinal infarcts visible as ill-defined pale yellow to white areas |
| | Flame haemorrhages | Retinal bleeds caused by high blood pressure |
| 4* | Grade 3 changes + | |
| | Hard exudates | Yellow, lipid-rich speckles from resolved retinal oedema |
| | Optic disc oedema | Swelling of the optic disc † |

*Consistent with accelerated hypertension. Vision is impaired when the macula is involved.

†Reserve the term papilloedema for when optic disc swelling is induced specifically by increased intracranial pressure.

**Table 4.1** Hypertensive retinopathy: grades and descriptions

### Interpretation of findings

At this stage, it is unclear whether or not Mrs Johnson has hypertension. However, she is at high risk of developing cardiovascular disease and complications.

**Case 2** *continued*

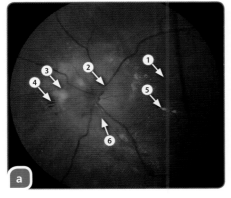
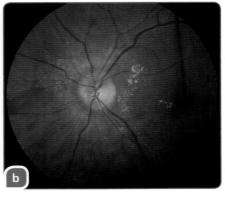

**Figure 4.1** (a) Features of all 4 grades of hypertensive retinopathy (see **Table 4.1**). Stage 1: ①, 'silver wiring' and arterial attenuation. Stage 2: ②, arteriovenous nipping. Stage 3: ③, 'cotton wool spots'; ④, flame haemorrhages. Stage 4: ⑤, hard exudate; ⑥, optic disc oedema. (b) After treatment with antihypertensive medication, the optic disc oedema and flame haemorrhages have resolved and the silver wiring appears to have improved, but the hard exudate persists. Courtesy of Mr Nachiketa Acharya.

## Hypertension management in diabetes

Mrs Johnson visits her GP for her annual diabetes review. Her blood pressure is 170/95 mmHg

Your blood pressure is high

I feel fine. Is it a problem?

Yes, especially with diabetes. It can cause serious problems like strokes. We need to see if this is a 'one off' or a real problem

I've got this gadget fitted for a whole day ... and blood tests and an ECG at the hospital tomorrow.

Her GP arranges for her BP to be assessed at home with an ambulatory monitor

The monitor confirms high blood pressure

The doctor explains the diagnosis

But I feel fine!

Most people do, but it's important to lower it to reduce risks of heart disease, stroke, or even eye or kidney problems

You look like a new woman

.... your risk of dying, heart attack or stroke is over 43% in the next 10 years

If we can improve your BP and cholesterol, and you stop smoking, we can more than halve that

It's time I started taking my health more seriously

Oh.

Since I quit the fags and started losing weight, I feel like one! My blood pressure is improving already...

The doctor explains the risks of hypertension, and the benefits of drug treatment and lifestyle changes

Mrs Johnson starts aquarobics three times a week to help lose weight

**Case 2** *continued*

# Investigations

## Blood pressure monitoring

Further blood pressure measurements are necessary to diagnose hypertension. Ideally, these are done using an ambulatory blood pressure monitoring (ABPM) device for 24 h. The results will determine if the clinic blood pressure measurements represent true hypertension, white coat hypertension or spurious anomalous recordings.

## Cardiovascular risk

It is already clear from Mrs Johnson's family history, diabetes, smoking, poor diet, lack of exercise and age that her risk of cardiovascular disease is high. However, formal estimation of risk requires measurement of lipid concentrations.

## Assessment of target organ damage

Proteinuria is evidence of renal damage from diabetes, hypertension-induced damage to glomerular blood vessels, or both; it requires further investigation. Creatinine clearance or estimated glomerular filtration rate need to be tested, and formal measurement of proteinuria is necessary. A 12-lead electrocardiogram is done to look for evidence of left ventricular hypertrophy and signs of ischaemic heart disease. Fundoscopy has already been done.

## Investigation results and re-review

Mrs Johnson returns a week later with her results (**Table 4.2**). These are used to estimate her risk for cardiovascular disease by using an online risk calculator. Her age, gender, lipid concentrations (total cholesterol and high-density lipoprotein cholesterol), blood pressure, diabetic status, smoking status and activity level are entered.

| Investigation results | |
| --- | --- |
| Test | Result |
| Ambulatory blood pressure monitoring | 152/93 mmHg (daytime average) |
| Electrocardiography | Normal sinus rhythm |
| Urea and electrolytes | Sodium = 138 mmol/L (133–146 mmol/L); potassium = 4.6 mmol/L (3.5-5.3 mmol/L); urea = 5.9 mmol/L (2.5–7.8 mmol/L); creatinine 80 µmol/L (49–90 µmol/L) |
| Estimated glomerular filtration rate | 82 ml/min/1.73m² (60–89 consistent with chronic kidney disease stage 2; mildly impaired renal function) |
| Total cholesterol | 5.8 mmol/L (≤5 mmol/L) |
| High-density lipoprotein cholesterol | 1.16 mmol/L (≥1 mmol/L) |

**Table 4.2** Mrs Johnson's investigation results.

**Online cardiovascular risk calculators use data from a large number of people to estimate cardiovascular risk in a single person.** These tools are not perfect. However, they can be powerful because they show the risk patients face with and without intervention, in easily understood terms.

Physicians and patients can calculate risks and benefits together in clinic. This helps to motivate patients to positively change their lifestyle and to regard the diagnosis seriously.

Mrs Johnson's 10-year risk of death, stroke or heart attack is 43%. However, the risk calculator shows that if her systolic blood pressure is normalised to 120 mmHg, this figure decreases to 32%. If she also stops smoking, becomes more active and reduces her total cholesterol to <5.2 mmol/L, this reduces even further to 17%.

**Case 2** *continued*

## Diagnosis

The diagnosis is essential hypertension. Although Mrs Johnson's average waking blood pressure is not quite as high as her office blood pressure, it still indicates hypertension. In view of her age and the lack of suspicious symptoms or signs, there is no need to investigate further for secondary causes. A combination of drug therapy and lifestyle changes is required to reduce her blood pressure and the risk of cardiovascular disease, target organ damage and premature death.

# Essential hypertension

Essential hypertension, also known as primary or idiopathic hypertension, is increased systemic blood pressure in the absence of any identifiable pathological cause. It is the commonest type of hypertension, accounting for about 95% of all cases.

Descriptions of multiple ways of defining, diagnosing, categorising and managing hypertension have been published. There is broad overlap in the literature, but it is important to be aware of local policies and procedures when assessing and managing patients with hypertension.

## Definition

Hypertension is widely defined as persistent systolic blood pressure > 140 mmHg, diastolic blood pressure > 90 mmHg, or both. Ideal blood pressure is < 120/80 mmHg. The ranges 120–140 mmHg for systolic and 80–90 mmHg for diastolic are considered high normal. However, it is important not to be too dogmatic about these boundaries, because an individual patient's overall risk is determined by additional features, such as other cardiac risk factors and evidence of renal disease.

It is useful to grade hypertension severity **(Table 4.3)**, because this helps to guide the most appropriate treatment.

Most patients are assumed to have essential hypertension, because true secondary hypertension is rare (about 5% of cases).

| Stages of hypertension | | |
| --- | --- | --- |
| Condition | Systolic blood pressure (mmHg)* | Diastolic blood pressure (mmHg)* |
| Ideal | < 120 | < 80 |
| High normal blood pressure (pre-hypertension) | 120–139 | 80–89 |
| Stage 1 hypertension | 140–159 | 90–99 |
| Stage 2 hypertension | 160–179 | 100–109 |
| Stage 3 hypertension | ≥ 180 | ≥ 110 |
| Accelerated hypertension | Same as stage 3 hypertension but with signs of grade 3 or 4 retinopathy (Table 4.1 and Figure 4.1) | |

*Precise boundaries differ depending on the methods and guideline used.

**Table 4.3** Stages of hypertension

Hypertension with an underlying secondary cause (see page 206) is less common than essential hypertension. Secondary hypertension is suspected when hypertension:

- is resistant to therapy
- occurs at a young age
- is accompanied by features suggesting a secondary cause (see page 207)

**Treat patients not millimetres of mercury!**
An obese, diabetic patient who smokes and has blood pressure 139/98 mmHg is at higher risk than a healthy person with blood pressure 141/91 mmHg. The aim of treatment is to reduce blood pressure, but not in isolation: the ultimate goal is reduction of morbidity and mortality.

## Epidemiology

Cardiovascular disease causes a third of deaths worldwide, and hypertension is thought to account for at least half of them. Risk factors for hypertension are typically associated with a western lifestyle, but hypertension is a major problem in low- and middle-income countries **(Figure 4.2)**. Some of the highest rates of hypertension are in Africa, South America, Eastern Europe and South East Asia, with > 45% of adults affected. In contrast, the prevalence of hypertension in the USA, Western Europe and Australia is < 40%.

African–Caribbean populations have a higher prevalence of hypertension than white and Asian populations, in a ratio of about 3:2. In North America, the prevalence among African Americans is > 10% more than that in white people. Furthermore, among patients with hypertension, black people have a greater tendency to develop cardiovascular disease, especially stroke.

Under the age of 50 years, more men than women have hypertension. However, this distribution becomes roughly equal beyond the menopause.

## Aetiology

The pathogenesis of hypertension is multifactorial. Numerous genetic and environmental factors have been implicated. By definition, essential hypertension has no identifiable direct secondary cause. However, multiple personal and lifestyle factors are associated with hypertension, and some of these risk factors are modifiable **(Table 4.4)**.

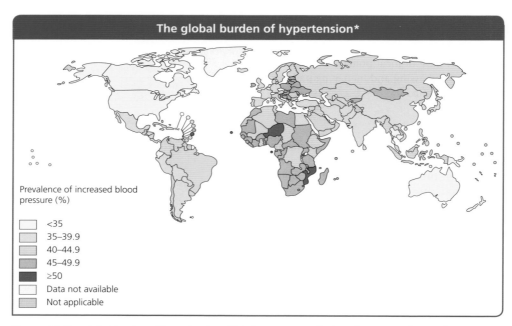

**The global burden of hypertension***

Prevalence of increased blood pressure (%)

- <35
- 35–39.9
- 40–44.9
- 45–49.9
- ≥50
- Data not available
- Not applicable

**Figure 4.2** The global burden of hypertension. High-income countries have lower prevalence of hypertension, and low- and middle-income countries have high prevalence. *Systolic blood pressure ≥140 mmHg and diastolic blood pressure ≥90 mmHg or using medication to lower blood pressure. Redrawn with permission from World Health Organisation (WHO). Raised blood pressure, 2008. Geneva: WHO, 2008. http://gamapserver.who.int/gho/interactive_charts/ncd/risk_factors/blood_pressure_prevalence/atlas.html. (Last accessed June 2014.)

## Risk factors for essential hypertension

| Modifiable | Non-modifiable |
|---|---|
| Obesity | Family history of hypertension |
| Increased salt intake | Advanced age |
| Excessive alcohol intake | African–Caribbean heritage |
| Sedentary lifestyle | Male gender (< 50 years) |
| Nicotine (smoking) | |

**Table 4.4** Modifiable and non-modifiable risk factors for essential hypertension

## Clinical features

Hypertension is asymptomatic in all but the most severe cases. Therefore diagnosis depends on clinical vigilance, ensuring that all adults have their blood pressure measured opportunistically.

Clinical history ascertains the duration and severity of hypertension. Modifiable and non-modifiable risk factors are identified, and responses to previous therapies (including any adverse reactions) are assessed. A family history is taken.

A full cardiovascular examination is done. It includes peripheral pulses, auscultation for carotid bruits, fundoscopy, calculation of body mass index and dipstick urinalysis.

Tailor history taking and examination to the individual patient. For example, signs of aortic coarctation should be sought in a young patient with severe upper body hypertension (see page 297). However, this would rarely be appropriate in an octogenarian with multiple risk factors for essential hypertension.

## Diagnostic approach

Each new diagnosis of hypertension requires significant, often lifelong, pharmacological treatment and lifestyle modification. Therefore hypertension should be diagnosed carefully and appropriately; the condition cannot be diagnosed from a single blood pressure reading.

If a reading of > 140/90 mmHg is obtained, measurement is repeated during the same consultation. If the second reading differs significantly from the first, measurement is repeated again. The lower of the latter two readings is documented as the blood pressure.

To establish the diagnosis of hypertension, it is important to use an ABPM device or home blood pressure recordings, if possible. ABPM recordings correlate more closely with the risk of target organ damage and the overall risk of cardiovascular disease. When ABPM or home monitoring is used, an average waking blood pressure > 130/85 is considered diagnostic of hypertension.

Ambulatory blood pressure monitoring provides more information about blood pressure than one-off or office measurements. Devices typically record blood pressure every 2 h over 24 h while the patient engages in their normal daily activities. Measurements of the average waking blood pressure are used to make decisions about treatment.

In home blood pressure monitoring, blood pressure recordings are taken by either the patient (using a semiautomated device) or another person. Blood pressure is measured with the patient at rest, in a seated position, several times daily over 5–7 days. Measurements are recorded in a blood pressure diary.

In normotensive patients, blood pressure is measured at least every 5 years. Patients with high normal blood pressure are monitored more closely, and their cardiovascular risk is calculated. A simple approach to diagnosis is shown in **Figure 4.3**.

## Investigations

Laboratory investigations are used to:

- help evaluate an individual patient's risk of developing cardiovascular disease
- look for evidence of target organ damage
- identify secondary causes

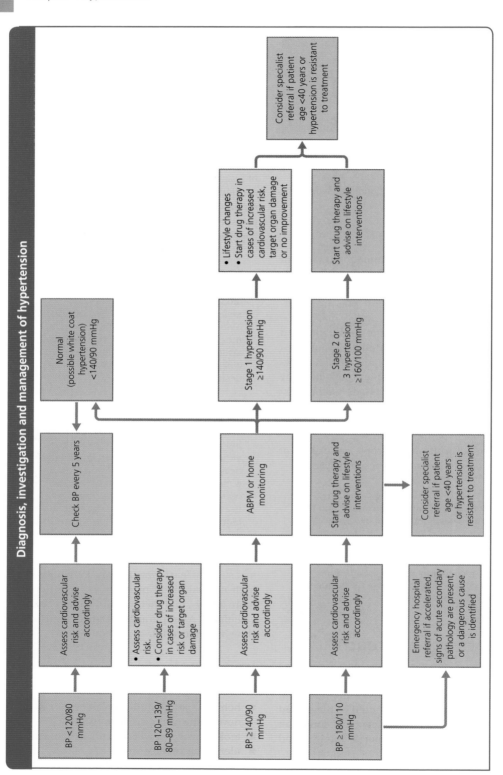

**Figure 4.3** An approach to the diagnosis, investigation and management of hypertension. Green, low concern; amber, moderate concern; red, high concern. ABPM, ambulatory blood pressure monitoring; BP, blood pressure.

## Investigations to help evaluate cardiovascular risk

The results of a fasting blood glucose test and a lipid profile help estimate cardiovascular risk. A high concentration of fasting blood glucose increases the risk, whereas normal results exclude diabetes. A lipid profile measures the concentration of total cholesterol, high-density lipoprotein cholesterol, low-density lipoprotein cholesterol and triglycerides.

## Investigations to find evidence of target organ damage

Target organ damage can be directly related to abnormally high blood pressure. The heart, eyes and kidneys are assessed, as summarised in **Table 4.5.** Target organ damage confers a greater risk of cardiovascular events and death, so patients with evidence of such damage require more aggressive blood pressure control and monitoring.

Cerebrovascular is commoner in older patients with hypertension. A cerebral computerised tomography or magnetic resonance imaging scan should be considered in those with memory problems.

## Investigations to identify secondary causes of hypertension

Secondary hypertension is less common than essential hypertension. However, investigations to identify a secondary cause are appropriate in selected cases, for example when the patient is young, has particularly high blood pressure or has hypertension that is resistant to treatment.

# Management

Hypertension is the most important risk factor for cardiovascular disease. All patients with hypertension require a formal estimation of their cardiovascular risk. The result influences choices regarding management of the condition. Informing patients of their individual cardiovascular risk also reinforces advice regarding lifestyle changes and sometimes improves adherence to drug therapy.

Patients with established cardiovascular disease, such as coronary artery disease, stroke and peripheral vascular disease, are automatically considered as high risk. For other patients, a 10-year cardiovascular risk > 20% is considered significant.

The ultimate goal of treatment is to reduce the risk of cardiovascular disease, death and target organ damage. To achieve this, both risk factor modification and blood pressure reduction are needed.

## Individualised treatment

Treatment decisions are guided by the patient's blood pressure and cardiovascular risk, and by any evidence of target organ damage. Consult local guidelines and protocols, but the general principles are as follows.

- Encourage all patients (those with normal, high normal and hypertension) to make positive modifications to their lifestyle to reduce their cardiovascular risk
- Patients with high normal blood pressure who are considered at high risk of cardiovascular disease or who have

| Investigations for target organ damage | | |
|---|---|---|
| Organ | Investigation(s) | Looking for |
| Heart | 12-lead electrocardiogram | Left ventricular hypertrophy and signs of coronary heart disease |
| Kidneys | Laboratory tests<br>urea and electrolytes<br>creatinine clearance<br>estimated glomerular filtration rate | Impaired renal function |
| | Dipstick urinalysis | Proteinuria (including microalbuminuria) and haematuria (signs of glomerular damage) |
| Eyes | Fundoscopy | Hypertensive retinopathy (**Table 4.1** and **Figure 4.1**) |

**Table 4.5** Investigations for target organ damage in hypertension

evidence of target organ damage are sometimes offered drug therapy

- Patients with isolated stage 1 hypertension (i.e. low cardiovascular risk and no target organ damage) are first advised to make lifestyle modifications; drug therapy is usually indicated if the response to these changes is suboptimal
- For all other hypertensive patients (i.e. those with stage 1 hypertension with increased cardiovascular risk or with target organ damage, as well as those with stage 2 or 3 hypertension), drug therapy and lifestyle modifications are required
- In patients with stage 3 hypertension, drug therapy is started immediately, without further blood pressure monitoring (ABPM or home monitoring) and regardless of cardiovascular risk or evidence of target organ damage

## Lifestyle changes

All patients with hypertension require counselling about how and why to modify their cardiovascular risk. The following lifestyle changes help decrease blood pressure.

- Reducing salt intake to < 6 g/day: excessive consumption of salt increases blood pressure, so patients should stop adding salt to their food and avoid eating processed foods, which contain added salt.
- Losing weight and exercising: obesity and a sedentary lifestyle predispose people to hypertension, but blood pressure is reduced in those who do 30 min or more of aerobic exercise on most days of the week
- Reducing alcohol intake: the amount of alcohol consumed correlates with blood pressure, and excessive alcohol consumption may antagonise pharmacological treatment, therefore men should aim to drink no more than 3 or 4 units (24–32 g) and women no more than 2 or 3 units (16–24 g) of alcohol per day
- Stopping smoking: advise all patients to stop smoking; nicotine replacement therapy helps some patients to do this

Referral for dietary advice, physical training or specialist smoking cessation services should also be considered.

The effects of these lifestyle changes extend beyond blood pressure control: successful weight loss and smoking cessation improve patient well-being and reduces the risk of many other diseases including respiratory disease and cancer.

## Medication

The following drugs are used to treat hypertension:

- angiotensin-converting enzyme (ACE) inhibitors (see page 158) and angiotensin II receptor blockers (see page 159)
- beta-blockers (see page 152)
- calcium channel blockers (see page 157)
- diuretics, chiefly thiazide and thiazide-like diuretics (see page 154)
- alpha-blockers (see page 156)

Patients should first be started on a single drug (step 1 therapy). If the response is suboptimal, the addition of a second (step 2) then a third (step 3) may be necessary.

Patients with hypertension that persists beyond step 3 (i.e. resistant hypertension) are referred to a hypertension specialist. Poor adherence is a common cause of apparently resistant hypertension. This problem is addressed by good patient education and ensuring that the prescription is a simple as possible.

Choice of drug is determined by:

- effects on blood pressure
- the patient's ethnicity
- patient age
- coexisting diseases
- previous adverse effects
- cost-effectiveness

The ability to appropriately balance these factors comes with experience. Follow local guidelines and protocols, but a useful strategy for the pharmacological treatment of hypertension is outlined in **Figure 4.4.**

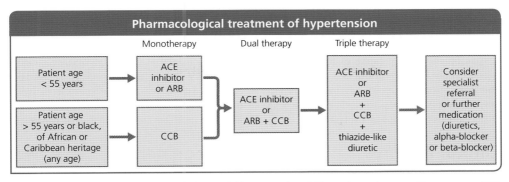

**Figure 4.4** Pharmacological treatment of essential hypertension. ACE, angiotensin-converting enzyme; ARB, angiotensin II receptor blocker; CCB, calcium channel blocker.

**Hypertension is more common in people of African or Caribbean ethnic origin.** Patients in this population also tend to have low-renin, salt-sensitive hypertension, which is less responsive to ACE inhibitor (or angiotensin II receptor blocker) or beta-blocker monotherapy. Therefore for these patients a calcium channel blocker or diuretic is usually a more suitable first-line agent. A renin–angiotensin system antagonist is usually reserved for second-line therapy.

**Vagal nerve stimulation and renal denervation are emerging as promising novel therapies for resistant hypertension.** Both work by influencing the balance between sympathetic and parasympathetic nervous activity. The vagal nerve is stimulated through a subcutaneous tunnelled wire connecting the carotid sinuses to a device delivering electrical impulses. In renal denervation, a catheter is used to ablate the renal sympathetic nerves in the renal arteries.

## Monitoring blood pressure targets

It is essential to monitor the patient's response to treatment. The clinic blood pressure can be used for this in most patients.

The aim of treatment is to normalise blood pressure (< 140/90 mmHg). However, blood pressure increases naturally with age, so the target for patients older than 80 years is < 150/85 mmHg. Tighter control (< 130/80 mmHg) benefits patients with diabetes, high cardiovascular risk or

renal dysfunction. However, this target can be difficult to attain and treatment is often limited by adverse effects, especially in the elderly.

## Complications

Hypertension manifests through its complications, which are usually caused by atherosclerotic damage to an organ system **(Table 4.6)**.

## Prognosis

In essential hypertension, prognosis is determined by the degree of target-organ damage and the level of cardiovascular risk. Every 20/10-mmHg increase in blood pressure is associated with a doubling of cardiovascular mortality.

| Complications of hypertension | |
|---|---|
| **Organ system** | **Complication(s)** |
| Cardiac | Left ventricular hypertrophy |
| | Diastolic heart failure |
| | Arrhythmia (especially atrial fibrillation) |
| | Coronary artery disease (myocardial infarction and angina) |
| Renal | Hypertensive nephropathy |
| | Renal insufficiency |
| | End-stage renal disease |
| Cerebral | Stroke |
| | White matter ischaemia with impaired cognition or dementia |
| | Hypertensive encephalopathy (at very high blood pressure) |
| Ophthalmic | Hypertensive retinopathy |
| | Reduced vision |

**Table 4.6** Complications of hypertension

# Secondary hypertension

A specific secondary cause of hypertension is identified in only about 5% of patients. The commonest cause of secondary hypertension is renal artery stenosis **(Figure 4.5)**. Other causes are listed in **Table 4.7.**

case-by-case basis. There are many causes of secondary hypertension. If a secondary cause is suspected but the specific cause is not obvious, a good general investigative work-up includes the tests listed in **Table 4.8.**

## Clinical features

The clinical features of the underlying cause help differentiate secondary hypertension from essential hypertension. Some of these features are listed in **Table 4.7.**

The clinical features arising directly from hypertension are similar to those of essential hypertension. However, secondary hypertension is more likely in cases of:

■ early-onset hypertension (<40 years)
■ unexpectedly severe hypertension
■ resistant hypertension

## Investigations

The choice of investigations should be tailored to clinical suspicion, on an individual

## Management

The aim of management of secondary hypertension is correction of the underlying cause. Therefore the treatments are as varied as the causes. Drug therapy, surgery or even renal dialysis may be used, depending on the cause. Antihypertensive medication is also required while the cause is being corrected; this therapy should continue if blood pressure does not normalise.

## Prognosis

In secondary hypertension, the prognosis is determined by that of the underlying cause. If the condition is promptly diagnosed and treated, and blood pressure decreases, the prognosis is usually good.

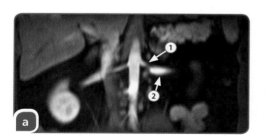 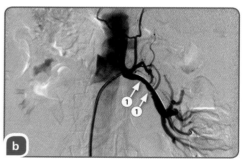

**Figure 4.5** Renal artery stenosis. (a) Magnetic resonance angiogram showing left renal artery stenosis ① and post-stenosis dilatation ②. (b) Invasive angiogram showing multiple stenoses in the left renal artery ①. The dark tube in the descending aorta is the catheter, which is injecting contrast dye (black) into the artery.

| Secondary causes of hypertension | | | |
|---|---|---|---|
| Category | Example(s) | Further information | Diagnostic test(s) |
| Renal | Chronic kidney disease | Chronic kidney disease of any cause (including hypertension itself) is the commonest secondary cause of hypertension. | Creatinine clearance or estimated glomerular filtration rate |
| | Polycystic kidney disease | Causes severe resistant hypertension. Most cases have autosomal dominant hereditability. Polycystic kidneys may be bilaterally palpable. | Renal ultrasound |
| Renovascular | Renal artery stenosis (atherosclerotic or rarely fibromuscular dysplasia) | Causes resistant hypertension occasionally associated with audible abdominal bruit. | Renal Doppler ultrasound, or CT or MRI angiography |
| Endocrine | Phaeochromocytoma | A catecholamine-secreting tumour associated with paroxysms of hypertension, flushing, tachycardia, anxiety and headaches. Rare but causes severe hypertension. | 24-h urinary collection for catecholamines or their metabolites* |
| | Primary hyperaldosteronism | Causes hypertension associated with hypokalaemia. The commonest cause is Conn's syndrome (aldosterone-secreting adenoma). | Serum potassium (to assess hypokalaemia) and aldosterone–renin ratio (which is increased)* |
| | Cushing's syndrome | Results from excessive exposure to corticosteroids. When caused by an ACTH-secreting pituitary tumour, it is known as Cushing's disease. Look for cushingoid appearance †. | 24-h collection of urine for measurement of cortisol, and dexamethasone suppression test* |
| Cardiovascular | Aortic coarctation | Congenital narrowing of the aorta, usually close to the arch. Causes upper body hypertension (sparing the lower body) and radiofemoral delay. | Echocardiogram or CT scan |
| Medications | Hormone replacement therapy, oral contraceptive pill, corticosteroids, mineralocorticoids and NSAIDs | Take a thorough drug history in all hypertensive patients to ensure all possible drug causes are identified | |
| Other substances | Alcohol, nicotine, liquorice and misused drugs | Excessive use is associated with hypertension. | |
| Other | Obstructive sleep apnoea | An increasingly common cause of hypertension associated with obesity. Morning headaches are common. A collateral history from a partner is useful. | Overnight sleep studies (oximetry and polysomnography) |
| | Pregnancy | Hypertension affects about 10% of pregnancies. | |

ACTH, adrenocorticotropic hormone; CT, computerised tomography; MRI, magnetic resonance imaging; NSAID, non-steroidal anti-inflammatory drug.

*CT or MRI are also used to identify tumours, when appropriate. † Features include facial puffiness (moon facies), central obesity (sparing the limbs), abdominal striae, atrophied skin and a buffalo hump (excess fat across the back of the neck).

**Table 4.7** Secondary causes of hypertension

| Investigating for secondary hypertension | |
|---|---|
| Type | Tests |
| Clinical examination | Body mass index |
| | Radiofemoral delay |
| | Abdominal bruit |
| Blood tests | Estimated glomerular filtration rate |
| | Parathyroid hormone |
| | Thyroid-stimulating hormone |
| | Calcium |
| | Potassium |
| | Aldosterone–renin ratio |
| 24-h urine collection | Cortisol |
| | Catecholamines |
| | Metanephrines |
| Imaging | Renal ultrasound (including Doppler) |
| Others | Sleep studies (if obese or history suggests obstructive sleep apnoea) |

**Table 4.8** Investigating for secondary hypertension

# Hypertension in other groups

The general principles of hypertension management are applicable to a wide variety of patient groups. However, certain features, in some groups, warrant specific discussion.

## Patients with white coat hypertension

In white coat hypertension, a patient's blood pressure is increased in the clinic but normal elsewhere. Because patients with this condition are hypertensive during visits to a physician, they are often diagnosed with hypertension and treated accordingly. However, white coat hypertension does not warrant drug therapy alone.

This highlights the importance of ABPM or home monitoring to confirm the diagnosis in apparent cases of stage 1 and 2 hypertension. Cardiovascular risk, patient education and lifestyle modification may still benefit patients, even in the absence of true hypertension.

## Elderly patients

Arteries become naturally less compliant (stiffer) with age, which increases systolic blood pressure (see page 75). However, age should not be a barrier to treatment, because it has been shown to benefit patients over 80 years of age.

Adverse drug effects, contraindications and polypharmacy-related interactions become more prevalent and problematic in older patients. Postural hypotension secondary to the use of antihypertensive medication is common. This adverse effect causes falls and reduced mobility or function, which are particularly troublesome and potentially dangerous for elderly patients.

## Patients with diabetes mellitus

Hypertensive patients with diabetes mellitus are at additional risk of cardiovascular disease, retinopathy, renal damage and peripheral neuropathy. The benefits of effective blood pressure control are greater in this group than in the general hypertensive population. Therefore more stringent blood pressure control is recommended for these patients, particularly those with evidence of target organ damage or increased cardiovascular risk. The blood pressure target for patients with diabetes is < 130/80 mmHg,40 but this is often difficult to achieve.

> **Renin–angiotensin system antagonists are good first–line therapeutic agents for patients with hypertension and diabetes, including the elderly and those with African-Caribbean heritage.** This is because both these disorders are associated with nephropathy, and these drugs are renoprotective.
>
> Elderly and African–Caribbean patients would not normally receive a renin–angiotensin system antagonist as first-line treatment for hypertension. In African-Caribbean patients, these drugs are used in combination with a diuretic or a calcium channel blocker to ensure renoprotection and effective blood pressure control (see page 205).

## Patients with coexisting diseases

As the population ages, the number of people with multiple coexisting diseases is increasing. The presence of a coexisting condition may affect the choice of antihypertensive drug. Certain classes of drugs provide combined benefit.

- Patients with hypertension and ischaemic heart disease: both conditions benefit from beta-blockers, ACE inhibitors and angiotensin II receptor blockers (see page 184).
- Patients with hypertension and heart failure: both conditions benefit from beta-blockers, ACE inhibitors, angiotensin II receptor blockers and potassium-sparing diuretics such as spironolactone and eplerenone (see page 247).

- Patients with hypertension and renal impairment: both conditions benefit from antagonists of the renin aldosterone system (ACE inhibitors, angiotensin II receptor blockers) which reduce blood pressure and proteinurea.

> **Metabolic syndrome is the association of central obesity, insulin resistance (and type 2 diabetes mellitus), hypertension and dyslipidaemia.** Diagnosis requires three of these conditions to be present.
>
> This increasingly prevalent syndrome is a powerful risk factor for cardiovascular disease and death. Between a quarter and a third of American and Western European adults are thought to be affected. The driving force behind this phenomenon appears to be increasing levels of obesity.

## Pregnant patients

More than 10% of pregnant women experience hypertension. This type of hypertension is a separate disease entity with unique pathophysiology.

Hypertension in pregnancy requires management by a specialist. It is diagnosed, investigated and treated differently from essential hypertension.

The condition is usually benign, but it increases the risk to mother and baby. Hypertension is the presenting feature of dangerous obstetric conditions such as pre-eclampsia and eclampsia. Drug therapy is limited by fetal risk, but options include beta-blockers (labetolol), methyldopa and hydralazine.

## Patients with hypertensive emergencies

Hypertensive emergencies include accelerated hypertension and hypertension associated with the following conditions:

- encephalopathy (usually > 200/110 mmHg)
- left ventricular failure

- myocardial ischaemia or infarction
- aortic dissection
- cerebral haemorrhage

Phaemochromocytoma hypertensive crisis is also an emergency.

Hypertensive emergencies require urgent and closely controlled blood pressure reduction in a secondary care setting. When blood pressure is very high (> 220/120 mmHg) or associated with dangerous secondary pathology, intravenous glyceryl trinitrate or labetolol are used to reduce blood pressure.

The aim is to bring systolic blood pressure below 220 mmHg or diastolic blood pressure below 120 mmHg (or both) over 1–2 h, and then < 160/100 mmHg over the next 12–24 h.

## Answers to starter questions

1.  Some studies have found that up to 50% of patients with hypertension do not take their medication properly. A combination of factors are likely to be responsible. Hypertension is usually asymptomatic; patients feel well and therefore may not understand why they need to take medication. Hypertensive medications can cause side effects and treatment can make patients feel worse, rather than better. Many patients do not understand the seriousness of their condition and are therefore not motivated to take medications. Medication adherence is improved with better patient education and counselling.

2.  Hypertension is usually an asymptomatic condition so patients are unaware of their raised blood pressure. Diagnosis relies upon clinicians being alert and remembering to check blood pressure opportunistically.

3.  Patients do not usually die directly from hypertension but of its complications and clinical sequelae. Reducing blood pressure does help to reduce risk but it is more effective to consider the patient as a whole and aim to reduce their risk of developing cardiovascular disease. This requires attention to other risk factors such as smoking and control of diabetes and hyperlipidaemia.

4.  The three key strategies are to: lower blood pressure with lifestyle changes and medication; reduce the risk of cardiovascular disease by risk factor modification and limit target organ damage.

5.  Urgent secondary care treatment is required for accelerated hypertension, very high blood pressure resulting in acute secondary pathology (e.g. optic disc swelling or encephalopathy) and when a dangerous cause, such as phaeochromocytoma, is suspected.

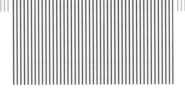

# Chapter 5
# Arrhythmias

## Starter questions

Answers to the following questions are on page 233.

1. Why does high blood pressure often accompany a low heart rate?
2. Why might a pacemaker and heart rate-limiting drugs be considered in the same patient?
3. In certain arrhythmias, such as atrial fibrillation, restoring normal sinus rhythm may not be the primary goal. Why is this?
4. Is installing automatic external defibrillators in public places effective?

## Introduction

Arrhythmia is an abnormality of heart rate or rhythm. In the healthy heart, the generation, conduction and propagation of electrical activity occurs in a controlled and orderly manner (see page 34). Disturbance at any point may result in arrhythmia.

Arrhythmias are a large and heterogeneous group of conditions. Some cause benign nuisance symptoms only, but others can result in syncope, cardiac arrest and death.

Arrhythmias are often paroxysmal, which makes diagnosis difficult. Furthermore, there is sometimes little correlation between symptom severity and the seriousness of the underlying problem. Symptoms of benign arrhythmias may be deeply distressing for some patients, and conditions causing fatal arrhythmia may be asymptomatic until cardiac arrest.

It is useful to divide arrhythmias by rate (into bradycardias and tachycardias) and electrophysiologically (nature of the electrical abnormality) because these are the two most important factors influencing prognosis and management.

Arrhythmia does not necessarily indicate a primary cardiac problem. Even in a healthy heart, abnormalities of rate or rhythm occur:

- as a normal physiological response to exercise, sleep or illness
- secondary to the effects of non-cardiac disease
- secondary to the use of certain drugs (prescribed and non-prescribed)

When a non-cardiac cause is identified, treatment focuses primarily on correcting the underlying problem.

# Case 3 Lethargy and fainting

## Presentation

Mr Gordon is a 72-year-old retired decorator with a long medical history of hypertension and type 2 diabetes mellitus, for which he takes diltiazem (see page 157) and metformin. He is seen in the outpatient clinic and gives a 4-week history of lethargy. He has 'fainted' several times, and says that 'something just isn't right'. He felt well until 4 weeks ago.

## Initial interpretation

Syncope (fainting) is a red flag symptom, because it may indicate an adverse prognosis. However, syncope can be caused by a number of cardiogenic and non-cardiogenic conditions. More information is needed about its nature and frequency. A collateral history from a witness would be helpful, if possible.

## Further history

Mr Gordon explains that he has fainted four times in the past month. He has felt close to fainting, but did not (presyncope) many more times. He lacks energy and is tired all the time.

No witness is available to talk to, but Mr Gordon says that his daughter told him that when he 'faints' he loses consciousness for only a few seconds before quickly returning to normal. He has fainted while sitting in his armchair, and on two occasions he has fainted from standing, when he bruised and cut his limbs and head.

## Examination

Mr Gordon's blood pressure is increased, with a wide pulse pressure at 170/85 mmHg. His radial pulse rate is only 32 beats/min and is regular. His jugular venous pressure is not elevated, but every few seconds a large venous pulsation rises

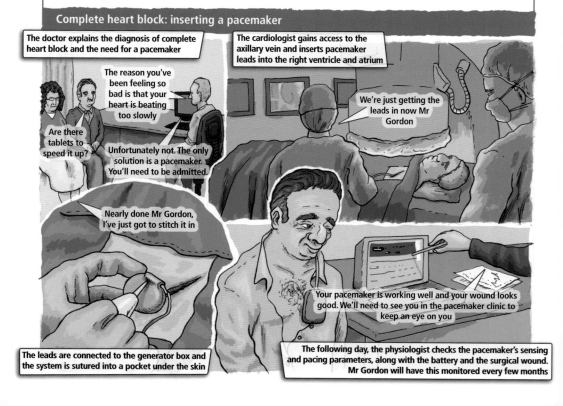

Complete heart block: inserting a pacemaker

**Case 3** *continued*

up both sides of his neck. He has a strong, non-displaced apex beat. The remainder of the cardiovascular and neurological examination is normal.

## Interpretation of findings

Prompt recovery from loss of consciousness favours syncope over seizure. Mr Gordon has a marked bradycardia. Therefore syncope is likely to be secondary to cerebral hypoperfusion caused by reduced cardiac output.

Mr Gordon has been syncopal even while sitting, which makes reflex or orthostatic hypotension unlikely. The occasional, large venous pressure waves indicate atrioventricular dissociation. Given the other features of his medical history and clinical examination, complete heart block is the likely cause of his symptoms.

## Investigations

Blood tests are done to check thyroid function and serum electrolytes. Hypothyroidism and serum electrolytes abnormalities are both recognised causes of bradycardia.

An urgent electrocardiogram (ECG) immediately shows that the heart rhythm is abnormal (**Figure 5.1**).

> **In complete heart block, the ventricles receive no electrical stimulus from the atria.** To avoid ventricular asystole and death, the heart's inbuilt failsafe mechanism takes over. Endogenous ventricular pacemakers begin to pace the heart. However, because of the nature of the ventricular tissues, the rhythm is slow and can be unstable (see page 44).

## Diagnosis

The ECG confirms complete heart block, warranting Mr Gordon's admission to hospital under the care of a cardiology team until a permanent pacemaker is fitted. In the meantime, his diltiazem is withheld (because it is a rate-limiting calcium channel blocker) and his heart rhythm is monitored in a specialist unit.

The following day, the permanent pacemaker is implanted (see page 164). Mr Gordon certainly must not drive until adequately treated and asymptomatic for ≥ 4 weeks.

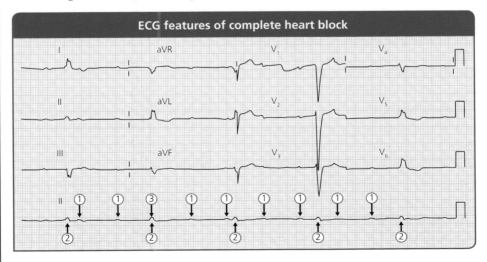

**ECG features of complete heart block**

**Figure 5.1** Electrocardiographic features of complete heart block. QRS complexes ② and P waves ① are both regular but occur at different rates and are dissociated from each other. The QRS complexes are broad. ③ points to a 'hidden' P wave occurring at the same time as a QRS complex.

# Case 4 Postoperative shortness of breath and palpitations

## Presentation

Mrs Bennett, aged 48 years, is recovering from an elective cholecystectomy (gall bladder removal), which was done 24 h previously. She has developed pneumonia and was started on antibiotics earlier the same day. The nurses report that she has become short of breath and has tachycardia at a rate of 156 beats/min. Her blood pressure is 110/68 mmHg, slightly lower than what is normal for her (125/75 mmHg). Her other observations are stable, and she has an oxygen saturation of 98% on room air.

## Initial interpretation

Shortness of breath and tachycardia are consistent with the diagnosis of pneumonia. However, the sudden change in symptoms and the jump in heart rate suggest that an arrhythmia has developed. Further assessment is needed to determine the cause.

## Further history

Mrs Bennett says that she suddenly became more short of breath and has had a 'fluttering' sensation in her chest ever since. She has not experienced chest discomfort, syncope or presyncope.

## Examination

Mrs Bennett is febrile (37.9°C) and clammy. She has an irregularly irregular heart rhythm at a rate of 163 beats/min. However, her jugular venous pressure is not elevated, and her heart sounds are normal.

The audible heart rate is slightly higher than the rate palpated at the radial pulse. Blood pressure is stable at 110/68 mmHg. A dull percussion note is heard, as well as coarse inspiratory crepitations at the left lung base.

## Interpretation of findings

The pyrexia and chest signs are completely consistent with the pneumonia, for which Mrs Bennett is already receiving treatment. However, the irregular pulse suggests atrial fibrillation. The speed of the ventricular response (163 beats/min) is likely to have caused the change in symptoms.

The pulse deficit is the difference between the audible and palpable rates. It occurs because weaker beats are not always palpable at the wrist.

## Investigations

Mrs Bennett's preoperative 12-lead ECG showed normal sinus rhythm (**Figure 5.2a**). However, a new ECG is devoid of P waves, and although the QRS complexes are of normal width and duration, the rate is much higher and the rhythm is chaotic (**Figure 5.2b**).

Blood tests results (**Table 5.1**) reflect Mrs Bennett's pneumonia, with increased white blood cell count and inflammatory markers. Serum urea and electrolytes are normal.

## Diagnosis

The clinical features and context suggest a diagnosis of atrial fibrillation, which the ECG confirms. Atrial fibrillation often complicates systemic illness. In this case, the cause is pneumonia, so the primary treatment is antibiotics.

Once the pneumonia resolves, her heart may spontaneously revert back to sinus rhythm without intervention. Mrs Bennett's symptoms may require short-term rate control with a beta-blocker, calcium channel blocker or digoxin to help her feel more comfortable.

**Case 4** *continued*

## ECG features of atrial fibrillation

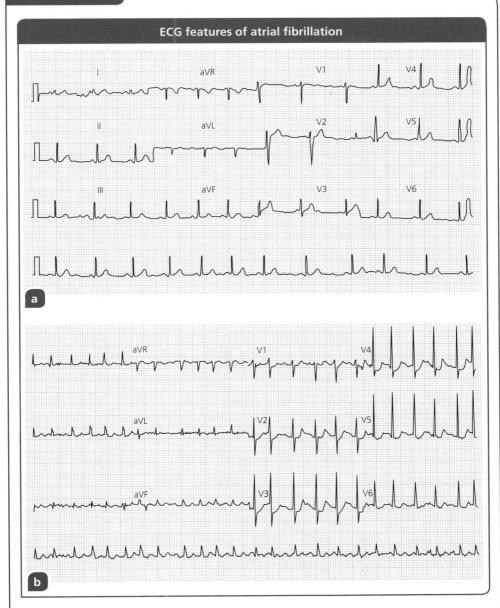

**Figure 5.2** (a) Mrs Bennett's pre-operative ECG showing sinus rhythm (b) Atrial fibrillation. The narrow QRS complexes are irregularly irregular. P waves are absent.

If the atrial fibrillation persists beyond 48 h, anticoagulation must be considered to reduce the risk of thromboembolic disease; this is the chief concern in cases of atrial fibrillation.

**Case 4** *continued*

| Mrs Bennett's blood test results | | | |
|---|---|---|---|
| **Haematology** | | | **Normal range** |
| Haemoglobin | Hb | 135 g/L | 115–165 |
| White cell count | WCC | 17.9 x10$^9$/L | 3.6–11.0 |
| Neutrophils | Neut | 15.8 x10$^9$/L | 1.8–7.5 |
| Lymphocytes | Lymph | 2.0 x10$^9$/L | 1.0–4.0 |
| Platelets | Plts | 201 x10$^9$/L | 140–400 |
| **Inflammatory markers** | | | **Normal range** |
| Erythrocyte sedimentation rate | ESR | 28 mm/hr | 3–9 |
| C-reactive protein | CRP | 68 mg/L | <10 |
| **Biochemistry** | | | **Normal range** |
| Sodium | Na$^+$ | 135 mmol/L | 133–146 |
| Potassium | K$^+$ | 3.9 mmol/L | 3.5–5.3 |
| Urea | Ur | 6.1 mmol/L | 2.5–7.8 |
| Creatinine | Cr | 62 µmol/L | 49–90 |

**Table 5.1** Mrs Bennett's blood tests results. Her white cell count (neutrophils) and inflammatory markers (ESR and CRP) are elevated, consistent with pneumonia.

# Mechanisms of arrhythmia

The mechanisms of arrhythmia genesis and propagation are aberrations of the normal electrophysiological processes described in chapter 1 (see page 34).

## Conduction block

Any disease which disrupts electrical conduction may reduce conduction velocity or block conduction altogether causing bundle branch block, bradycardia or heart block (see pages 129–130 and 217–218). Ischaemia and infarction are the commonest causes of conduction block, but infiltrative diseases, (e.g. amyloid) surgery or drug effects may also be involved. The nature and location of the block determines the clinical significance. This can be diagnosed from the rhythm and QRS morphology on the ECG. Drugs that reduce AVN conduction velocity (e.g. Ca$^{2+}$ channel blockers, beta blockers and digoxin) should be avoided in patients with significant conduction deficit.

## Ectopic beats

When increased cellular automaticity (see page 40) causes an ectopic site to discharge prematurely it results in an extra or ectopic beat. Occasional ectopic beats are a normal phenomenon. However, ischaemia, electrolyte derangement, sympathetic activation, myocardial stretch and certain drugs disrupt the resting membrane potential, alter ion channel function and cause more frequent ectopic beats. The more distal the ectopic focus, the less coordinated the conduction throughout the myocardium. Ectopic beats originating from the atria, therefore, cause an abnormal P wave morphology whereas those originating from the ventricles result in a broad QRS complex with abnormal morphology on the ECG trace.

# Re-entry

Re-entry occurs when electrical activation does not conduct via the normal pathways but instead follows an alternative, abnormal circuit which loops back on itself to form a 're-entry' circuit. Re-entry is a common cause of arrhythmia **(Figure 5.3)**. Re-entry circuits require:

■ a circuit of tissue around which a wave of depolarisation can travel

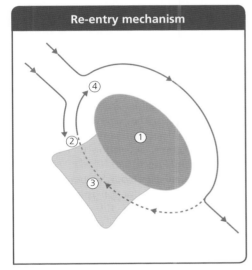

**Figure 5.3** The mechanism of re-entry. An electrical wave front arrives at an area of scar tissue ①. The wave front is blocked on one side by an area of unidirectional block ②. On the other side, the wave conducts normally around the scar and continues onwards, but conducts retrogradely through the area of unidirectional block ③. This wave front is held up by slow conduction (dashed line). Slow conduction allows the myocardium at ④ to become excitable again (absolute refractory period ended) and the wave front continues around the re-entry circuit.

■ an area within this circuit that only allows conduction in a single direction, i.e. unidirectional block
■ specific conduction and refractory properties, so that conduction through the circuit is slow enough to allow the distal myocytes time to repolarise (i.e. become excitable again), but rapid enough to ensure it depolarises the distal tissue before the next normally-conducted beat

If these conditions are met, a wave of depolarisation can cycle perpetually around the re-entry circuit taking over control of the rhythm. Re-entry is a cause of tachyarrhythmias such as supraventricular tachycardia and ventricular tachycardia. Timing is critical – the difference between conduction being too quick or too slow can be very slight. Therefore, any factor which influences conduction velocity and/or the refractoriness of myocardial tissues, influences the initiation and termination of re-entry arrhythmias.

# Triggered activity

Arrhythmia is also caused by oscillations in the membrane potential which occur during repolarisation. These fluctuations are known as early after depolarisations (EADs) during phase 3, and delayed after depolarisations (DADs) during phase 4 (see page 37). EADs are more common if phase 3 repolarisation is prolonged, for example in long QT syndrome or with certain drugs. DADs are more common when there is an increase in cytoplasmic $Ca^{2+}$ concentration, as occurs in sympathetic activation. Should a fluctuation in membrane potential reach the threshold potential, it will trigger an action potential and thus a heartbeat. If this occurs recurrently, an arrhythmia ensues. Torsade de pointes is an example of an arrhythmia caused by after depolarisations (see pages 266 and 358).

# Bradyarrhythmia

Bradyarrhythmia is an inappropriately slow ventricular rhythm. Bradycardia is any ventricular rate <60 beats/min. The difference between bradycardia and bradyarrhythmia therefore lies in the appropriateness of a given rhythm. Bradycardia and bradyarrhythmia reflect a reduction in either electrical activity or conduction. Bradycardia may occur as a normal physiological response during rest or sleep (i.e. sinus bradycardia).

The causes of bradyarrhythmia are numerous, but clinical features, diagnostic approach, investigations and management are similar.

> **Avoid being dogmatic about cut-off points for bradycardia.** A heart rate of 58 beats/min is unlikely to cause any more of a problem than one of 61 beats/min. Consider the individual patient, their age, health and physical fitness, and decide if the rate is inappropriately low for them. A resting heart rate of 44 beats/min may be normal for a professional cyclist but may cause profound symptoms for a 76-year-old woman with advanced emphysema and heart failure.

# Aetiology

**Table 5.2** lists some common non-cardiac causes of bradycardia. Cardiac bradyarrhythmia syndromes include sinus node disease, heart block, atrial fibrillation and chronotropic incompetence.

| Non-cardiac causes of bradycardia and bradyarrhythmia | |
| --- | --- |
| Physiological | Sleep |
| | Athletic training (increased vagal tone) |
| Drug effects | Beta-blockers |
| | Calcium channel blockers (dihydropyridine class) |
| | Amiodarone |
| Metabolic | Hypothyroidism |
| | Hypothermia |
| Electrolyte disturbance | Deranged potassium |
| | Deranged calcium |
| | Deranged magnesium |
| | Deranged sodium |
| Others | Increased intracranial pressure |
| | Obstructive sleep apnoea |

**Table 5.2** Common non-cardiac causes of bradycardia and bradyarrhythmia

## Sinus node disease

In sinus node disease, the sinus node fails to pace the heart appropriately. The result is a plethora of atrial arrhythmias, including:

- sinus pauses
- sinus tachycardia
- sinus bradycardia
- atrial tachycardia
- chronotropic incompetence (see page 218)
- atrial fibrillation

The combination of bradycardia and atrial tachycardias in the same patient, on different occasions, is known as tachy–brady syndrome and suggests sinus node disease. Sinus node disease is also known as sinus node dysfunction and sick sinus syndrome.

## Heart block

This condition results from impaired conduction between the atria and the ventricles. Heart block is categorised into 1st, 2nd and 3rd degrees, according to its severity **(Table 5.3** and **Figure 5.4)**.

In complete heart block, the absence of atrioventricular conduction results in atrioventricular dissociation. This means that the atria and ventricles will, by chance, occasionally contract synchronously. When this happens, atrial systole occurs against a closed tricuspid valve, causing blood to reflux back up the jugular veins (i.e. cannon waves).

> **Complete heart block is always treated seriously, because of the risk of asystole.** The slower the ventricular escape rate and the broader the QRS complexes, the more unstable the rhythm. Urgent specialist referral is needed for all cases of complete heart block.

## Atrial fibrillation

If the patient has atrial fibrillation, the ventricular response will be fast, slow or normal (see page 229).

## Chronotropic incompetence

This condition occurs when a patient's heart rate is normal at rest but fails to rise in response

## Degrees of heart block

| Degree | Electrocardiographic features | Treatment |
|---|---|---|
| 1st | Prolonged PR interval | Conservative |
| 2nd | Mobitz type I: prolonging PR interval, culminating in a dropped ventricular beat (QRS complex) | Conservative |
| | Mobitz type II: regularly more than one P wave to each QRS complex in a 2:1, 3:1 or 4:1 ratio; higher levels of block and variable block are also possible | Permanent pacemaker if symptomatic * |
| 3rd (complete) | Complete atrioventricular dissociation: regular P waves, regular QRS complexes but no association between the two | Permanent pacemaker * |

**Table 5.3** Degrees of heart block. (* if a reversible cause has been excluded.)

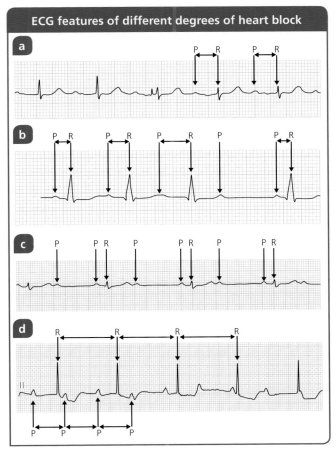

**ECG features of different degrees of heart block**

**Figure 5.4** Electrocardiographic features of different degrees of heart block. (a) 1st-degree heart block: a prolonged but constant PR interval. (b) 2nd-degree heart block (Mobitz type 1, Wenckebach block): progressive prolongation of the PR interval culminates in a dropped QRS complex. (c) 2nd-degree heart block (Mobitz type 2). In this case there are two P waves to each QRS complex, i.e. 2:1 block. (d) 3rd-degree (complete) heart block: dissociated atrial and ventricular activity.

to exercise or physiological stress. Therefore it is often diagnosed with exercise ECG testing.

Chronotropic incompetence causes symptoms on exertion and is occasionally the first sign of another bradyarrhythmia. If it is sufficiently symptomatic, a permanent pacemaker should be considered.

## Pathophysiology

Conditions that reduce automaticity (see page 40) or cause infiltration or fibrosis of the conduction tissues cause bradycardia. They include:

- age-related fibrosis

- ischaemic heart disease
- myocardial infiltration (sarcoidosis and amyloidosis)
- rheumatoid conditions (systemic lupus erythematosus and rheumatoid arthritis)
- congenital heart disease
- hyperthyroidism
- electrolyte disturbance

## Clinical features

Bradycardia causes palpitations, light-headedness and dizziness (non-vertiginous). More severe bradycardia results in collapse and syncope.

During bradyarrhythmia, the heart rate is slow. Significant symptoms are rare unless the heart rate is < 45 beats/min. Blood pressure is often increased in the early stages.

Hypotension, cerebral hypoperfusion (resulting in confusion) and shock indicate cardiovascular decompensation. This is a late and dangerous development in bradyarrhythmia.

## Diagnostic approach

Diagnosis is made by ECG and therefore relies on 'catching' the arrhythmia when it occurs. This is simple if the patient happens to be symptomatic at the time. However, bradycardia is often paroxysmal, which makes diagnosis difficult.

## Investigations

All patients require basic blood tests to exclude a biochemical cause for bradycardia. Hypothyroidism may cause symptomatic bradycardia, as can electrolyte disturbance (**Table 5.2**).

Electrocardiography during symptoms is vital. A 12-lead ECG may suffice but prolonged ambulatory ECG monitoring may be needed to catch the arrhythmia, if it is infrequent. For in-patients, a period of cardiac monitoring may provide the required evidence.

## Management

Asymptomatic bradycardia is usually treated conservatively, unless there is a compelling reason to insert a permanent pacemaker, such as complete heart block. The strategy for managing symptomatic bradycardia is as follows.

1. Identify and correct any reversible causes, including the use of certain drugs
2. If reversible causes have been excluded or corrected but the problem persists, insert a permanent pacemaker

### Medication

Rate-limiting medications are withheld during symptomatic bradyarrhythmia.

### Device therapy

The only definitive treatment for symptomatic bradyarrhythmia is insertion of a permanent pacemaker (see page 164). The pacemaker's generator box can be removed or changed relatively simply, but the pacing wires fix into the ventricular myocardium. Removal is technically challenging and carries a significant risk of morbidity and mortality. Therefore a permanent pacemaker is inserted only if:

- reversible causes have been excluded
- it is proven beyond reasonable doubt that the patient's symptoms are secondary to bradycardia
- any infection is eradicated before insertion (to minimise the risk of device-related infection)

**Figure 5.5** shows methods for artificially pacing the heart. Complications of permanent pacemaker insertion are summarised in **Table 5.4**.

Antibradycardia devices are single- or dual-lead and have different responses to bradycardia (**Table 5.5**).

Commonly, only the first four code letters are used (see **Table 5.5**). Therefore:

- a VVIR pacemaker is a single-lead permanent pacemaker that paces the ventricle, senses the ventricle, is inhibited by sensing and responds to activity by increasing the pacing rate
- a DDDR permanent pacemaker is a dual-lead permanent pacemaker that both paces and senses the atria and ventricle, and inhibits or paces accordingly in a rate-responsive manner

## Methods of artificially pacing the heart

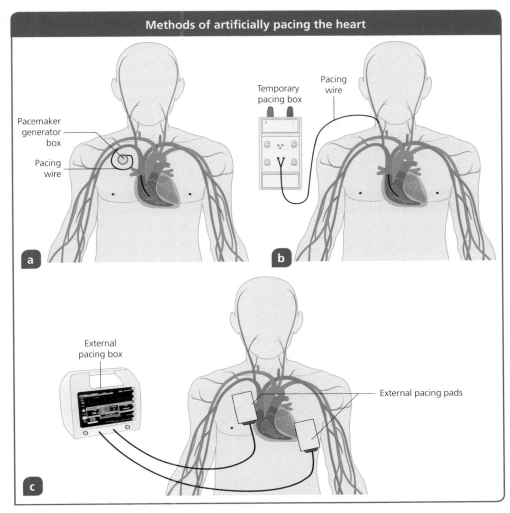

**Figure 5.5** Methods used to increase heart rate in unstable bradycardia. (a) Permanent pacemaker system. The lead is inserted into a vein and advanced through the superior vena cava, right atrium and tricuspid valve. The lead tip is fixed into the right ventricular myocardium at the apex. The generator box is placed into a subcutaneous pocket. (b) Temporary transvenous pacing. A wire is inserted into the right ventricular apex (under X-ray imaging) through either the jugular, subclavian or femoral vein. The wire is then connected to an external pacing box outside the body. (c) Transcutaneous pacing. Electrical activity is delivered to the heart through pads on the chest wall. This is uncomfortable but can be life-saving in an emergency.

## Emergency and interim treatment

When severe bradycardia causes acute cardiac instability, transcutaneous pacing (pacing pads, **Figure 5.5c**), transvenous pacing or an intravenous drug infusion (e.g. atropine or isoprenaline, see pages 42 and 51) is used to increase heart rate. These temporary measures stabilise patients until a permanent pacemaker can be inserted.

Temporary transvenous pacing involves inserting a pacing wire into the right ventricular apex through a central vein and pacing the heart from an external power box. It is usually used as a bridge to permanent pacemaker insertion in unstable patients.

If ischaemia is excluded, an intravenous infusion of a drug that increases heart rate (a positive chronotrope) can be used to stabilise the patient's condition until pacing is possible.

## Complications of pacemaker insertion

| Complication | Context |
|---|---|
| Pneumothorax | Occurs if the lung pleura is damaged during insertion |
| Bleeding | Post-procedural bleeding can result in a pocket haematoma (usually managed with a compression dressing) |
| Perforation | Can result in cardiac tamponade (see page 358) which requires emergency drainage |
| Infection | Treatment involves long courses of intravenous antibiotics. If this is unsuccessful, the device may need to be explanted and replaced. |
| Lead displacement | A more common complication that causes device malfunction (rectified by repositioning the leads) |

**Table 5.4** Complications of pacemaker insertion

## Standard nomenclature for antibradycardia pacemakers

| I | II | III | IV | V |
|---|---|---|---|---|
| Chamber-paced | Chamber-sensed | Response to sensing | Rate responsiveness | Multisite pacing |
| O (none) | O (none) | O (none) | O (none) | O (none) |
| A (atrium) | A (atrium) | T (triggers pacing) | R (rate-responsive) | A (atrium) |
| V (ventricle) | V (ventricle) | I (inhibits pacing) | | V (ventricle) |
| D (dual, A&V) | D (dual, A&V) | D (T&I) | | D (dual) |

**Table 5.5** Standard nomenclature for antibradycardia pacemakers. This table explains the letter codes used to name pacing device.

Positive chronotropic drugs used for this purpose include isoprenaline (a β-adrenergic agonist) and atropine (an anticholinergic drug). They are used in specialist units with cardiac monitoring facilities.

> **Guideline documents regarding indications for insertion of a permanent pacemaker are long and complicated.** However, they can be summarised in two words: symptomatic bradycardia. The patient must have both symptoms and bradycardia, and the former should be a consequence of the latter.

- Sinus arrest – temporary cessation of sinoatrial node impulse formation. When this occurs, there is an absence of atrial activity (i.e. P waves) on the ECG. Pause length is independent of the normal P-P interval
- Sinoatrial arrest – transient failure of conduction across the atrial myocardium. The pauses are the length of two or more normal P-P intervals
- Atrio-ventricular (AV) block – if conduction through the AV node is temporarily blocked, atrial depolarisation (P waves) will not be followed by

## Cardiac pauses

A cardiac pause is a transient cessation in cardiac electrical activity (**Figure 5.6**). This results in a pause in cardiac output which is often symptomatic. Symptoms include palpitations, transient light-headedness and occasionally syncope. Causes of cardiac pauses include:

### ECG showing a cardiac pause

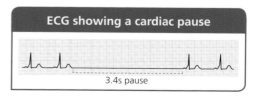

3.4s pause

**Figure 5.6** Electrocardiogram showing a 3.4s cardiac pause. The rest of the electrocardiogram shows normal sinus rhythm.

ventricular depolarisation. A pause in cardiac output therefore occurs before either AV conduction is restored or a ventricular escape rhythm occurs

> Holter ECG monitoring is usually accompanied by a 'patient symptom diary', where patients keep a record of any symptoms they experience throughout the duration of the monitoring period. This allows clinicians to interpret the results of the investigation in the context of knowing exactly when symptoms occur.

Pauses are best identified with Holter monitoring (see page 132) in tandem with a diary of symptoms. The clinical features, diagnostic approach and management are similar to those for other bradyarrthmias.

Waking pauses lasting over 3 s are considered significant and require further investigation, especially when the patient has other symptoms.

# Tachyarrhythmias

Tachyarrhythmias are abnormal heart rhythms >100 beats/min. They are divided according to the width/duration of the QRS complex into:

- narrow complex tachycardia (QRS ≤120 ms)
- broad complex tachycardia (QRS >120 ms)

Narrow QRS complexes reflect organised, efficient electrical activity originating above the atrioventricular node. Heartbeats originating from below the atrioventricular node result in disorganised, delayed depolarisation and hence broad QRS complexes. Therefore:

- narrow complex tachycardias are also known as supraventricular tachycardias and are usually benign in isolation
- broad complex tachycardias usually indicate a ventricular origin, and are more unstable than supraventricular tachycardias.

## Supraventricular tachycardias

Supraventricular tachycardias occur in healthy and diseased hearts and can be symptomatic or asymptomatic. In an otherwise healthy heart, this type of tachycardia is largely a benign problem but can be a nuisance for patients. Modern invasive catheter-based treatments offer a high chance of a cure (see page 163).

## Epidemiology

Supraventricular tachycardias affect about 0.2% of the population.

## Aetiology

Narrow complex tachycardias are subdivided by the nature of the electrical abnormality.

### Atrioventricular nodal re-entry tachycardia

This is the most common cause of supraventricular tachycardia; it accounts for about 80% of cases. The condition is caused by a small re-entry circuit involving the atrioventricular node and the surrounding atrial tissue.

The electrocardiographic characteristics of atrioventricular nodal re-entry tachycardia are shown in **Figure 5.7**. Although the underlying abnormality is present from birth, clinical features usually manifest in adulthood.

### Atrioventricular reciprocating tachycardia

This type of tachycardia occurs when electrical signals conduct abnormally between the atria and ventricles. Normally, the atria are electrically insulated from the ventricles, and the atrioventricular node is the only electrical connection (see page 20). Accessory pathways are abnormal connections between the atria

## ECG features of atrioventricular node re-entry tachycardia

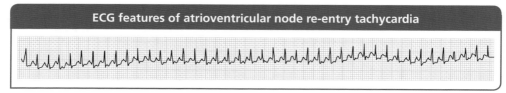

**Figure 5.7** Electrocardiographic features of atrioventricular node re-entry tachycardia. Note the tachycardia and narrow QRS complexes.The atria and ventricles depolarise almost synchronously. As a result, the P waves are hidden inside the QRS complexes.

and the ventricles. They may conduct in either direction: from atrium to ventricle or from ventricle to atrium.

Accessory pathways cause arrhythmia if they allow an abnormal circuit to bypass the sinoatrial node and 'take over' the rhythm. If the circuit conducts down the atrioventricular node and septum in a forward direction, the atrioventricular reciprocating tachycardia is orthodromic and results in a narrow complex tachycardia (**Figure 5.8**). Conduction in the reverse direction is antidromic, and because ventricular depolarisation occurs in the wrong direction, a broad complex tachycardia results.

Accessory pathways are present from birth. Clinical features tend to manifest in childhood or adolescence.

## Wolf–Parkinson–White syndrome

This condition occurs when an accessory pathway results in ventricular pre-excitation (**Figure 5.9**).

## Atrial flutter

This arrhythmia is characterised by a rapid atrial rate: about 300 beats/min. In typical atrial flutter, there is a re-entry circuit in the right atrium, involving the cavotricuspid isthmus, atrial septum and crista terminalis. This gives rise to the classic sawtooth appearance of atrial flutter on ECG (**Figure 5.10**).

Atrial flutter increases the risk of stroke. Therefore thromboprophylaxis should be considered, as it is in cases of atrial fibrillation (see page 231).

## Atrial tachycardia

This type of tachycardia arises from increased automaticity, a macro or micro re-

### ECG features of atrioventricular reciprocating tachycardia

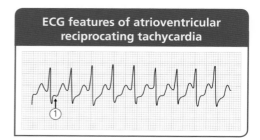

**Figure 5.8** Electrocardiographic features of orthodromic atrioventricular reciprocating tachycardia. Note the fast rate and narrow complexes. The atria are depolarised by the ventricles through an accessory pathway. The result is a subtle retrograde P wave after the QRS ① indenting the ST segment. Antidromic atrioventricular reciprocating tachycardias result in a broad complex tachycardia.

### ECG features of Wolff–Parkinson–White syndrome

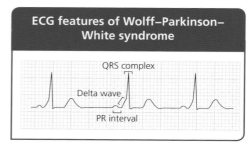

**Figure 5.9** Electrocardiographic features of Wolff–Parkinson–White syndrome. The short PR interval and slurring of the QRS upstroke (delta wave) indicate early ventricular depolarisation through the accessory pathway during sinus rhythm.

entry circuit, or both, elsewhere in the atria. It causes a narrow complex tachycardia with an abnormal P wave morphology.

## Atrial fibrillation

Unlike other supraventricular tachycardias,

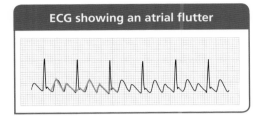

**ECG showing an atrial flutter**

**Figure 5.10** Electrocardiogram showing an atrial flutter. Note the sawtooth baseline (green) and narrow complex tachycardia (100 beats/min). There are three atrial flutter waves to every conducted QRS. Only two flutter waves are clearly visible; the third is mostly hidden within the QRS complex.

atrial fibrillation causes an irregularly irregular rhythm (see page 229).

# Clinical features

Narrow complex tachycardias may be asymptomatic or cause palpitations. Patients describe the palpitations as fast and regular or as a 'fluttering' in the chest. They may complain of shortness of breath or fatigue. Ischaemic chest pain and low blood pressure indicate compromise of the cardiovascular system. When this occurs, urgent direct current cardioversion (DCCV) is required (see page 356).

Rarely, persistent supraventricular tachycardia itself induces heart failure by tiring the myocardium; this is termed tachycardiomyopathy. However, tachycardiomyopathy develops slowly over several weeks or months. Arrhythmia is much more commonly the consequence rather than the cause of heart failure.

> **Supraventricular tachycardias are generally benign rhythms, but 'pre-excited atrial fibrillation' is potentially very dangerous.** This condition occurs when an accessory pathway conducts atrial fibrillation from the atria to the ventricles. Pre-excited atrial fibrillation can quickly degrade into ventricular fibrillation (i.e. cardiac arrest). It is important not to give these patients drugs that block the atrioventricular node, because this increases conduction though the accessory pathway.

# Diagnostic approach

Diagnosis relies on capturing the supraventricular tachycardia on an ECG and matching the electrical abnormality with patient symptoms. A 12-lead ECG may suffice, but ambulatory monitoring is usually required for identifying paroxysmal arrhythmias.

# Investigations

Once supraventricular tachycardia has been diagnosed, investigations are used to identify the cause. An echocardiogram is necessary to exclude structural heart disease and to assess cardiac function. Thyroid function and urea and electrolytes are checked, because hyperthyroidism and electrolyte derangement are common reversible precipitants of supraventricular tachycardia. An electrophysiological study may be required to identify the underlying electrical abnormality or mechanism.

# Management

Supraventricular tachycardias causing cardiovascular instability are treated with urgent synchronised DCCV (see page 356). The optimal management of supraventricular tachycardia is determined by the cause. For example, atrial flutter responds well to DCCV, but medication or an ablation procedure is usually required to reduce the chance of recurrence.

## Vagal manoeuvres

Vagal stimulation sometimes terminates a supraventricular tachycardia quickly and simply. Physical manoeuvers that achieve this include:

- the Valsalva manoeuvre (asking the patient to cough, bear down or blow hard into a 10-mL syringe)
- carotid sinus massage (but first exclude carotid bruit)

## Medication

Atrioventricular node re-entry tachycardias and atrioventricular reciprocating tachycardias are terminated, and the frequency of attacks reduced, by drugs that block atrioventricular node conduction. These drugs include beta-blockers and calcium channel blockers.

However, drugs that block atrioventricular node conduction are avoided if ventricular pre-excitation is evident (e.g. in Wolf–Parkinson–White syndrome), because they encourage conduction across the accessory pathway. Instead, class 1 (flecanide, propafenone or disopyramide) or class 3 drugs (amiodarone) are favoured, because they reduce conduction across the accessory pathway.

Atrial flutter and atrial tachycardia respond poorly to drug therapy.

## Catheter ablation

Drug therapy reduces the risk of paroxysms of supraventricular tachycardia. However, ablation eradicates the abnormal underlying circuit.

Ablation, either cryotherapy or radiofrequency, is delivered through intracardiac catheters. The aim is to break the abnormal circuit or electrical focus by creating a scar in the myocardial tissue. Long term curative success rates for ablation are high (> 95%).

## Prognosis

Patients should be reassured that although supraventricular tachycardia may be worrying and difficult to treat, the prognosis in most cases is excellent.

> **Always consider atrial flutter if the ventricular rate is 150 beats/min.** In atrial flutter, the atrial rate is always about 300 beats/min. This is too fast for 1:1 atrioventricular node conduction. Ventricular rate usually occurs with 2:1 (150 beats/min), 3:1 (100 beats/min) or 4:1 (75 beats/min) atrioventricular block. Drugs that block the atrioventricular node are used to control the ventricular rate (**Figure 5.10**).

## Ventricular tachycardia

Ventricular tachycardia is a broad complex tachycardia originating from a ventricular focus. It is defined as ≥3 successive ventric-

ular beats occurring at a rate of >100 beats/min. It is more malignant than supraventricular tachycardia, because it may cause ventricular fibrillation, cardiac arrest and death.

The electrocardiographic hallmark of ventricular tachycardia is a regular broad complex tachycardia. However, in some cases broad complex tachycardia reflects an underlying supraventricular tachycardia with abnormal conduction. For example, the combination of atrial flutter with bundle branch block produces a regular broad complex tachycardia on the ECG.

Torsades de pointes ('twisting of the points') is a form of polymorphic ventricular tachycardia in which the QRS complexes appear to twist around an imaginary baseline axis (**Figure 5.11**).

> **Ventricular tachycardia is regular.** Whenever a broad complex tachycardia has an irregularly irregular rhythm, think of atrial fibrillation with a fast ventricular response and abnormal electrical conduction (i.e. left or right bundle branch block).

## Aetiology

Monomorphic ventricular tachycardia results from an abnormal re-entry circuit, in most cases precipitated by myocardial scarring (e.g. from ischaemic heart disease). Any condition associated with an abnormality of the ventricular myocardium (fibrosis, infiltration or cardiomyopathy) increases the risk of ventricular tachycardia. Conditions such as arrhythmogenic right ventricular cardio-

### ECG showing torsade de pointes

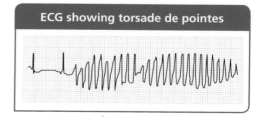

**Figure 5.11** Electrocardiogram showing torsade de pointes, a broad complex tachycardia. The complexes appear to twist around the baseline.

myopathy, Brugada syndrome and long QT syndrome also cause ventricular tachycardia. These are covered in Chapter 10.

Torsades de pointes occurs secondary to prolongation of the QT interval. It is therefore associated with the long QT syndromes, hypokalaemia and hypomagnesaemia, as well as the use of amiodarone, erythromycin and methadone.

> **Ventricular rhythms with a rate between 60–100 beats/min are referred to as accelerated idioventricular rhythms.** Rates slower than this are usually escape rhythms seen in bradyarrhthmia. Accelerated idioventricular rhythms are commonly associated with myocardial reperfusion following treatment for myocardial infarction. In this context they are usually benign, self-limiting and resolve spontaneously.

## Clinical features

Ventricular tachycardia may be classified as:

- pulsed (palpable pulse) or pulseless (no palpable pulse)
- non-sustained (< 30 s) or sustained (> 30 s)
- monomorphic (with a consistent QRS appearance; **Figure 5.12**) or polymorphic (with a frequently changing QRS appearance; **Figure 5.11**)

The condition is poorly tolerated and rarely asymptomatic. Syncope indicates a poorer prognosis. Other symptoms include:

- palpitations
- presyncope
- symptoms of heart failure in sustained ventricular tachycardia

The history should also include symptoms of associated conditions, such as ischaemic heart disease and heart failure. A family history of arrhythmia or sudden cardiac death is also important.

In ventricular tachycardia with a palpable pulse, the pulse is rapid and weak. Pulseless ventricular tachycardia presents with cardiac arrest. Signs of potential causes or complications should also be sought.

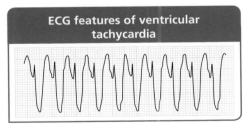

**ECG features of ventricular tachycardia**

**Figure 5.12** Electrocardiographic features of ventricular tachycardia, a regular broad complex tachycardia.

## Diagnostic approach

It is often difficult to discern ventricular tachycardia from a supraventricular tachycardia with abnormal conduction. Both conditions give rise to a regular broad complex tachycardia. About 85% of regular broad complex tachycardias are caused by ventricular tachycardia. In patients with known structural heart disease (including heart failure or ischaemic heart disease), about 95% of broad complex tachycardias are caused by ventricular tachycardia.

The following electrocardiographic features support a diagnosis of ventricular tachycardia (over supraventricular tachycardia with abnormal conduction).

- Very broad QRS: > 160 ms
- Extreme axis: –90° to −180°
- Concordance: all chest lead complexes are positive or all are negative
- Fusion beats: produced when a sinus beat fuses with a ventricular beat
- Capture beats: produced when a sinus beat 'captures' the ventricles to produce occasional 'normal'-looking beats
- Bizarre QRS morphology
- Atrioventricular dissociation: regular P and QRS complexes but at different rates

In cases of doubt, the arrhythmia should be treated as ventricular tachycardia until proven otherwise.

## Investigations

The aims of investigations are:

- To make a diagnosis: this is usually done with a 12-lead or ambulatory ECG

- To identify the cause: echocardiography or cardiac magnetic resonance imaging may show functional impairment or structural abnormalities, and coronary angiography may be used to diagnose coronary artery disease
- To stratify risk: risk is determined by the presence or absence of structural heart disease, including heart failure and ischaemic heart disease
- To make an electrophysiological diagnosis: the mechanism of the arrhythmia is often elucidated at an electrophysiological study

## Management

Emergency synchronised DCCV is required for any patient whose condition is compromised (e.g. hypotension or ischaemia) in any way (see page 356). Once sinus rhythm has been restored, the focus moves towards identifying and correcting the cause, if possible. This process commonly requires the alleviation of ischaemia or optimising the treatment of heart failure.

All patients with torsades de pointes need urgent DCCV to restore sinus rhythm. Correction of magnesium or potassium deficiency, or both, in addition to cessation of any QT-prolonging drugs reduces recurrence.

### Medication

In patients with a structurally abnormal heart, drugs (e.g. amiodarone or beta-blockers) are used to reduce the frequency of ventricular tachycardia. Beta-blockers and aldosterone antagonists may improve prognosis in the context of heart failure.

In patients whose heart is structurally normal, drug therapy is sometimes the only management necessary.

### Surgery

If the electrophysiological study identifies an appropriate target, catheter ablation is possible for monomorphic ventricular tachycardia. Although success rates (about 60-75%) are lower than those for supraventricular tachycardia, they are higher for cases associated with a structurally normal heart.

### Device therapy

Implantable cardioverter defibrillators (ICDs) are used for secondary prevention in patients with ventricular tachycardia or ventricular fibrillation causing syncope or cardiac arrest. ICDs are used as primary prevention in patients with a high-risk condition such as severe heart failure (see pages 164 and 248).

These devices do not reduce the frequency of ventricular arrhythmia, but they restore sinus rhythm when it occurs. The decision to use an ICD must be considered carefully, and insertion should follow full discussion with the patient, because of the significant associated complications and impact on quality of life.

### Prognosis

The key determinant of prognosis in ventricular tachycardia is the presence or absence of underlying structural heart disease, including coronary heart disease and heart failure. Ventricular tachycardia in a structurally normal heart has a much better prognosis than that in a structurally abnormal heart. ICD insertion in patients with a structurally abnormal heart has been shown to reduce mortality.

## Ventricular fibrillation

In ventricular fibrillation, the ventricular myocardium is devoid of any coordinated electrical or mechanical activity. Cardiac output ceases. Ventricular fibrillation always results in cardiac arrest (**Figure 5.13**). Therefore ventricular fibrillation requires emergency DCCV, otherwise asystole and death quickly ensue (see page 356).

Patients who survive a ventricular fibrillation cardiac arrest and those deemed at high risk of ventricular fibrillation are treated with an ICD.

**ECG features of ventricular fibrillation**

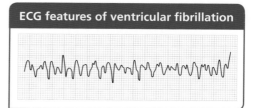

**Figure 5.13** Electrocardiographic features of ventricular fibrillation. The rhythm, polarity and magnitude are completely irregular.

# Atrial fibrillation

Atrial fibrillation is an irregular, often rapid rhythm where the atria fail to contract: efficiently, regularly or in coordination with the ventricles. It is the commonest cardiac arrhythmia. It is classed according to duration:

- paroxysmal (< 7 days)
- persistent (> 7 days)
- permanent (> 7 days and resistant to therapy)

The condition can be:

- lone, with no identifiable cause
- valvular, i.e. associated with valve disease (often prosthetic or rheumatic valve disease)
- secondary to other cardiac or non-cardiac disease

Depending on ventricular response rate, atrial fibrillation results in bradycardia, tachycardia or a normal rate.

In most patients, the biggest concern is the increased risk of thromboembolic disease, especially stroke.

## Epidemiology

The prevalence of atrial fibrillation increases with age. The condition affects 1% of the general population but up to 10% of those over 80 years old. Atrial fibrillation is commonly asymptomatic, so it often remains undiagnosed.

## Aetiology

Atrial fibrillation is more common in people with other illnesses, especially those associated with increased atrial pressure. Hypertension is the commonest predisposing condition, followed by heart failure, ischaemic heart disease, valvular heart disease and thyroid disease. Excess alcohol consumption and drug misuse also predispose to atrial fibrillation. The condition is also common in the acutely unwell or perioperative patients.

## Pathophysiology

Atrial stress induces chronic myocardial, electrical and biochemical changes, which are thought to be central to the initiation and propagation of atrial fibrillation. It is increasingly appreciated that in many patients, particularly those with paroxysmal atrial fibrillation, the initiating electrical stimuli emanate from the pulmonary veins. This is the rationale behind pulmonary vein ablation therapy.

Fibrillation is a pattern of rapid, unsynchronised and chaotic electrical activity. Atrial fibrillation is characterised by the absence of any coordinated electrical or mechanical atrial activity. Electrical activity is conducted to the ventricles through the conducting tissues but in an irregular, haphazard manner. Therefore the ventricular response rate is determined by the conductivity of the atrioventricular node and the His and Purkinje tissues.

## Clinical features

The clinical features of atrial fibrillation are usually determined by the ventricular response rate. The clinical features of tachycardia and bradycardia are described on page 220. Atrial fibrillation with normal ventricular rate may be asymptomatic or symptomatic with palpitations, lethargy, chest pain and dyspnoea. As well as questions about symptoms, the history should inquire about:

- predisposing factors (e.g. family history, hypertension and lung disease)
- stroke and bleeding risk
- complications (e.g. heart failure and thromboembolic disease)

An irregularly irregular pulse is found on examination. Atrial fibrillation often remains silent, so its presenting feature can be a stroke.

Check blood pressure (for hypertension) and for signs of other predisposing conditions. Also examine for signs of complications such as heart failure or thromboembolic disease (i.e. stroke).

> **There is no such thing as 'fast' or 'slow' atrial fibrillation.** Atrial fibrillations are always fast. It is the ventricular response rate that can be fast, slow or normal in rate. It is better to say that a patient has 'atrial fibrillation with a fast/slow/controlled ventricular response rate', for example.

## Diagnostic approach

Permanent atrial fibrillation is easily and quickly diagnosed by palpating an irregularly irregular pulse rhythm and doing an ECG (**Figure 5.2**). Paroxysmal atrial fibrillation usually requires Holter monitoring to catch a paroxysm.

> **The left atrial appendage is where blood clots tend to form in atrial fibrillation.** A transoesophageal echocardiogram is needed to identify a clot here, because this region is not well visualised in a transthoracic study.

## Investigations

Multiple investigations are necessary in atrial fibrillation (**Table 5.6**). Transoesophageal echocardiography is done to identify

or exclude left atrial clot if DCCV is being considered in atrial fibrillation beyond 48 h and before 6 weeks of anticoagulation is complete. This is because cardioversion can cause clot to dislodge, embolise and cause stroke.

## Management

The key aims of management are to reduce the risk of thromboembolic disease, control the ventricular rate and alleviate symptoms.

> **Online calculators and mobile device applications** are useful for quickly estimating the risk of stroke and bleeding (e.g. with the $CHA_2DS_2$-VASc and HAS-BLED scores).

### Anticoagulation

Atrial fibrillation increases the risk of stroke fivefold. Oral anticoagulant therapy decreases this risk by nearly two thirds. For most patients, reducing the risk of thromboembolic disease is the single most important aim of treatment.

The risk of bleeding must be balanced against the benefits of anticoagulation in the individual patient.

- The $CHADS_2$ score and the $CHA_2DS_2$-VASc score are used to estimate the annual risk of stroke in patients with atrial fibrillation (**Table 5.7**)
- The HAS-BLED score estimates the major bleeding risk in patients receiving warfarin (**Table 5.8**).

> **Novel oral anticoagulant drugs such as the factor Xa inhibitors apixaban and rivaroxaban and the thrombin inhibitor dabigatran appear to be as effective as warfarin in preventing venous thromboembolism in patients with atrial fibrillation.** These drugs also have improved safety profiles. They are an attractive option, because, unlike warfarin, blood monitoring is unnecessary.

| Investigations in atrial fibrillation | |
|---|---|
| Investigation | Reason |
| Thyroid function tests | To exclude hyperthyroidism, a potentially reversible cause |
| Coagulation screen | Required for patients considered for anticoagulation |
| Urea and electrolytes | To exclude electrolyte derangement, a potential reversible cause |
| Liver function tests | To exclude derangement (potential reversible cause) and also useful when considering anticoagulation |
| Echocardiography | To exclude structural heart disease |

**Table 5.6** Investigations used in atrial fibrillation

| CHA$_2$DS$_2$-VASc score for estimating stroke risk in atrial fibrillation | | | |
|---|---|---|---|
| Risk factors | Criteria | Category | Score if yes* |
| Congestive heart failure | Signs, symptoms or imaging evidence of reduced left and /or right ventricular failure | Yes or no | 1 |
| Hypertension | Blood pressure >140 mmHg systolic and/or >90 mmHg diastolic on at least 2 occasions or taking antihypertensive medication | Yes or no | 1 |
| Age | | <65 years | 0 |
| | | 65–74 years | 1 |
| | | ≥75 years | 2 |
| Diabetes mellitus | Fasting glucose level ≥7.0 mmol/L or taking treatment on diabetic medication | Yes or no | 1 |
| Stroke | Previous history of stroke, transient ischaemic attack or thromboembolic disease previously? | Yes or no | 2 |
| Vascular disease? | History of ischaemic heart disease, peripheral vascular disease, arterial and /or venous thrombosis | Yes or no | 1 |
| Sex | Female | Yes or no | 1 |

*A total score of 0 indicates low annual stroke risk. Higher scores reflect increased risk. For example, total scores of 1, 2 and 3 equate to annual stroke risk of 1.3%, 2.2% and 3.2% respectively. A total score of 6 equates to a risk of 9.8%.

**Table 5.7** The CHA$_2$DS$_2$-VASc score for estimating risk of stroke in patients with atrial fibrillation.

| HAS-BLED score for estimating bleeding risk | | |
|---|---|---|
| Category | Criterion | Score* |
| Hypertension | Uncontrolled (systolic blood pressure > 160 mmHg) | 1 |
| Abnormal renal function | Dialysis, renal transplant or creatinine > 200 mmol/L | 1 |
| Abnormal liver function | Cirrhosis; bilirubin over twice the normal range; or AST, ALT and ALP over three times the normal range | 1 |
| Stroke | History of stroke, particularly lacunar infarcts | 1 |
| Bleeding | History of bleeding or anaemia, or predisposition to bleeding | 1 |
| Labile INRs | Difficult, unstable control, with high INRs | 1 |
| Elderly | Age ≥ 65 years | 1 |
| Drugs | | |
|   Alcohol | ≥ 8 units/week | 1 |
|   Antiplatelet therapy or NSAIDs | Concomitant use of antiplatelet therapy or NSAIDs (including aspirin) | 1 |

* Higher scores reflect increasing risk of bleeding. A total score of ≥ 3 indicates higher risk (≥ 3.7 bleeds per 100 patient-years). Bleeding risk should be balanced against the risk of stroke when considering oral anticoagulation therapy in patients with atrial fibrillation.

ALP, alkaline phosphatase; ALT, alanine aminotransferase; AST, aspartate aminotransferase; INR, international normalised ratio; NSAID, non-steroidal anti-inflammatory drug.

**Table 5.8** The HAS-BLED score for estimating the risk of major bleeding in patients on oral anticoagulation therapy

## Rate control

Depending on contraindications and intolerances, beta-blockers, calcium channel blockers and digoxin are all used to control heart rate. A single-agent approach is best, but a second agent can be added if control is suboptimal.

Digoxin is reserved for more sedentary patients because, unlike other agents, it does not allow the heart rate to rise (physiologically) during exercise. The initial target is maintenance of a resting heart rate ≤ 110 beats/min.

## Management of acute atrial fibrillation

If atrial fibrillation causes significant cardiovascular compromise, emergency DCCV is required, regardless of the duration of atrial fibrillation (see page 356). If the atrial fibrillation is secondary to systemic illness, treatment is targeted at the underlying cause. If the atrial fibrillation persists after the cause has been alleviated, DCCV is considered after ≥ 6 weeks of effective anticoagulation.

## Management of paroxysmal atrial fibrillation

The frequency of paroxysms can be reduced by beta-blockers, class 1C drugs (flecanide or propafenone) or class 3 drugs (amiodarone or dronedarone). However, these drugs are limited by contraindications, complications and lack of efficacy (see page 150).

Direct current cardioversion is used to restore sinus rhythm from a paroxysm of atrial fibrillation, but reversion back to atrial fibrillation is common. Because of the risk of inducing stroke, cardioversion is avoided if the atrial fibrillation lasts > 48 h. DCCV is done only if ≥ 6 weeks of full anticoagulation has been achieved, or if a transoesophageal echocardiogram excludes intracardiac clot.

Isolation of the pulmonary veins by catheter ablation is a newer treatment, which provides long-term relief from atrial fibrillation in some patients. However, a significant proportion of patients require repeat procedures to achieve optimal control.

Some patients respond well to a pill-in-the-pocket strategy. A drug (usually a beta-blocker, flecanide or propafenone) is taken promptly when atrial fibrillation symptoms begin. The aim is to chemically cardiovert the patient into sinus rhythm without the need to seek further help.

## Permanent atrial fibrillation

By definition, sinus rhythm cannot be restored in permanent atrial fibrillation with oral antiarrhythmic therapy. The primary aim is to reduce the risk of thromboembolic disease. Rate control is needed if the ventricular response is fast.

## Surgery and device therapy

During heart surgery, surgeons occasionally deliberately scar the atria with either a scalpel or diathermy and electrically cardiovert the heart into sinus rhythm. This Cox maze procedure provides long-term relief from atrial fibrillation for some patients.

Left atrial occluder devices can be implanted into the left atrium to incarcerate a clot in the left atrial appendage. More robust evidence is required before these catheter-delivered devices become mainstream treatment options.

## Prognosis

The prognosis for atrial fibrillation is good as long as the risk of thromboembolism is minimised and the rate is controlled appropriately.

# Answers to starter questions

1. Bradycardia (heart rate <60 bpm) allows more time for diastolic ventricular filling and thus more ventricular stretch. This increases the stroke volume and widens the pulse pressure (see Chapter 1, page 49). This compensatory measure can maintain an acceptable cardiac output. Eventually, these mechanisms become exhausted and decompensation results in hypotension and shock, a worrying sign in bradycardic patients.

2. Patients on rate-limiting drugs can develop symptomatic bradycardia. Usually, the drug is discontinued or substituted because the risks associated with taking them outweigh the benefits. However, sometimes it is decided that the benefits are such that the drug is continued and a pacemaker implanted to protect against bradycardia. This is often referred to as a 'pace and block' strategy. An example is a patient experiencing both tachy- and bradyarrhythmias in whom taking rate-limiting drugs will limit the tachycardias but exacerbate the bradycardia.

3. Large clinical trials have failed to show that restoring sinus rhythm in atrial fibrillation has prognostic benefit, but there is definitely benefit in anticoagulating patients at risk of stroke or other thromboembolic complications. The key treatment aims are therefore to manage the thromboembolic risk, control rate and control symptoms.

4. Many cardiac arrests are due to ventricular fibrillation or ventricular tachycardia. The only effective treatment is prompt defibrillation. However, most out of hospital cardiac arrests occur in public places and affect those not known to be at risk. Automatic external defibrillators (AEDs) are portable electronic devices which detect and shock ventricular tachycardia/ventricular fibrillation. They are designed to be used by trained first responders and laypeople. In some countries, they are being installed in public areas at great cost and when used appropriately they do save lives. However, the clinical and cost-effectiveness is dependent on placement in areas with a high density of both potential victims and resuscitators.

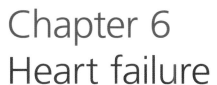

# Chapter 6
# Heart failure

## Starter questions

Answers to the following questions are on page 251.

1. What conditions can mimic heart failure?
2. Can heart failure be reversed?
3. Can any lifestyle changes help the treatment of heart failure?
4. Why do treatments for systolic heart failure not work for diastolic heart failure?
5. Is heart failure a single organ disease?

## Introduction

Heart failure is a combination of symptoms and signs resulting from impairement of the heart's ability to pump blood efficiently. It has a large number of causes. More than a single organ disease, it is a multifaceted syndrome that causes psychological, musculoskeletal, haematological, pulmonary, endocrine, endothelial, renal and hepatic dysfunction.

Diagnosis depends on the presence of symptoms such as dyspnoea and signs such as oedema. Heart failure is classified by:

■ time (acute versus chronic)
■ anatomy (right versus left-sided)
■ physiology (systolic versus diastolic dysfunction)

■ aetiology (ischaemic versus non-ischaemic)
■ genetics (inherited versus acquired)
■ cardiac versus non-cardiac aetiology (low output versus high output)

Non-invasive cardiac imaging modalities (see page 134) such as echocardiography are used to assess the pumping and relaxing properties of the heart. The results of imaging studies are used to calculate the ejection fraction, which gives a measure of the heart's systolic contractile function. The ejection fraction is calculated by dividing the stroke volume (the volume ejected with each heartbeat) by the end-diastolic volume:

$$\text{stroke volume} = \text{end-diastolic volume} - \text{end-systolic volume}$$

$$\text{ejection fraction} = \text{stroke volume} / \text{end-diastolic volume}$$

The ejection fraction is the volume of blood ejected with each heartbeat, expressed as a percentage of the end-diastolic volume.

The ejection fraction is >50% in healthy adults. In patients with heart failure, the ejection fraction is used to divide the condition into two types, which each affect 50% of patients:

- heart failure with reduced ejection fraction (HFREF)
- heart failure with preserved ejection fraction (HFPEF).

## Case 5 Breathlessness at night, ankle swelling and cough

### Presentation

Mr Moxon, aged 65 years, presents to his local emergency department complaining of 6 months of nocturnal breathlessness and cough. He thought he had been experiencing a run of heavy colds. However, he attends the emergency department after his wife noticed that his legs had begun to swell.

### Initial interpretation

Mr Moxon has three common presenting complaints: shortness of breath, leg swelling and cough. Only a few conditions could cause all three simultaneously, such as respiratory, renal or liver failure.

### Shortness of breath

Is the breathlessness new? Is it getting worse? Is it just at night or during the day too? Does it come on with exertion, the cold or heavy meals? How many pillows does he use? Does the cough wake him?

Other information, for example regarding wheeze, chest pain and dizziness, is also relevant when considering differential diagnoses. These include ischaemic heart disease, chronic obstructive pulmonary disease (COPD) and pulmonary embolus.

### Leg swelling

When did this come on? Is it on one or both sides? Did it start after injury or surgery? Has it happened before? How far does it extend up the leg/s, and is it worsening?

Bilateral leg swelling is usually secondary to a systemic process such as drug effects, abdominal mass, obesity or failure of the heart, kidneys or liver. Unilateral leg oedema is usually caused by a local process such as infective cellulitis, deep venous thrombosis or trauma.

### Cough

When does the cough occur? Is it productive? If so, what is the colour and consistency of the sputum?

Possible differential diagnoses include infection, drug side-effect, malignancy and anxiety.

### Patient's agenda

It is important to determine why Mr Moxon has visited the emergency department today. He may be worried that he has something serious. Identifying this involves a discussion of his ideas, concerns and expectations.

**Case 5** *continued*

Paying attention to the patient's agenda is essential in a patient-centred approach and for synchronising their agenda with the clinician's. The ICE mnemonic can be used.

- Ideas: what does the patient think is going on, and why? (For example, they may attribute their cough to lung cancer)
- Concerns: what are the patient's worries, and why? (For example, they may think that without treatment they will die)
- Expectations: what do they want? (For example, reassurance, a diagnosis or a referral)

## History

The illness started 6 months ago with what seemed like a heavy cold. However, this increased in intensity to a cough producing a white froth. Mr Moxon is not short of breath during the day, but he has begun to have difficulty lying flat in bed and wakes up breathless during the night.

He had reassured himself that his illness could not be too serious or involve his heart, because of the absence of chest pain. However, he started to worry when his legs began to swell. Mr Moxon denies any palpitations, fever, weight loss or other symptoms. Mr Moxon's medical history includes:

- myocardial infarction
- coronary artery bypass graft
- hypertension
- hypercholesterolaemia
- type 2 diabetes mellitus

Since his coronary artery bypass graft 5 years ago, he has had no further angina attacks and has not needed to use his glyceryl trinitrate spray.

In terms of family history, Mr Moxon is an only child. His parents are both living; his father, now in his nineties, has dementia, and his mother, in her eighties, is his father's main carer. Mr Moxon is married and has two children, both of whom are well.

The drug history includes aspirin, atenolol, simvastatin, metformin and gliclazide. He is allergic to penicillin. He is a retired bank clerk and does not smoke or drink alcohol.

His systems review is unremarkable.

## Interpretation of history

Mr Moxon has multiple risk factors for heart failure, including ischaemic heart disease, hypertension and diabetes. He is unlikely to have COPD, because he has never smoked nor worked in a dusty environment (e.g. a coal mine).

Despite feeling increasingly unwell, the absence of chest pain had reassured Mr Moxon. This is not uncommon; patients often become preoccupied with one symptom and ignore others. The absence of chest pain suggests that the symptoms are not ischaemic in origin, and this is supported by the lack of symptomatic relief by glyceryl trinitrate. The frothy white sputum strongly suggests the presence of pulmonary oedema.

Symptoms specific to heart failure include:

- paroxysmal nocturnal dyspnoea (waking up breathless during the night)
- orthopnoea (the inability to lay flat because of the resulting breathlessness)

Both symptoms result from gravity redistributing fluid to the lungs when the patient is recumbent causing pulmonary congestion.

## Examination

Mr Moxon has a heart rate of 110 beats/min and a blood pressure of 100/80 mmHg. His jugular venous pressure is raised at 8 cm, and his capillary refill time is 1.5 s. His respiratory rate is 20 breaths/min and oxygen saturation 94% on room air.

**Case 5** *continued*

A laterally displaced apex beat is found on precordial palpation. On auscultation of the chest there are crepitations and reduced air entry at the lung bases but normal heart sounds with no added sounds. Pitting peripheral oedema is present up to the thighs. Mr Moxon is apyrexial. Abdominal examination reveals mild ascites and tender hepatomegaly.

## Interpretation of findings

The tachycardia and hypotension indicate that Mr Moxon has a reduced stroke volume due to impairment of the left ventricular function. The increase in heart rate compensates for the reduction in stroke volume in order to maintain an adequate blood pressure. His jugular venous pressure is abnormally high, a result of right ventricular impairment and elevated central venous pressure. This could be a consequence of left ventricular impairment which elevates pulmonary pressures increasing right ventricular afterload. At present, there is adequate compensation to maintain peripheral tissue perfusion as noted by his normal capillary refill time. The crepitations suggest pulmonary oedema, and the reduced air entry suggests pleural effusions. Left sided heart failure causes increased back pressure in the pulmonary circulation, causing pulmonary oedema. When both ventricles are impaired (biventricular or congestive cardiac failure), the right ventricle cannot clear blood from the systemic venous circulation either. This manifests as peripheral oedema and an elevated jugular venous pressure. It also causes swelling of the liver (hepatomegaly) and ascites.

The displaced apex beat suggests that the left ventricle is dilated which is consistent with heart failure.

## Investigations

The working diagnosis is congestive cardiac failure as a consequence of ischaemic heart disease. A chest X-ray is performed to look for signs of left ventricular failure, and shows pulmonary oedema (**Figure 6.1**). An electrocardiogram to rule out silent myocardial ischaemia shows sinus tachycardia.

Blood tests are performed to rule out other diagnoses such as renal failure or contributing factors such as anaemia. The liver function test results are consistent with hepatic congestion (elevated transaminases, hyperbilirubinaemia and hypoalbuminaemia) but the other results are normal.

## Diagnosis

The symptoms and signs are consistent with a diagnosis of acute-on-chronic HFREF. The likely cause is ischaemic heart disease causing left ventricular systolic dysfunction which has progressed to congestive (biventricular) heart failure.

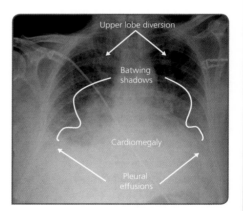

**Figure 6.1** Chest X-ray showing signs of pulmonary oedema. (perihilar, batwing shadows). The increased cardiothoracic ratio (where the cardiac silhouette is >50% of the total width of the lungs) indicates cardiomegaly. Pleural effusions are a common sign but have many non-cardiac causes.

**Case 5** *continued*

Mr Moxon is moved to the coronary care unit for monitoring, intravenous diuretics and echocardiography to investigate the nature and severity of the heart failure.

# Case 6 Breathlessness on exertion, and ankle swelling

## Presentation

Ms Lewis, aged 35 years, presents to her general practitioner (GP) with increasing breathlessness over the past few days. She also mentions that her shoes are becoming tighter and wonders if her ankles have begun to swell.

## Initial interpretation

Both symptoms have multiple potential causes, but together the possibilities are pulmonary embolus (pulmonary hypertension) or renal, hepatic or cardiac failure. It is necessary to ascertain when the symptoms started, how they have progressed and their effects on daily activities, as well as to ask if Ms Lewis has thoughts as to what may be causing her symptoms.

## History

A week ago, Ms Lewis had a flu-like illness and took time off work because of fatigue.

### Diagnosis of heart failure

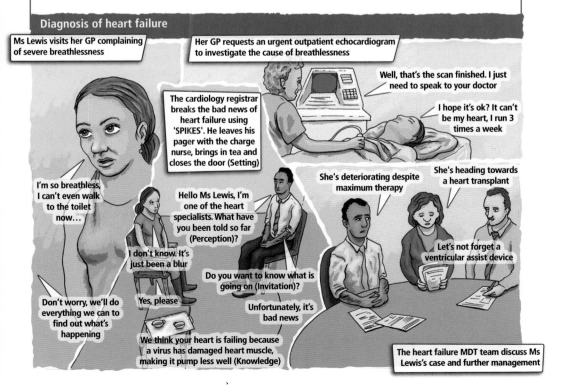

At first, she was just slightly more breathless when running with her dog. However, she is now breathless walking from the kitchen to her living room.

Her other medical history is unremarkable. Her parents, who are in their fifties, and her brother, who is in his thirties, are all fit and well. She takes no regular medications and has no drug allergies.

Ms Lewis does not smoke. Weekly, she drinks two to four glasses of wine and goes running three to five times. She works as a teacher at a primary school and is single.

Nothing unusual is noted in her systems review.

## Interpretation of history

Ms Lewis's dyspnoea is severe and has progressed rapidly to New York Heart Association (NYHA) functional class 3 (**Table 6.3**). She has no risk factors for ischaemic heart disease, but she has had a recent flu-like illness. The short space of time between that illness and the onset of heart failure symptoms makes viral myocarditis a possibility.

There is no family history of any inherited cardiac diseases. Ms Lewis has not travelled recently. She takes no regular medications and does not drink alcohol to excess. Therefore idiopathic dilated cardiomyopathy, pulmonary embolus and drug- or alcohol-induced cardiomyopathy are less likely (see page 330).

As a runner, she is used to breathlessness during exercise, so breathlessness on minimal exertion is concerning. She needs urgent specialist assessment.

## Examination

Ms Lewis's blood pressure is 110/75 mmHg; heart rate, 100 beats/min; temperature, 37°C; and capillary refill time, 3 s. Her apex beat is not palpable. However, her jugular venous pressure is elevated at 9 cm. Her first and second heart sounds are normal, but a 3rd heart sound is heard, as well as bibasal lung crepitations. There is bilateral mild pedal oedema.

## Interpretation of findings

The apex beat is impalpable in half of normal patients, so this finding may not be significant. During auscultaiton of the praecordium, the 3rd heart sound (see page 114) is a result of rapid ventricular filling in the presence of volume overload and is heard at the start of diastole ('lub-dedub'). Dyspnoea is sensitive for, and ankle oedema specific to, heart failure. The presence of tachycardia suggests the heart is not pumping effectively.

There is evidence of both pulmonary and peripheral systemic oedema.

- Pulmonary oedema causes inspiratory crepitations on chest ausculsations and suggests left ventricular failure
- Peripheral oedema is indicative of right sided failure

These findings suggest that both sides of the heart are involved (congestive cardiac failure).

## Investigations

Ms Lewis is referred for an urgent echocardiogram. This shows biventricular dilatation and severe biventricular systolic dysfunction, with a left ventricular ejection fraction of only 15%. Therefore she is admitted by the cardiology team for urgent care.

## Diagnosis

Ms Lewis has acute HFREF which is likely to be a result of viral myocarditis. Ms Lewis is treated acutely with intravenous diuretics, nitrates and non-invasive ventilation.

# Chronic heart failure

Chronic heart failure is a syndrome of clinical features, usually with a gradual onset, due to impairment of the heart's ability to pump blood. To function optimally, the heart must fill and eject blood efficiently; impairing either causes heart failure.

Ventricular contraction impairment causes systolic dysfunction and reduced ejection fraction, known as heart failure with reduced ejection fraction (HFREF). Impairment of ventricular relaxation (filling) causes diastolic impairment, which is known as heart failure with a preserved ejection (HFPEF) and causes 50% of cases.

Heart failure is also categorised according to which side of the heart is affected: right or left. Congestive cardiac failure is when there is evidence of both right and left ventricular dysfunction (biventricular failure).

The American Heart Association-American College for Cardiology classification of heart failure categorises the disease progression (**Table 6.1**).

| Classification of heart failure progression | | |
|---|---|---|
| Stage | Pathophysiology | Description |
| A | High risk without structural heart disease or symptoms | Type 2 diabetes mellitus<br>Hypertension<br>Obesity<br>Ischaemic heart disease<br>Family medical history |
| B | Structural heart disease without signs or symptoms | Left ventricular hypertrophy<br>Previous myocardial infarction<br>Left ventricular systolic dysfunction |
| C | Structural heart disease with current or prior symptoms | Clinical heart failure |
| D | Refractory heart failure requiring specialist intervention | Transplant<br>Organ support<br>Palliation |

**Table 6.1** The American Heart Association–American College of Cardiology classification for the progression of heart failure

## Epidemiology

Heart failure affects 1% of people in Europe. The condition has a 5-year survival rate of 50%; worse than many cancers. It is the most common cause of hospitalisation in the over 65s, and is responsible for over 5% of hospital admissions in the UK.

In the UK, the cost of the management of heart failure accounts for almost 2% of the annual National Health Service budget. Half of patients are readmitted within 6 months, and the average hospital stay is 7 days. Therefore it is unsurprising that chronic heart failure is so costly.

The average age of diagnosis is 76 years. HFREF is more common in men and HFPEF in women.

The **SPIKES** mnemonic is a useful framework for breaking any kind of bad news to a patient:

Setting: ensure the environment is private and comfortable for the patient and minimise interruptions.

Perception: determine what the patient understands about their condition and how much they want to know.

Invitation: ask if the patient wants to know the details of the problem.

Knowledge: give the patient information in clear, concise stages. Check the patient understands what is being said at each stage.

Emotions: identify and respond emphatically to any emotions unearthed by the bad news.

Strategy and summary: conclude and outline the plan of action

## Aetiology

Any significant mechanical, structural or electrical cardiac abnormality can cause heart failure, as can many non-cardiac disorders which increase the physiological demand on the heart, such as haematological, endocrine, inflammatory, infective and malignant disease processes. The most common cause of chronic heart failure is ischaemic heart disease. Causes of heart failure are listed in **Table 6.2**.

HFREF and HFPEF share much of their aetiology. The commonest cause of HFREF is ischaemic heart disease and the most common risk factor for HFPEF is hypertension. Other HFPEF risk factors include diabetes, obesity, age, renal impairment and lung disease.

# Prevention

All cardiac patients should be encouraged to improve their lifestyle. Cardiovascular risk is reduced by smoking cessation, regular exercise and maintaining a healthy weight.

Primary prevention of chronic heart failure comprises early recognition of, and interventions to reduce, cardiovascular risk factors such as type 2 diabetes mellitus, obesity and hypercholesterolaemia. The aim is to reduce the risk of ischaemic heart disease, which causes HFREF, and left ventricular hypertrophy, which leads to HFPEF.

Once ischaemic heart disease or left ventricular hypertrophy manifest, early recognition and intervention are implemented to reduce futher ischaemic injury and prevent adverse remodelling of the myocardium.

# Pathogenesis

Different mechanisms underlie the pathogenesis of heart failure, depending on whether the ejection fraction is reduced or preserved.

## Heart failure with reduced ejection fraction

HFREF is caused by an abnormality of systolic contraction. Myocardial infarction leads to cell death, tissue necrosis and scar formation. Scar tissue does not contribute to the pumping action of the heart, so stroke volume is reduced (left ventricular systolic dysfunction). Furthermore, at rest the cardiac muscle does not have an optimal length–tension relationship, because of the Frank–Starling law (**Figure 6.2;** see page 50).

Increasing venous return increases preload, which in turn stretches the myocardium. Myocardial stretching increases the number of actin–myosin interactions, which increases end-diastolic volume and thus stroke volume. However, after a certain point, increasing venous return serves only to pathologically overstretch the myocardium beyond its optimum length–tension relationship, which reduces its contractile force. In heart failure the raised pulmonary and systemic venous pressure contribute to this pathological over-stretching.

## Heart failure with preserved ejection fraction

HFPEF is caused by an abnormality of myocardial relaxation. Chronically increased

| Causes of heart failure | | | |
|---|---|---|---|
| Cause | Example | Ventricle | Incidence |
| Coronary artery disease | Myocardial infarction | Left >right | Common |
| Arrhythmia | Atrial fibrillation | Both | Common |
| Valvular dysfunction | Mitral regurgitation | Left >right | Common |
| Lifestyle | Obesity | Left >right | Common |
| Pulmonary disease | Pulmonary embolus | Right | Intermediate |
| Idiopathic | Dilated cardiomyopathy | Both | Intermediate |
| Infective | Viral myocarditis | Both | Rare |
| Infiltrative diseases | Amyloidosis | Both | Rare |
| Autoimmune disease | Hyperthyroidism | Both | Rare |
| Inherited/ congenital | Atrial septal defect | Left/ right/ both* | Rare |
| Adverse drug effect | Bleomycin chemotherapy | Both | Rare |
| Physiological state | Post-partum cardiomyopathy | Both | Rare |

*Depending on specific abnormality. Common = 30-50% of cases, intermediate 10–30%, rare <10%.

**Table 6.2** Causes of heart failure: examples, predominant ventricle affected and incidence.

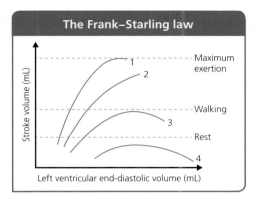

**Figure 6.2** The Frank–Starling law. ①, normal during exercise; ②, normal at rest; ③, heart failure; ④ cardiogenic shock. In healthy individuals (1 and 2) this shows the contractile force of the heart (stroke volume) responds to increases in venous return (end-diastolic volume). This does not occur adequately in patients with heart failure (3 and 4).

left ventricular afterload as a consequence of hypertension leads to compensatory left ventricular hypertrophy. The hypertrophy creates a thick ventricular wall and a small ventricular cavity. Furthermore, increased stiffness and reduced compliance mean that the left ventricular myocardium fails to relax during diastole (left ventricular diastolic dysfunction).

There may also be an active process of myocardial fibrosis caused by subclinical microvascular ischaemia. This process results in increased left ventricular end-diastolic pressure, inadequate filling of the ventricle, and reduced stroke volume (and therefore cardiac output). This is significant, because about 70% of ventricular filling occurs passively during ventricular diastole.

## Compensation

Both HFREF and HFPEF reduce cardiac output (**Figure 6.3**). This effect leads to up-regulation of the sympathetic nervous system and the renin–angiotensin–aldosterone system. Up-regulation of these systems increases cardiac output, total peripheral resistance, and blood pressure and thus maintains tissue perfusion. These changes first serve to augment the function of the failing heart, but eventually they hasten its decline (**Figure 6.4).**

## Clinical features

The clinical features of chronic heart failure reflect the pathophysiological changes (**Figure 6.5** and **Table 6.4**). Symptoms include:

- ankle swelling
- lightheadedness
- lethargy
- weight loss
- low mood

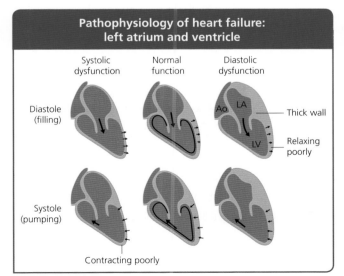

**Figure 6.3** Heart failure pathophysiology in the left atrium and ventricle: difference between systolic and diastolic dysfunction. In systolic dysfunction (HFREF) there is reduced contraction of the heart during systole and in diastolic dysfunction (HFPEF) there is reduced relaxation of the heart during diastole, both lead to reduced stroke volume. Ao, aorta; LA, left atrium; LV, left ventricle.

## Pathophysiology of heart failure

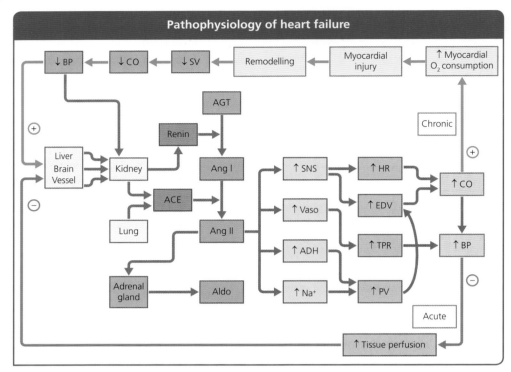

**Figure 6.4** Pathophysiology of heart failure. ACE, angiotensin-converting enzyme; ADH, antidiuretic hormone; AGT, angiotensinogen; Aldo, aldosterone; Ang I, angiotensin I; Ang II, angiotensin II; BP, blood pressure; CO, cardiac output; EDV, end-diastolic volume; HR, heart rate; PV, plasma volume; SNS, sympathetic nervous system; SV, stroke volume; TPR, total peripheral resistance; Vaso, vasoconstriction.

Right and left-sided heart failure differ in their presentation (**Table 6.5**):

- Right-sided heart failure: failure to clear blood returning from the systemic circulation. The rise in systemic venous pressure causes peripheral oedema and elevated the jugular venous pressure
- Left-sided heart failure: increased pressure in the left atrium and the pulmonary circulation. This causes pulmonary congestion with dyspnoea, orthopnoea and paroxysmal nocturnal dyspnoea

There may also be symptoms and signs that identify the underlying cause. Many of these features are non-specific and common making it difficult to differentiate heart failure from other causes of dyspnoea.

The NYHA classification of heart failure grades the severity of breathlessness experienced by the patient during physical activity, from I (no limitation) to IV (breathless at rest) (**Table 6.3**).

### NYHA classification of heart failure

| Class | Symptoms | Example |
|---|---|---|
| I | None | Normal activity |
| II | Mild | Breathless on incline |
| III | Moderate | Comfortable at rest |
| IV | Severe | Breathless at rest |

**Table 6.3** New York Heart Association functional classification of heart failure

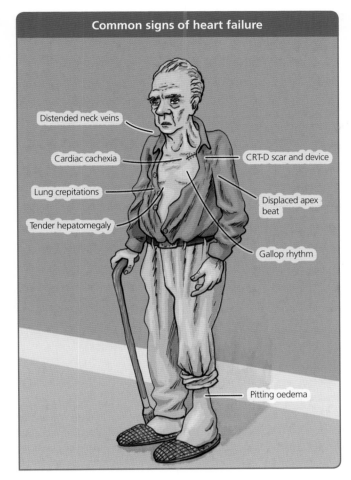

**Figure 6.5** Common signs of heart failure.

Common signs of heart failure

- Distended neck veins
- Cardiac cachexia
- Lung crepitations
- Tender hepatomegaly
- CRT-D scar and device
- Displaced apex beat
- Gallop rhythm
- Pitting oedema

**Pulmonary oedema does not always indicate cardiac disease.** Non-cardiogenic causes include high altitude, (a result of acute pulmonary hypertension) decreased plasma oncotic pressure (a result of low albumin) and increased alveolar capillary permeability (e.g. acute respiratory distress syndrome).

## Diagnostic approach

Heart failure is diagnosed using the history and examination findings. It is not a definitive diagnosis; the underlying aetiology, risk factors and aggravating factors need to be identified and treated where possible.

## Investigations

All patients require ECG, chest X-ray, blood tests and echocardiography. Investigations are used to support the diagnosis, determine underlying aetiology and guide prognosis.

### Electrocardiography

Common abnormalities include:

- evidence of ischaemic heart disease; Q waves, T wave inversion, bundle branch block
- left ventricular hypertrophy; especially in HFPEF
- prolonged QRS duration (bundle branch block); as a marker of prognosis
- rhythm abnormalities; atrial fibrillation, paroxysmal ventricular arrhythmias

## Symptoms and signs of heart failure

| Symptom | Sensitivity (%) | Specificity (%) |
|---|---|---|
| Orthopnoea | 21 | 81 |
| Oedema | 23 | 80 |
| Paroxysmal nocturnal dyspnoea | 33 | 76 |
| Dyspnoea | 66 | 52 |
| Signs | Sensitivity (%) | Specificity (%) |
| Tachycardia | 7 | 99 |
| Raised jugular venous pressure | 10 | 97 |
| Third heart sound | 31 | 95 |
| Peripheral oedema | 10 | 93 |
| Crepitations | 13 | 91 |

**Table 6.4** Symptoms and signs of heart failure. Sensitivity is the ability to identify a condition correctly and specificity the ability to exclude a condition correctly.
Adapted from Harlan WR, et al. Chronic congestive heart failure in coronary artery disease: clinical criteria. Ann Intern Med 1977; 86:133–138.

## Chest X-ray signs of heart failure

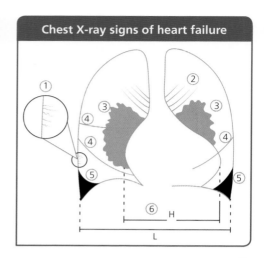

**Figure 6.6** Chest X-ray features of heart failure: ① Kerley B lines ② upper lobe venous diversion ③ ill-defined peri-hilar (batswings) shadowing ④ fluid in the oblique and horizontal fissures ⑤ pleural effusions ⑥ increased cardiothoracic ratio, where the width of the heart shadow (H) is >50% of the width of the lung fields (L).

## Right and left-sided heart failure

| Symptom or sign | Right-sided heart failure | Left-sided heart failure |
|---|---|---|
| Peripheral oedema | Prominent | Not prominent |
| Oedema | Systemic | Pulmonary |
| Organomegaly | Liver | Cardiac |
| Raised jugular venous pressure | Prominent | Not prominent |
| Dyspnoea | Not prominent | Prominent |
| Gastrointestinal | Prominent | Not prominent |

**Table 6.5** Symptoms and signs of right-sided and left-sided heart failure

A normal ECG makes the diagnosis of heart failure unlikely.

## Chest X-ray

Signs of heart failure are visible (**Figures 6.1** and **6.6**). These findings can also support a diagnosis such as pulmonary fibrosis or COPD.

## Blood tests

Blood tests are performed for a variety of reasons such as assessing severity and ruling out other causes (**Table 6.6**). For example, concentrations BNP increase with the severity of heart failure and fall with successful treatment, while anaemia is an alternative cause of dyspnoea.

## Echocardiography

Transthoracic echocardiography should be performed as soon as heart failure is suspected to:

- measure the ejection fraction to distinguish HFREF from HFPEF
- assess for valve disease
- measure chamber dimensions
- identify left ventricular hypertrophy

## Other tests

Other tests useful in assessing heart failure include:

- 6 minute walk test; used to objectively assess functional capacity and monitor

| Blood tests used in heart failure | |
|---|---|
| Blood test | Purpose |
| Full blood count | Anaemia causes high-output heart failure |
| Urea and electrolytes | Assess renal function |
| Liver function tests | Abnormalities reflect congestion (right-sided failure) |
| Thyroid function tests | Check for hypo-/hyperthyroidism |
| Lipids | Hyperlipidaemia causes ischaemic heart disease |
| Glucose | Check for diabetes |
| Natriuretic peptides | BNP elevated in heart failure |

**Table 6.6** Common blood tests used in the diagnosis and assessment of heart failure

response to therapy
- Cardiopulmonary exercise testing; used to assess exercise capacity and predict outcome in patients with heart failure, it asses the pulmonary, cardiovascular and skeletal muscle systems in combination and is used in those being considered for heart transplantation.
- Coronary angiography; used to diagnose coronary artery disease, the commonest cause of HFREF
- Cardiac MRI; high resolution functional imaging modality used to assess ventricular volumes and wall thickness, cardiac chamber dimensions, ventricular systolic function and demonstrate myocardial ischaemia. It may also support the cause of heart failure by revealing myocardial scar location or infiltrative disease.

> **Echocardiograms that show normal systolic function do not exclude heart failure.** Patients with normal systolic function can still have severe valve disease, severe diastolic dysfunction, pericardial disease or high output heart failure.

## Management

A heart failure management plan should be agreed with a heart failure team, including a cardiologist and specialist nurse. The major aims of management are to:

- treat the underlying cause
- improve prognosis
- improve quality of life
- reduce symptoms
- reduce aggravating factors

This is achieved by a combination of lifestyle modifications, pharmacological and device therapy.

### Lifestyle modification

All patients should be encouraged to improve their lifestyle. This includes:

- Exercise: in stable patients regular, structured, aerobic exercise is safe. This improves functional capacity and quality of life, and reduces morbidity and hospitalisation. This is best achieved through a tailored rehabilitation programme which offers education and psychological support
- Alcohol: abstinence is vital in alcohol-related cardiomyopathy and all patients should drink in moderation
- Smoking: all patients should stop smoking
- Salt and water restriction: useful in advanced heart failure. Typical targets are <1.5 L/day of fluid and <6 g/day of salt
- Vaccination: against influenza (annually) and pneumococcus (once only)
- Driving: patients should be aware of the legal driving restrictions, especially those with large goods or passenger carrying licenses (see page 318)

### Pharmacological management

Pharmacological management aims to improve prognosis, reduce symptoms and target the underlying cause. Treatments that improve prognosis antagonise the pathogenic neurohumoral responses activated in HFREF, i.e. drugs that antagonise the renin-angiotensin-aldosterone and sympathetic nervous systems.

#### HFPEF

There are currently no treatments that improve prognosis in HFPEF. Treating the underlying cause involves aggressive management of hypertension, tight diabetes control, weight reduction and lipid control. Symptomatic control involves diuretics to reduce fluid retention and beta-blockers to reduce heart rate and increase diastole.

### HFREF

First-line therapy for all patients with HFREF is beta-blockers and an ACE inhibitor. In the long-term patients are monitored and have their medication monitored by their local doctor (see page 365).

### Symptomatic management

Thiazide and loop diuretics are used in all symptomatic stages of heart failure to relieve symptoms of fluid retention and congestion, with their doses titrated according to symptom severity. Dosing increments should be monitored for deterioration in renal function or electrolyte derangement. Digoxin is used to control ventricular rate in patients with atrial fibrillations and for symptom relief in advanced heart failure with severe symptoms. Some calcium channel blockers (e.g. amlodipine) are used to control blood pressure but negatively inotropic agents such as diltiazem and verapamil are avoided.

> Depression is three times more common in patients with heart failure and correlates with disease severity and a significantly reduced quality of life.
>
> Patients often do not volunteer information leading to a diagnosis of depression so physicians need to be aware so that the condition can be treated.

> In severe systolic heart failure, contrast imaging of the ventricle can show sluggish blood movement; this phenomenon is called 'spontaneous contrast'. This may seem like an indication to prescribe anticoagulants to prevent clotting. However, there is no evidence to support their routine use in heart failure in patients with normal sinus rhythm.

### Devices

Over the past decade, advances in implantable devices have improved the prognosis for some patients with heart failure. These devices include cardiac resynchronisation therapy and implantable cardioverter defibrillators. However, they are reserved for specific HFREF patients with evidence of ventricular dyssynchrony or who are at increased risk of life-threatening ventricular arrhythmias (see page 164).

## Surgery

Valve repair or replacement surgery is considered in patients with significant primary valve disease and coronary artery bypass graft surgery in those with severe or multi-vessel ischaemic heart disease. Patients who are markedly symptomatic despite maximal medical therapy, such as those with NYHA class 3 or 4 heart failure, are also considered for surgery. Surgery may include:

- mitral valve repair for mitral regurgitation
- left ventricular restoration
- insertion of a left ventricular assist device (**Figure 6.7**)
- heart transplant

Heart transplant is the gold standard treatment in chronic heart failure and the only curative option. It is contraindicated in the elderly, those with renal failure, irreversible

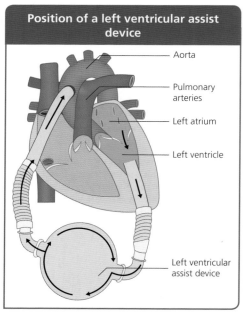

**Position of a left ventricular assist device**

- Aorta
- Pulmonary arteries
- Left atrium
- Left ventricle
- Left ventricular assist device

**Figure 6.7** A left ventricular assist device in situ.

pulmonary arterial hypertension and other non-cardiac severe disease.

## Prognosis

Heart failure has a poor prognosis that is worse than many cancers. Around 35% of patients with a new heart failure diagnosis will die within 12 months with a further 10% mortality in subsequent years. Around half will die within 5 years of diagnosis. Patients who are severely symptomatic with a poor prognosis can be offered palliative care (see page 368).

# Acute heart failure

Acute heart failure is a sudden onset of symptoms and signs as a result of impaired cardiac function.

## Epidemiology

Patients are typically in their mid seventies. Around 30% present with no history of cardiac dysfunction. Two thirds of patients are known to have ischaemic heart disease, and one third have diabetes, chronic kidney disease, COPD or atrial fibrillation.

## Aetiology

Acute heart failure occurs in two ways:

1. It develops suddenly (de novo heart failure), e.g. myocardial infarction, acute valvular dysfunction, arrhythmia, cardiac tamponade
2. As a result of chronic heart failure (acute-on-chronic heart failure) when the mechanisms maintaining cardiac output become overwhelmed. Causes include: negatively inotropic drugs, poor adherence to medication, significant illness (e.g. intercurrent infection, anaemia, thyrotoxicosis) and thyroid dysfunction

## Prevention

Hospital admission can be prevented through multiple measures, which include:

- frequent monitoring of disease progression
- encouraging medication adherence
- detecting and treating arrhythmia as early as possible
- managing intercurrent illnesses (e.g. pneumonia) aggressively and involving appropriate specialists in the management

of common comorbidities (e.g. chronic kidney disease)

## Clinical features

Patients present with fatigue, oedema, cough and breathlessness with significant orthopneoa (the most severe symptom). Clinical signs include tachycardia, increased respiratory rate, hypertension (**Table 6.7**) and a third heart sound (gallop rhythm). Severe presentations are usually secondary to predominantly left-sided failure causing pulmonary oedema which causes reduced oxygen saturations and inspiratory crepitations on chest auscultation. Patients often have signs of right-sided decompensation including elevated jugular venous pressure and peripheral oedema. It is important to elicit signs reflecting fluid status and tissue

| Blood pressure in acute severe *de novo* heart failure | | |
|---|---|---|
| Blood pressure | Prevalence (% of cases) | Signs |
| High (> 150 mmHg) | 50 | Symptoms with abrupt onset (hours or days) |
| Normal (120–149 mmHg) | 40 | Symptoms with gradual onset (days or weeks) |
| Low (91–119 mmHg) | 9 | Hypoperfusion |
| Very low (< 90 mmHg) | 1 | Cardiogenic shock |

**Table 6.7** Blood pressure in patients with acute severe *de novo* heart failure

perfusion because these guide treatment (**Table 6.8**).

ECG changes are non-specific (typically tachycardic), but chest X-rays demonstrate signs of pulmonary oedema. An urgent echocardiogram is considered in all patients, especially in those with new-onset heart failure to help identify the cause.

> **Cardiogenic shock occurs when the heart is unable to pump enough blood for the body's most basic physiological needs.** It is defined as systolic blood pressure < 90 mmHg in the presence of one of the following low urine output, poor peripheral perfusion, confusion or serum lactate > 2.0 mmol/L.

> **Hippocrates (c.400 BC) was the first person to describe heart failure.** He noted how the 'flesh is consumed and becomes water ... the feet and legs swell; the thighs melt away.' This text also describes the 'cardiac cachexia' of chronic heart failure: the loss of muscle, fat and bony mass as a result of a combination of chronic inflammation, deconditioning, chronic breathlessness and a catabolic state.

## Management

Haemodynamic state and clinical stage determine therapy (**Table 6.8**).

The patient is moved to an appropriate place, such as a coronary care unit or high-dependency unit. Initial management includes drugs that reduce the cardiac preload and afterload by inducing vasodilation and pulmonary capillary pressure:

- an intravenous loop diuretic to remove excess fluid
- intravenous morphine to reduce stress and to venodilate
- intravenous glyceryl trinitrate to vasodilate and to accommodate excess fluid
- cessation of administration of inappropriate drugs (e.g. NSAIDs)
- inotropes to augment cardiac output when a reversible cause of cardiogenic shock is identified

| Management of acute heart failure | |
|---|---|
| Haemodynamic state | Treatment |
| Wet and cold | Vasodilators and additional diuretics |
| Wet and warm | Diuretics and additional vasodilators |
| Cold and dry | Ionotropes and intra-aortic balloon pump |
| Warm and dry | The aim for all patients with heart failure |

**Table 6.8** Treatment of patients with acute heart failure in various haemodynamic and clinical states Wet, signs of fluid overload. Dry, absence of these. Cold, signs of reduced tissue perfusion. Warm, absence of these.

Initial non-pharmacological management includes:

- sit patient upright to improve ventilation-perfusion matching
- oxygen if patient is hypoxic (saturation <94%)
- stop intravenous fluids (except in acute right ventricular failure)
- non-invasive ventilation with continuous positive airways pressure (CPAP) in patients with pulmonary oedema and significant dyspnoea and hypoxia
- monitoring urea, electrolyte, urine output and daily patient weights (i.e. fluid balance)
- restrict fluid intake is restricted to 1.5 L/day
- invasive ventilation is patients with respiratory failure who fail to improve with treatment

Once a patient has stabilised, they should be commenced on chronic heart failure therapy. However, if these drugs are started too early, they can cause rapid deterioration of cardiac and renal function.

> **Oxygen is not given to patients with normal oxygen saturation (94–98%).** There is no evidence to support such treatment, despite it seeming like common sense that all breathless patients need oxygen.

# Answers to starter questions

1. Heart failure can be mimicked by conditions that cause symptoms of breathlessness, fatigue or oedema, such as ischaemic heart disease, chronic obstructive pulmonary disease, pulmonary embolus, malignancy, renal and liver failure. Sometimes they co-exist. A thorough history and examination helps to differentiate the cause, e.g. fever, recent travel, unilateral leg swelling, weight loss, haemoptysis and jaundice are all unlikely in heart failure.

2. In rare cases, heart failure is reversible. Certain insults such as tachycardia, alcohol and cytotoxic drugs (e.g. Herceptin) can lead to a nonischaemic dilated cardiomyopathy. If the tachycardia is treated, the alcohol intake reduced or cytotoxic drugs stopped, then this can lead to stabilisation, or improvement, of ventricular systolic function over weeks to months. This reinforces the concept that heart failure is a syndrome and that its cause must be identified and treated.

3. Certain lifestyle changes can help treat heart failure. Regular exercise helps prevent loss of skeletal muscle mass and function which can improve symptoms and quality of life. In more advanced disease, salt and water restriction help to reduce fluid overload. Strict control of risk factors such as smoking cessation and reducing alcohol consumption can prevent further deterioration in cardiac function. In patients with alcohol induced cardiomyopathy, 50% have normalisation of cardiac function following alcohol cessation. Halving salt intake reduces hospital readmission rates and delays deterioration in symptoms. Risk of mortality is reduced in those who undergo two months of a structured, tailored exercise program.

4. Drugs used for systolic heart failure (HFREF) do not have a similar efficacy in patients with diastolic heart failure (HFPEF) because the underlying processes behind each syndrome are different. For example, left ventricular hypertrophy, microvascular ischaemia and fibrosis cause diastolic heart failure whereas macrovascular ischaemia, infarction, scarring and fibrosis cause systolic heart failure. This suggests that new classes of drugs for diastolic heart failure are needed. Potential mechanisms to target include those that improve myocardial relaxation, reduce the burden of fibrosis or lead to regression of myocardial hypertrophy.

5. Heart failure is not a single organ disease but rather a multifaceted syndrome that can lead to dysfunction of the vascular endothelium and thyroid gland, vitamin D deficiency, secondary hyperparathyroidism, reduction in slow-twitch skeletal muscle fibres, elevated C-reactive protein and uric acid, proteinuria and disruption to haematopoiesis. It is important to be mindful of these systemic effects, how they impact on patients' symptoms and how they can lead to misdiagnosis during routine investigations.

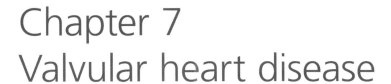

# Chapter 7
# Valvular heart disease

## Starter questions

Answers to the following questions are on page 282–283.

1. How is valve disease treated?
2. What can go wrong after valve replacement surgery?
3. What patient factors influence valve replacement surgery?
4. Why should patients being considered for valve surgery undergo a left heart catheter study?
5. What are the consequences of right and left sided valve disease?
6. Does a normal transthoracic echocardiogram exclude endocarditis?

# Introduction

In valvular heart disease, the cardiac valves become:

- stenosed (stiffened, leading to restricted forward flow through the narrowed valve orifice)
- regurgitant (leaky, allowing reverse flow)
- both stenosed and regurgitant

The most common major valve problem is aortic stenosis. It is closely followed by mitral regurgitation.

The long-term consequence of untreated left-sided valve disease is left ventricular dysfunction, pulmonary arterial hypertension or both.

Historically, rheumatic fever was the leading cause of valve disease worldwide. It remains the leading cause in low- and middle-income countries. However, in high-income countries age-related degeneration is now responsible for most cases of valve disease.

Over 10% of people aged 70 years or older are affected by valve disease. This compares with less than 1% of those younger than 40 years.

Surgical valve repair or replacement is the only definitive treatment for a stenosed or regurgitant valve. However, judging the optimal timing for surgery is challenging. If the intervention is left too late, irreversible heart failure and pulmonary arterial hypertension result. On the other hand, surgery carries risks, and prosthetic valves may fail in time, so intervening too early increases the likelihood of the need for redo surgery.

Infective endocarditis damages the structure, integrity and function of cardiac valves. Without adequate, early antibiotic treatment, it is a devastating and rapidly fatal illness.

# Case 7 Chest pain on exertion

## Presentation

Mr Vivek Singh, a 72-year-old retired steelworker, is seen in the chest pain clinic. He gives a 4-month history of slowly progressive chest discomfort and breathlessness. His symptoms always accompany exertion and have not occurred at rest. He is a non-smoker, has type 2 diabetes mellitus and has no personal or family history of coronary artery disease.

## Initial interpretation

In the context of Mr Singh's age, gender and diabetic history, his symptoms of exertional chest discomfort and breathlessness strongly suggest coronary artery disease. At this point, without any additional information, this is the most likely diagnosis. Other possible diagnoses include a primary lung disorder, aortic stenosis, a musculoskeletal chest wall problem or anxiety (see page 87 for causes of chest pain).

## Further history

Mr Singh describes the discomfort as a 'heaviness' in the centre of his chest. Light work is still possible, but he is no longer able to do anything heavy in his garden. The discomfort does not radiate anywhere else, and it resolves at rest.

His blood pressure is measured every year or so, and he remarks that his general practitioner has commented that it has been 'slightly low if anything'. The referral letter mentions a heart murmur. On further questioning, Mr Singh reports having had similar symptoms for well over a year, but they have become much worse over the past 4 months.

## Examination

Mr Singh has a regular heart rate of 80 beats/min, and his blood pressure is 107/86 mmHg. The upstroke of his carotid pulse is slow. His jugular venous pressure is not visible while he reclines at 45°. He has a left ventricular heave. His second heart sound is quiet in the aortic area.

A loud ejection systolic murmur is heard across the precordium and radiates into the carotid arteries. A less obvious decrescendo diastolic murmur is heard at the left sternal edge when Mr Singh sits forwards. His breath sounds are vesicular, and his chest is otherwise clear. No peripheral oedema is present.

## Interpretation of findings

Mr Singh has a narrow pulse pressure and a slow rising pulse, both of which are signs of aortic stenosis. This possibility is supported by the left ventricular heave and the nature of the ejection systolic murmur.

The diastolic murmur is consistent with some degree of aortic regurgitation. Aortic regurgitation commonly coexists with aortic stenosis. However, in the absence of any other specific signs, the regurgitation appears to be of secondary importance to the stenosis.

## Case 7 continued

Coronary artery disease remains possible. However, the physical findings mean that aortic stenosis is the most likely underlying problem.

> **Not all ejection systolic murmurs indicate aortic stenosis.** Aortic valve sclerosis (calcific thickening of mobile valve leaflets) can cause a harsh-sounding murmur in the absence of significant stenosis. Pulmonary stenosis also gives rise to an ejection systolic murmur but this is rare.

## Investigations

Mr Singh's blood tests and chest X-ray are unremarkable. His electrocardiogram (ECG) shows sinus rhythm but meets the criteria for left ventricular hypertrophy.

His echocardiogram confirms mild left ventricular hypertrophy (**Figure 7.2**), mild left ventricular dilatation but with good systolic function. The aortic valve is trileafleted but heavily calcified, and the leaflets appear immobile. The transvalvular velocity is 4.93 m/s and the peak pressure gradient (the difference between left ventricular and aortic pressure) is 97 mmHg, suggesting severe aortic stenosis (**Figure 7.2**). There is also a mild jet of aortic regurgitation.

## Diagnosis

Mr Singh has symptomatic severe aortic stenosis. The mild aortic regurgitation is of little importance. The left ventricular function is preserved, but it is worrying that the left ventricle has started to dilate.

Mr Singh is then referred for a coronary angiogram (to identify coexisting coronary artery disease) and to the cardiac surgeons for consideration for aortic valve replacement. This procedure will be with or without coronary bypass surgery, depending on the results of angiography.

# Case 8  Flu-like symptoms

## Presentation

Mrs Renata Capello, a 28-year-old mature student, presents to the emergency department with a 7-day history of cold sweats, muscle aches and pains, and lack of energy. She had taken her own temperature, which had reached 38°C. She was previously fit and well. Her only medical history is an 'innocent' heart murmur she has had since childhood.

## Initial interpretation

Mrs Capello describes the typical symptoms of a fever. Her symptoms are non-specific. She is diagnosed with a viral illness, given advice, reassured and allowed home.

## History

Mrs Capello re-presents 72 h later, her condition having deteriorated. She is hardly eating anything. The cold sweats are much worse at night. She wakes up drenched and has to change her bedclothes. She says that she has never felt as ill as this, and is particularly worried because she has recently developed unsteadiness when she walks. She appears to be slurring her words slightly.

**Case 8** *continued*

## Interpretation of history

The duration of the illness and marked deterioration go against influenza. The drenching night sweats and general malaise imply that a significant infective illness is likely. The unsteadiness and dysarthria indicate a neurological deficit, specifically a cerebellar lesion. The acute nature of this development suggests a vascular cause.

The combination of fever and neurological deficit mean that a central nervous system infection needs to be considered; examples are abscess, meningitis and encephalitis. However, infective endocarditis is also a concern, because the acute neurological deficit may indicate that a vegetation (an infected mass attached to the valve) has embolised to the brain.

## Further history

Mrs Capello denies any neck stiffness, photophobia or headache. Therefore meningitis, intracranial abscess and encephalitis are unlikely. She has had no recent foreign travel and has not injected any drugs. She now remembers that about 4 weeks ago she had a tooth removed by her dentist.

She knows little about her heart murmur. Her mother told her she had had it since childhood, and that the family physician had reassured them.

## Examination

She is cool and clammy to touch, and is febrile. From observation from the end of the bed, she looks ill and weak. She has splinter haemorrhages under her fingernails and has enlarged, tender cervical

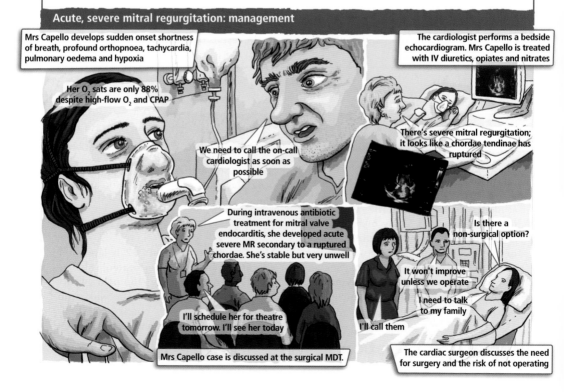

Acute, severe mitral regurgitation: management

Mrs Capello develops sudden onset shortness of breath, profound orthopnoea, tachycardia, pulmonary oedema and hypoxia

Her O₂ sats are only 88% despite high-flow O₂ and CPAP

We need to call the on-call cardiologist as soon as possible

The cardiologist performs a bedside echocardiogram. Mrs Capello is treated with IV diuretics, opiates and nitrates

There's severe mitral regurgitation; it looks like a chordae tendinae has ruptured

During intravenous antibiotic treatment for mitral valve endocarditis, she developed acute severe MR secondary to a ruptured chordae. She's stable but very unwell

Is there a non-surgical option?

It won't improve unless we operate

I need to talk to my family

I'll schedule her for theatre tomorrow. I'll see her today

I'll call them

Mrs Capello case is discussed at the surgical MDT.

The cardiac surgeon discusses the need for surgery and the risk of not operating

lymph nodes. She has tachycardia at a rate of 115 beats/min, and her blood pressure is 105/68 mmHg.

Jugular venous pressure is not elevated. She has a mid-systolic murmur that radiates into her left axilla; it is louder on expiration than on inspiration. She has bibasal inspiratory crepitations and is dyspnoeic.

Neurological examination confirms dysarthria and right-sided ataxia (intention tremor, past-pointing and impairment of rapid, alternating movements, i.e. dysdiadochokinesis). Mrs Capello falls to the right when she tries to walk.

# Interpretation of findings

The fever and tender lymphadenopathy imply an underlying infective illness. Splinter haemorrhages can be secondary to trauma. However, this is unlikely considering Mrs Capello's occupation and lifestyle.

The nature, timing and radiation of the murmur are consistent with mitral valve prolapse and mitral regurgitation. Bibasal crepitations and breathlessness suggest that she has developed heart failure with pulmonary congestion. The focal neurological deficit implies cerebellar stroke and, given the context, septic embolisation is likely.

In summary, she has signs and symptoms of infection, splinter haemorrhages, a cardiac murmur and a recent history of dental surgery. Bacterial infective endocarditis is now at the top of the differential diagnosis list. Tachycardia, hypotension and focal neurological deficit point to advanced disease complicated by heart failure and embolisation.

# Investigations

Chest X-ray shows pulmonary congestion, and ECG reveals sinus tachycardia with bifid P waves. White cell count is increased (neutrophils, $18 \times 10^9$/L), C-reactive protein is 124 mg/L and erythrocyte sedimentation rate is 65 mm/h. The rest of the blood tests are unremarkable.

A urine dipstick test is positive for blood and protein, and a urine sample is sent for microscopy, culture and sensitivity. Three paired blood culture samples have already been sent to the microbiology laboratory.

The on-call cardiologist carries out echocardiography. The echocardiogram shows anterior mitral valve leaflet prolapse and a moderate, posteriorly directed regurgitation jet with a 0.9-cm vegetation on the mitral valve. The left atrium is dilated. Computerised tomography of the head confirms right cerebellar infarction.

# Diagnosis

Mrs Capello has infective endocarditis. Formal diagnosis is made according to the Duke criteria (see page 280). Identification of the causative organism through the blood culture results would help guide treatment.

Mitral valve prolapse is often a benign condition. However, in this case it appears to have provided the focus for infection. The precipitating event was probably the recent dental surgery.

Intravenous antibiotics and specialist care on the cardiology unit are required. Furthermore, transoesophageal echocardiography is necessary to further assess the mitral valve. The case should be discussed with the cardiac surgeons as soon as possible, with a view to mitral valve surgery.

Mrs Capello is treated with intravenous antibiotics as an inpatient on the coronary care unit. 36 hours later she deteriorates suddenly. She develops tachypnoea, profound orthopnoea, tachycardia, pulmonary oedema and hypoxia. She is seen by the on-call cardiology doctor who performs

**Case 8** *continued*

a bedside echocardiogram which shows torrential mitral regurgitation (worse than before) secondary to a ruptured chordae tendinae (a consequence of the endocarditis). She is treated with continuous positive airway pressure (CPAP), intravenous diuretic, nitrate and opiates. Her condition stabilises. Her case is urgently discussed by the cardiothoracic surgical multi-disciplinary team and the surgeons schedule her for emergency valve surgery.

# Aortic valve disease

In aortic valve disease the aortic valve becomes stenosed, regurgitant or both. It also affects the function of the left ventricle and the pulmonary circulation.

## Aortic stenosis

Aortic stenosis occurs when the aortic valve orifice is narrowed, obstructing forward blood flow through the valve during systole. The normal aortic valve is trileafleted, with an orifice area of 3–4 cm$^2$ (adjusted for body surface area).

Aortic stenosis usually remains asymptomatic until the valve area is reduced to < 1.5 cm$^2$. Before that happens, the only sign of disease may be a murmur.

## Types

Aortic stenosis is categorised according to cause and severity. Although clinical history and physical examination provide important information, the most objective method of determining severity is echocardiography.

Valve lesions are categorised into mild, moderate or severe according to clinical and echocardiographic findings. 'Trivial' changes are considered non-significant. It is useful to be aware of the key markers of severe disease. **Table 7.1** outlines the clinical and echocardiographic markers of severe valve disease.

## Epidemiology

Aortic stenosis is the commonest significant valve lesion in high-income countries. Its prevalence continues to rise in line with the ageing of the population. Degenerative aortic stenosis affects about 2% of people aged > 65 years, 3% of those aged > 75 years and 4% of those aged > 85 years.

## Aetiology

Aortic stenosis may be idiopathic (cause unknown) or have a specific cause.

- Age-related degenerative aortic stenosis usually manifests from the 6th or 7th decade (**Figure 7.1**). Age is the most significant risk factor, but others include smoking, hypercholesterolaemia, diabetes mellitus, hypertension and renal impairment.
- Congenital bicuspid aortic valve is common and accounts for about half of surgical aortic stenosis cases. Bicuspid aortic valve affects about 1–2% of the general population, and men are twice as likely as women to have the condition. Bicuspid aortic valve usually presents from the 5th decade of life.
- Rheumatic aortic valve disease is increasingly rare in high-income countries, but it is common in low- and middle-income countries and people who have migrated from them. The mitral valve is coaffected in almost all cases.

| Markers of severe aortic and mitral valve disease | | |
|---|---|---|
| Lesion | Clinical markers | Echocardiographic markers |
| Aortic stenosis | Slow rising pulse | Valve area $< 1$ $cm^2$ |
| | Narrow pulse pressure | Peak transvalvular velocity $> 4$ m/s |
| | Left ventricular heave | Mean pressure gradient $> 40$ mmHg |
| | Thrill | Peak pressure gradient $>64$ mmHg |
| | Soft S2 | |
| Aortic regurgitation | Collapsing pulse | Regurgitant jet width $> 60\%$ of left ventricular outflow tract width |
| | Wide pulse pressure | Neck of regurgitant jet $> 6$ mm |
| | Thrill | Pandiastolic flow reversal in descending aorta |
| | Soft S2 | Regurgitant fraction $> 50\%$ |
| | Long duration murmur (except in acute severe aortic regurgitation) | Dilating left ventricle |
| Mitral stenosis | Long duration mid-diastolic murmur | Mitral valve area $< 1$ $cm^2$ |
| | Tapping apex | |
| | Diastolic thrill | Mean pressure gradient $> 10$ mmHg |
| Mitral regurgitation | Basal lung crepitations | Neck of regurgitant jet $> 7$ mm |
| | Laterally displaced apex | Dense triangular Doppler signal |
| | | Systolic pulmonary vein flow reversal |
| | | Regurgitant fraction $> 50\%$ |
| | | Dilating left ventricle |

*Left ventricular failure and pulmonary arterial hypertension are clinical and echocardiographic markers of severity for all left-sided valve lesions.

**Table 7.1** Clinical and echocardiographic markers of severe aortic and mitral valve disease

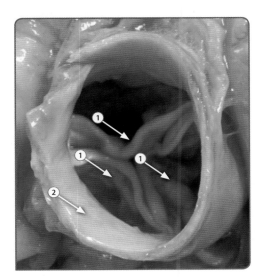

**Figure 7.1** Senile calcific aortic stenosis at post-mortem: looking down the aorta ② to a thickened trileafleted aortic valve with nodular calcific deposits that restrict movement of the leaflets ①.

- Rare causes and associated conditions include Paget's disease of the bone, systemic lupus erythematosus, connective tissue diseases and hyperparathyroidism.

Subaortic valve stenosis (left ventricular out-flow tract) and supra-aortic valve stenosis (aortic narrowing) mimic aortic stenosis but are considered separate conditions.

## Prevention

Risk factors for aortic valve degeneration are similar to those for coronary artery disease. Risk factor modification has positive effects on the incidence of symptomatic coronary artery disease, but no definite effect on aortic stenosis has been shown in prospective trials. More work is needed in this area before any sound recommendations are made.

## Pathogenesis

Calcific aortic valve degeneration is an indolent process involving leaflet microtrauma, chronic inflammation, lipid deposition and osteoblastic calcium deposition (**Figure 7.2**). Turbulent blood flow accelerates the process.

Aortic stenosis increases outflow resistance, and this results in compensatory left ventricular hypertrophy. Hypertrophy stiffens the walls of the left ventricle, increases oxygen demand, reduces blood flow and induces diastolic left ventricular impairment. Eventually, left ventricular systolic dysfunction ensues. Left ventricular dysfunction results in reduced cardiac output, increased left ventricular and left atrial pressures, and, ultimately, pulmonary arterial hypertension (**Figure 7.3**). Eventually, the failing left ventricle begins to dilate. It is important that surgical intervention precedes decompensation as the later pathophysiological consequences of aortic stenosis are irreversible.

## Clinical features

Aortic stenosis has a long, asymptomatic latent period, during which the patient remains at low risk of serious complications. The key symptoms are included in **Table 7.2**. Symptoms usually start when the valve orifice area reaches about < 1.5 cm$^2$. Symptoms accompany exertion, when the heart attempts to increase flow (cardiac output) across the stenotic valve.

Surgery must be considered when symptoms begin. Therefore a detailed history is essential.

Clinical signs of aortic stenosis include:

- slow-rising, low-volume carotid pulse
- narrow pulse pressure
- heaving apex beat
- quiet or absent aortic second heart sound
- ejection systolic murmur, loudest at the aortic area, radiating into the carotid arteries and loudest on expiration
- aortic thrill (in severe cases)

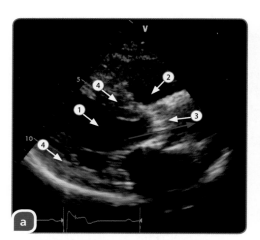

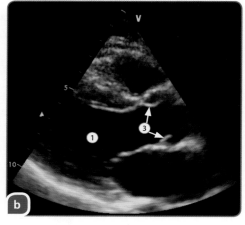

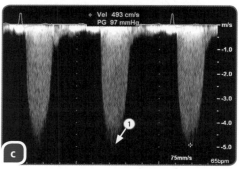

**Figure 7.2** Severe aortic stenosis. (a) Heavily calcified aortic valve with restricted valve cusp movement and hypertrophied left ventricular myocardium secondary to the aortic stenosis ④. Blue arrow, direction of systolic blood flow. ①, left ventricular cavity; ②, right ventricle; ③, heavily calcified aortic valve; (b) Normal aortic valve for comparison. The valve is in the open position during systole. (c) Doppler trace through the aortic valve. ①, significantly increased velocities indicating severe disease.

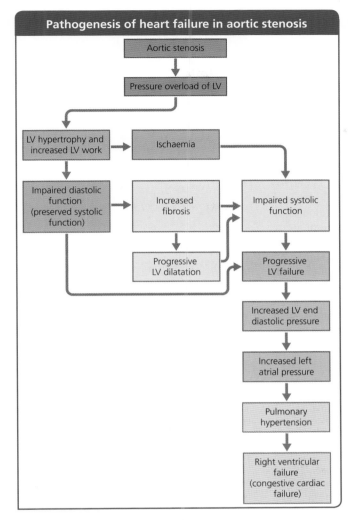

**Figure 7.3** The pathogenesis of heart failure, pulmonary arterial hypertension and right heart failure in aortic stenosis. The purple and amber colours indicate increasing severity and irreversibility. LV, left ventricle.

A thrill is a rare clinical sign. It reflects a loud murmur (intensity graded ≥ 4/6). A thrill is like the sensation when the hand is placed on a cat's body while it is purring.

| Key symptoms of aortic stenosis | |
| --- | --- |
| Symptom | Details |
| Dyspnoea and fatigue | Diastolic impairment resulting from stiffened hypertrophied left ventricular myocardium |
| Angina | Oxygen supply–demand mismatch |
| | Increased coronary small vessel resistance |
| | Many patients with aortic stenosis have coexisting coronary artery disease |
| Presyncope or syncope | Stenosis restricts cardiac output, causing relative cerebral hypoperfusion |
| Heart failure symptoms | Systolic heart failure reflects irreversible change, and improvement with surgery may be limited |

**Table 7.2** Key symptoms of aortic stenosis in increasing order of severity

The severity of aortic stenosis cannot be inferred from the volume of the murmur. Loud murmurs may occur with minimal or no significant stenosis. Late in the natural history of aortic stenosis, when the left ventricle is failing and flow is reduced, the murmur becomes quiet. A slow-rising pulse, heaving apex beat, associated thrill or signs of pulmonary arterial hypertension are markers of severe aortic stenosis.

## Diagnostic approach

Aortic stenosis is usually diagnosed in a patient with symptoms or after the incidental finding of a heart murmur in an asymptomatic patient. Transthoracic echocardiography is used to confirm the diagnosis and grade the level of valve dysfunction.

## Investigations

The principal electrocardiographic feature of aortic stenosis is left ventricular hypertrophy which occurs secondary to the increased afterload. Transthoracic echocardiography is used to diagnose, grade and monitor aortic stenosis. Echocardiographic features of aortic stenosis are listed in **Table 7.3. Figure 7.2** shows echocardiograms from a patient with aortic stenosis. Echocardiography is also used to identify abnormalities of other valves and for consequences of aortic stenosis, such as heart failure and pulmonary hypertension.

**Aortic stenosis may appear severe but have a lower than expected pressure gradient due to reduced blood flow velocity.** 'Low-flow' aortic stenosis occurs secondary to either a critically severe stenosis or heart failure or both. Response to exercise or an inotrope (e.g. dobutamine) as part of a stress echocardiogram helps differentiate between the former (flow increases) and latter (no increase in flow), and is an important investigation in those being considered for surgery.

All patients being considered for surgical intervention undergo left heart catheterisation (see page 138). This is because coronary artery disease is common in patients with aortic stenosis, and coronary artery bypass graft (CABG) (see pages 165 and 184) can be done during the same operation, if needed. Additionally, during the procedure, catheter measurement of the left ventricular–aortic pressure gradient can be done in order to assess stenosis severity. The greater the gradient, the more severe the stenosis.

| Echocardiographic features of aortic stenosis ||
|---|---|
| Echo mode | Purpose |
| Standard two-dimensional echocardiography | To assess: <br> ■ left ventricular wall thickness <br> ■ valve shape <br> ■ left ventricular function <br> ■ left ventricular dimensions <br> ■ valve calcification <br> ■ valve dimensions |
| Doppler echocardiography | To assess: <br> ■ systolic blood flow velocity (and therefore pressure gradient) across the valve – for grading stenosis severity |
| M mode | To assess: <br> ■ patency and mobility of the valve cusps |

**Table 7.3** Some echocardiographic features of aortic stenosis

## Management

Valve replacement is the only definitive treatment for aortic stenosis. Correctly timing intervention is the main challenge.

### Medication

Medical therapy is a palliative measure because no drug therapy has been shown to prevent or delay progression of aortic stenosis.

Medication is often needed for coexisting hypertension or associated conditions such as angina and heart failure, which occur as a consequence of aortic stenosis. Because cardiac afterload (see page 52) is effectively fixed by the stenosed aortic valve, profound hypotension can be precipitated by antihypertensive drugs such as angiotensin-converting enzyme (ACE) inhibitors (see page 158). Furthermore, patients with advanced disease can become preload dependent (see page 50) and quickly deteriorate (acute reduction in cardiac output) if given preload reducing drugs such as venodilators (e.g. nitrates). Although these drugs are not absolutely contraindicated, caution and regular clinical review are required when they are used.

## Surgical aortic valve replacement

The commonest valve operation is aortic valve replacement. It is indicated when severe aortic stenosis gives rise to symptoms. Aortic valve replacement is also considered for asymptomatic patients with severe aortic stenosis if they require cardiac surgery, such as CABG, for another condition. Surgery for asymptomatic patients remains controversial but is considered if left ventricular function starts to deteriorate.

Prosthetic valves are either mechanical or biological.

- Mechanical valves are prosthetic devices designed to replicate natural valvular function
- Biological valves are most commonly xenografts; they are formed from animal tissue usually of porcine or bovine origin

In the Ross procedure, a patient's own pulmonary valve is explanted and used to replace the diseased aortic valve. This autograft procedure is used in infants and children.

Mechanical valves are durable. However, patients require lifelong anticoagulation to prevent thrombus formation over non-biological material which causes valve malfunction and occlusion.

Biological valves are not prone to thrombus occlusion, so patients do not need anticoagulation beyond the first 3 months after surgery.

However, these valves are less durable than mechanical ones and often require re-do surgery within 10–15 years (**Figure 7.4a**).

All types of prosthetic valve are susceptible to general wear and tear over time, failure, infection (**Figure 7.4**) and dehiscence.

**Scars and sounds provide valuable information during clinical examination.**

- A patient with a **midline sternotomy** scar has usually had valve surgery, CABG (or both) or surgery to correct a congenital anomaly

- A **vein-harvesting scar** (over the path of the saphenous vein, see page 32) on either leg is because the patient has probably had CABG

- **Mechanical valves** give an audible click that is sometimes even heard from the end of the bed

- **Biological valves** may sound normal or slightly crisp when they close; they are more difficult to detect clinically

## Percutaneous therapy

Until recently, open surgical aortic valve replacement was the only definitive treatment for aortic stenosis. However, transcatheter aortic valve implantation (TAVI) now offers a less invasive approach.

In TAVI, a bioprosthetic valve mounted inside a mechanical frame is delivered through a catheter to the aortic root (**Figure 7.5**). Various approaches are used: transfemoral, transaortic, trans-subclavian, transcarotid and transapical

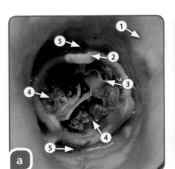
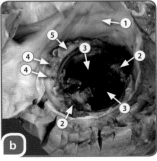

**Figure 7.4** Failure of prosthetic aortic valve replacement surgery. Both images are post mortem specimens looking down the aorta onto the valve. (a) Calcification and degeneration of a bioprosthetic valve. ① Ascending aorta; ② suture ring; ③ deformation of one of the valve cusps; ④ calcification and degeneration; ⑤ sutures holding the valve in place. (b) Infective endocarditis on a mechanical valve. ① Ascending aorta; ② vegetation; ③ tilting metallic disc leaflets; ④ sutures; ⑤ suture ring.

## Transcatheter aortic valve implantation

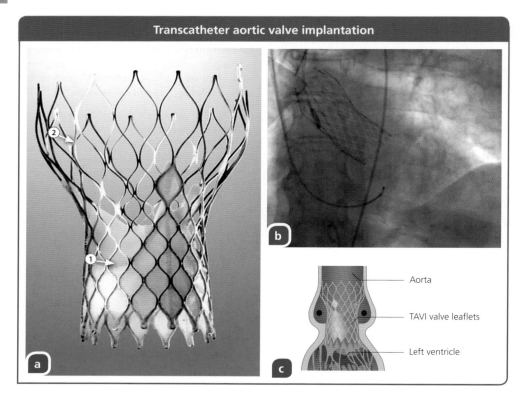

Aorta

TAVI valve leaflets

Left ventricle

**Figure 7.5** Transcatheter aortic valve implantation (TAVI). (a) Stent-mounted TAVI valve. ① Pericardial valve leaflets (just seen) inside. ② Nitonol self-expand frame. (b) A fluoroscopic image (taken during the insertion procedure) of the corevalve bioprosthesis just after deployment in the aortic root of a patient with severe aortic stenosis. (c) Position of the valve relative to the valve cusps and aorta.

(via the left anterolateral chest wall). The delivery catheter is usually delivered through a large vascular sheath of 5–8 mm in diameter. For comparison, most coronary stents are delivered via sheath of only 2 mm diameter.

First generation TAVI devices are self-expanding or balloon expanding, but multiple other technologies have been introduced to permit smaller vascular access, reduction of paraprosthetic aortic regurgitation and repositioning. Self-expanding prostheses extend from the left ventricular outflow tract into the aortic root. The fully expanded frame allows the bioprosthetic valve leaflets to function in a supra-annular position, maximising the area of the prosthetic valve orifice. Balloon expanding valves are intra-annular.

TAVI is less invasive than conventional surgery; conscious sedation is increasingly used. The 30-day mortality rate is 3–5%. Procedural risks include stroke, bleeding, myocardial infarction and vascular damage. Mild post-TAVI aortic regurgitation is common (about 50%) but is clinically significant in about 13%.

The results of TAVI are comparable to those of aortic valve replacement in surgically high-risk patients, and they are superior to medical therapy in patients who are unsuitable for aortic valve replacement. Other work has shown that TAVI can be superior to surgery in high risk but operable patients. TAVI is currently targeted to inoperable or high risk patients, but as experience with this new technique is gained, the number of patients in whom it is indicated is likely to increase.

## Prognosis

For asymptomatic patients with mild-moderate aortic stenosis, prognosis is good. The presence of symptoms is associated with a poorer outcome which is nearly normalised by surgery (**Table 7.4**).

| Prognosis for patients with severe aortic stenosis | |
|---|---|
| Patient group | Mortality rate |
| With no symptoms | Good |
| With symptoms of angina | 50% at 5 years |
| With symptoms of syncope | 50% at 3 years |
| With symptoms of heart failure | 50% at 2 years |
| After surgery | nearly normal |

**Table 7.4** Prognosis for patients with severe aortic stenosis. Surgery should ideally be performed once symptoms develop but before the left ventricle starts to fail

| Diseases that can predispose to aortic regurgitation | |
|---|---|
| Disease category | Examples |
| Diseases causing disruption of the aortic root | Aneurysm or dissection |
| Connective tissue diseases | Marfan's syndrome |
| | Ehlers–Danlos syndrome |
| | Osteogenesis imperfecta |
| Inflammatory diseases | Rheumatoid arthritis |
| | Ankylosing spondylitis |
| | Large artery vasculitides |

**Table 7.5** Diseases predisposing to aortic regurgitation

> The pathophysiological consequences of valvular heart disease depend on whether it is stenotic or regurgitant. Stenosis causes pressure overload and hypertrophy of the feeding chamber, whereas regurgitation results in volume overload and dilatation.

# Aortic regurgitation

Aortic regurgitation occurs when an incompetent aortic valve allows blood to leak back into the left ventricle during diastole.

## Epidemiology

The prevalence of aortic regurgitation increases with age. About 10% of the general population have some degree of aortic regurgitation, but only 10% of these cases are significant enough to warrant medical attention. Degenerative valve disease is the primary cause of aortic regurgitation in high-income countries.

## Aetiology

Valve degeneration can be caused by:

- leaflet degeneration
- aortic root dilatation
- prolapse of the valve cusps

All of which may contribute to valvular incompetence. Infective endocarditis, bicuspid aortic valve and previous rheumatic fever accelerate this process.

Diseases that predispose to aortic regurgitation are listed in **Table 7.5.**

# Pathogenesis

Aortic regurgitation results in increased left ventricular end diastolic volume. The left ventricle becomes volume overloaded, and stroke volume increases to compensate for this and to maintain cardiac output.

Chronic aortic regurgitation results in left ventricular dilatation. During the compensated phase, patients often remain asymptomatic. However, this phase is temporary and eventually the left ventricle fails.

> Valvular regurgitation is normally a slowly progressive problem accompanied by ventricular remodelling and physiological compensation (see page 49) which maintains cardiac output. However, in acute severe regurgitation, the there is insufficient time to compensate. Cardiovascular decompensation, tachycardia, heart failure and pulmonary oedema quickly ensue. Causes of acute aortic regurgitation include endocarditis and aortic dissection. Causes of acute mitral regurgitation include endocarditis and rupture of the chordae or papillary muscle apparatus.

# Clinical features

Clinical signs often precede symptoms in aortic regurgitation.

## History

After a long latent period, patients with moderate to severe aortic regurgitation complain of dyspnoea, paroxysmal nocturnal dyspnoea and orthopnoea, i.e. symptoms of left ventricular failure. Regurgitation of blood into the left ventricle reduces diastolic blood pressure in the aortic root. This reduces coronary perfusion pressure (see page 69), predisposing patients to angina.

## Examination

Increased stroke volume and low diastolic pressure cause a wide pulse pressure, which gives rise to a multitude of eponymously named clinical signs (**Table 7.6**).

Left ventricular dilatation causes a laterally displaced apex beat.

The murmur associated with aortic regurgitation is heard best at the left sternal edge, with the patient leaning forwards on expiration. It occurs in early diastole in a decrescendo pattern, and often lasts the whole of diastole in severe aortic regurgitation.

The longer the duration of the murmur, the more severe the aortic regurgitation. However, in acute severe aortic regurgitation, the murmur is short as the left ventricular pressure elevates quickly reducing the pressure gradient.

An additional ejection systolic murmur (i.e. a flow murmur) often results from increased stroke volume, even in the absence of aortic stenosis.

The initially wide pulse pressure narrows as the left ventricle fails.

> **A murmur indicates turbulent blood flow**. This can be caused by a normal flow of blood over an abnormal valve or an abnormally high flow of blood across a normal valve. The latter is a flow murmur, and is heard in patients with high cardiac output states such as sepsis, anaemia and thyrotoxicosis.

> **Aortic regurgitation and aortic stenosis frequently coexist**. This results in mixed atrioventricular disease and mixed clinical signs. However, one pathology usually predominates.

# Diagnostic approach

History and examination are important. Echocardiography is used to confirm the diagnosis and grade severity.

## Investigations

Two-dimensional echocardiography is used to measure aortic root and left ventricular dimensions. The technique is also used to assess the mechanism of aortic regurgitation by identifying evidence of leaflet degeneration, leaflet prolapse and poor coaption.

Doppler analysis is used to measure the size and volume of the regurgitant jet. The results provide clues as to the severity of aortic regurgitation (**Figure 7.6**).

## Management

The only definitive treatment for aortic regurgitation is valve replacement surgery. Patients with mild or moderate aortic regurgitation should be monitored episodically in the outpatient clinic.

| Eponymous clinical signs of aortic regurgitation | |
| --- | --- |
| Clinical sign | Description |
| Corrigan's pulse | Collapsing pulse, brisk upstroke and prompt collapse |
| De Musset's sign | Head nodding in time with pulse |
| Quincke's sign | Pulsating nail bed capillaries |
| Traube's sign (pistol shot femoral arteries) | Systolic and diastolic murmur heard over the femoral arteries |
| Müller's sign | Pulsating uvula |

**Table 7.6** Eponymous clinical signs of aortic regurgitation

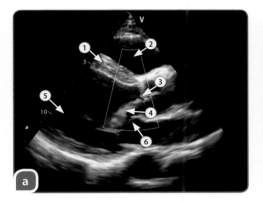
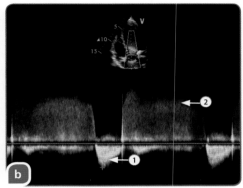

**Figure 7.6** Transthoracic echocardiogram in aortic regurgitation. (a) Two dimensional echo with colour Doppler showing a jet of aortic regurgitation ④ flowing back into the left ventricle ⑤ during diastole. The jet is impairing movement of the anterior mitral valve ⑥. ①, ventricular septum; ②, Right ventricle; ③, aortic valve. (b) Doppler trace through the aortic valve, showing both forward ① and regurgitant ② flow.

## Medication

Vasodilator therapy (e.g. angiotensin-converting enzyme inhibition and calcium channel blockers) is used to reduce cardiac afterload which decreases the transvalvular gradient and regurgitant volume, thus improving left ventricular function.

Afterload reduction is useful as a bridge to surgery and in patients who are unsuitable for surgery. Rate-limiting drugs (e.g. beta blockers and non-dihydropyridine calcium channel blockers) should be used with caution, because they prolong diastole and therefore the regurgitant phase.

## Surgical aortic valve replacement

Aortic valve replacement is considered in all patients with severe aortic regurgitation and one or more of the following:

- symptoms of New York Heart Association class II–IV heart failure
- left ventricular dilatation
- dilated aortic root

When the aortic root is dilated, aortic valve replacement plus aortic root graft is required.

## Percutaneous therapy

No percutaneous interventions are available for aortic regurgitation.

## Prognosis

Pre- and postoperative prognosis is chiefly determined by left ventricular function. Mortality is over 10 times higher in patients with an impaired left ventricle compared with those with normal left ventricular function. Therefore serial echocardiography is key to identifying the optimal time for surgery.

# Mitral valve disease

The mitral valve is more complex than the other cardiac valves. Mitral valve disease comprises mitral stenosis, mitral regurgitation and mitral prolapse.

## Mitral stenosis

Mitral stenosis is a slowly progressive disease with a long latent period lasting several decades. The normal mitral valve orifice area is 4–5 cm². In mitral stenosis, symptoms usually become apparent when this area is reduced to less than 2 cm².

## Epidemiology

The majority of cases of mitral stenosis are rheumatic in origin (**Figure 7.7**). Therefore mitral stenosis is increasingly rare in high-income countries.

> **The prevalence of mitral stenosis is decreasing, but it remains an examination favourite.** It is difficult to hear the murmur; listen carefully, for the mitral stenosis murmur in an elderly woman with seemingly lone atrial fibrillation. The murmur is often described as the 'absence of silence'. Remember to listen with the bell, in the left lateral position, over the apex and during expiration.

Rheumatic fever is complicated by mitral stenosis in twice as many women as men.

## Aetiology

Aside from rheumatic fever, congenital heart disease, mitral valve calcification and previous infective endocarditis increase the risk of mitral stenosis.

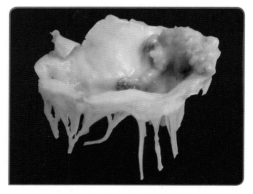

**Figure 7.7** Rheumatic mitral valve: calcified and fibrotic valve cusps with thickened chordae.

## Clinical features

Dyspnoea, fatigue, cough, orthopnoea and paroxysmal nocturnal dyspnoea are the chief symptoms of mitral stenosis. Palpitations are also common. Rarely, patients experience chest pain, caused by dilated pulmonary arteries as pulmonary arterial hypertension develops.

Symptoms and signs of mitral stenosis are exacerbated by conditions associated with increased blood flow, such as exercise and pregnancy.

Various signs should be sought in a patient with suspected mitral stenosis.

- A malar flush may be visible. Patients with severe mitral stenosis may develop a malar flush which is the appearance of flushed or rosy cheeks. The remainder of the face is usually pale with a subtle grey and/or blue tinge reflecting pulmonary hypertension, reduced blood flow to the face and cyanosis.
- The first heart sound may be palpable (a non-displaced, tapping apex beat) and is loud
- The key finding is a mid-diastolic murmur that has a low-pitched, rumbling character and does not radiate; this murmur is best heard with the bell of the stethoscope over the apex in the left lateral position during expiration
- Rarely, an opening snap is heard just after the second heart sound; this indicates valve mobility
- Signs of pulmonary arterial hypertension may also be identified (see page 270)

Most patients with mitral stenosis also have atrial fibrillation induced by atrial dilatation. Atrial fibrillation makes the interpretation of the heart sounds and murmur more difficult.

## Diagnostic approach

The diagnosis of mitral stenosis relies on clinical assessment complemented by electrocardiography, chest X-ray, echocardiography and invasive catheter studies.

# Investigations

The four main investigations used to detect mitral stenosis are listed in **Table 7.7**.

# Management

Asymptomatic patients with mild to moderate disease simply require monitoring, without any therapy. The aim of medical therapy is to control the ventricular rate if the patient is in atrial fibrillation, and to reduce the risk of thromboembolic disease.

Surgical valve repair or replacement is reserved for patients with severe symptomatic disease. Occasionally, patients with minimal or no symptoms are also considered for surgical intervention if there is evidence of increasing pulmonary artery pressure.

# Medication

Beta-blockers and rate limiting calcium channel blockers help to control heart rate in patients with atrial fibrillation with increased ventricular rate; slowing the heart rate maximises diastolic left ventricular filling time. Loop diuretics (e.g. frusemide) and venodilators (e.g. nitrates) help to ease pulmonary congestion.

Patients with atrial fibrillation receive anticoagulation. Anticoagulation is also indicated in those with mitral stenosis related thromboembolic disease, even in the context of sinus rhythm.

## Percutaneous therapy

Balloon valvuloplasty is a good non-surgical option for mitral stenosis with non-calcified,

| Investigations used in mitral stenosis | |
|---|---|
| Investigation | To identify |
| Electrocardiography | P wave mitrale (see page 126) reflecting left atrial enlargement |
| | Atrial fibrillation |
| Chest X-ray | Left atrial enlargement |
| | Pulmonary congestion |
| | Pulmonary oedema (in advanced cases) |
| Echocardiography# (**Figure 7.7**) | Left atrial dilatation |
| | Thickening, calcification, fusion of the mitral valve leaflets |
| Standard two-dimensional | Reduced mitral valve orifice area |
| Doppler | Increased transvalvular blood flow velocity during diastole, reflecting increased pressure gradient between left atrium and ventricle |
| | Assessment of pulmonary artery pressure |
| Three-dimensional | Aids surgical preoperative planning |
| Cardiac catheterisation | Estimates left atrial pressure |
| | A Swan–Ganz catheter (with balloon at the tip) can be 'floated' into a distal pulmonary artery branch through the right heart (usually accessed via the jugular vein):<br>■ Balloon inflation occludes blood flow<br>■ The pressure transduced from the tip equilibrates with the left atrial pressure, giving a surrogate measure of the pressure; this is known as the pulmonary–capillary wedge pressure*<br>■ Simultaneous catheter measurement of left ventricular pressure provides the mitral valve gradient, which reflects severity |

#Transthoracic echo is sufficient for surveillance in most cases but transoesophageal allows clearer assessment and is used for preoperative assessment.
*This method is used because the left atrium is difficult to access with a catheter.

**Table 7.7** Investigations in the diagnosis and assessment of mitral stenosis.

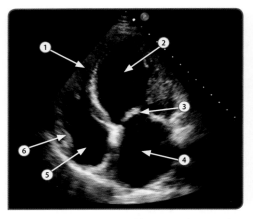 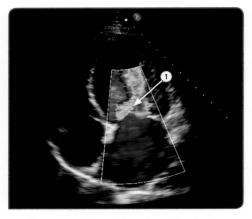

**Figure 7.8** Mitral stenosis. (a) Echocardiogram showing significant restriction of the mitral valve during diastole. ①, right ventricle; ②, left ventricle; ③,mitral valve with a very small orifice; ④, left atrium; ⑤, right atrium; ⑥, tricuspid valve. (b) Colour Doppler signal showing a central, high-velocity jet of blood flowing into the left ventricle through the mitral valve ①,indicating significant mitral stenosis.

pliable valve leaflets. Inflation of the balloon separates the fused valve leaflet commissures (i.e. commissurotomy) and restores the diastolic mitral valve orifice. This procedure is contraindicated in patients with left atrial thrombus, significant mitral regurgitation, calcified leaflets or fused subvalvular apparatus in order to minimise the risk of thromboembolic complications and iatrogenic mitral regurgitation.

The balloon catheter is usually delivered from the femoral vein to the left atrium through an atrial septal puncture. In carefully selected patients, recurrence is about 25% at 5 years. The most serious complication is severe mitral regurgitation.

## Surgery

Mitral valve repair or replacement is an option for those with severe symptomatic disease, in whom balloon valvuloplasty is contraindicated.

## Prognosis

Asymptomatic patients have a good prognosis: > 80% survival at 10 years. However, symptomatic mitral stenosis is associated with only 10% survival at 10 years, and mean survival is < 3 years if pulmonary arterial hypertension develops.

**Pulmonary arterial hypertension has many causes, but is often due to left-sided heart disease.** Pulmonary arterial hypertension is reversible if the cause is corrected early. However, the condition becomes irreversible and self-propagating over time, and has a poor prognosis. It causes strain on the right heart, resulting in:

■ a loud pulmonary second heart sound

■ a pulmonary regurgitation murmur

■ a right ventricular heave (reflecting right ventricular dilatation and failure)

■ tricuspid regurgitation (reflecting right ventricular dilatation and failure)

■ raised jugular venous pressure

■ peripheral oedema

# Mitral regurgitation

Mitral regurgitation occurs when blood leaks from the left ventricle into the left atrium during systole. The condition is common and results from a number of cardiac pathologies. Its natural history, management and prognosis depend on the cause. In most patients, mitral regurgitation is slowly progressive. Many cases never require intervention.

Rarely, acute severe mitral regurgitation occurs when the valve or sub-valve apparatus are suddenly damaged. This may result from myocardial infarction, infective endocarditis or chordal rupture.

Unlike chronic mitral regurgitation, the left ventricle and left atrium do not have time to accommodate the altered haemodynamic state. The result is a sudden decrease in cardiac output and acute onset severe pulmonary oedema.

> **Patients with acute severe mitral regurgitation need urgent surgical intervention.** The patient's condition should be stabilised with aggressive treatment with intravenous nitrates, diuretics, continuous positive airway pressure and intra-aortic balloon pump support as a bridge to emergency surgery.

## Types

There are two types of mitral regurgitation: primary and secondary (**Table 7.8**).

## Epidemiology

Trivial, non-significant mitral regurgitation is common. Significant regurgitation affects of about 1–2% of the population and affects men and women equally. It is more common in those with a history of cardiac disease.

## Aetiology

Primary mitral regurgitation is caused by conditions which directly affect the structure or function of the valve or valve apparatus such as infective endocarditis, rheumatic heart disease, mitral valve prolapse and congenital or inherited cardiac diseases. Secondary mitral regurgitation is caused by left ventricular dilatation (dilated cardiomyopathy, see page 330). Mitral regurgitation can also be idiopathic.

## Pathogenesis

Regurgitation of blood into the left atrium reduces forward flow (i.e. cardiac output). Blood regurgitating into the left atrium increases left ventricular preload. Therefore the left ventricle becomes volume-overloaded.

Chronically, the left atrium and left ventricle dilate to accommodate the increased volume. This ultimately leads to left ventricular failure and pulmonary artery hypertension.

## Clinical features

Many patients with mitral regurgitation remain asymptomatic for many years. A significant proportion never develop symptoms. Symptoms of mitral regurgitation include:

- lethargy and fatigue
- dyspnoea
- cough
- palpitations
- orthopnoea
- paroxysmal nocturnal dyspnoea

Clinical signs include:

- a laterally displaced apex beat (reflecting left ventricular dilatation)
- a soft first heart sound
- a pansystolic murmur (loudest at the apex and radiating into the left axilla; heard best on expiration)

| Primary and secondary mitral regurgitation | |
|---|---|
| Type | Description |
| Primary | Occurs secondary to disease directly affecting the mitral valve leaflets or subvalvular apparatus (chordae and papillary muscle) |
| Secondary (functional) | Occurs secondary to left ventricular dilatation, which stretches the mitral valve annulus and distorts the subvalvular apparatus |
| | May also occur if myocardial ischaemia causes papillary muscle dysfunction; this may present with varying severity because of the transient effects of ischaemia |

**Table 7.8** Primary and secondary mitral regurgitation

- signs of pulmonary arterial hypertension and pulmonary congestion (in advanced cases)
- irregularly irregular cardiac rhythm in atrial fibrillation (commonly complicates mitral regurgitation as a consequence of atrial stretch)

## Diagnostic approach

Diagnosis of mitral regurgitation normally follows identification of the characteristic pansystolic murmur at the apex. A thorough clinical assessment, including electrocardiography, chest X-ray and echocardiography, help confirm the diagnosis and grade severity.

## Investigations

A combination of ECG, chest X-ray and echocardiography are used in the diagnosis and assessment of mitral regurgitation.

- Electrocardiography may show P mitrale or atrial fibrillation
- Chest X-ray often demonstrates cardiomegaly, left atrial enlargement, and in uncompensated cases, pulmonary congestion or pulmonary oedema
- Transthoracic echocardiography is used to assess left atrial size, left ventricular dimensions and function, mechanism regurgitation (from assessment of the valve and sub-valve apparatus); Doppler mode is used to assess the velocity, size and direction of the regurgitant jet (**Figure 7.9**)
- Transoesophageal echocardiography is used in all preoperative cases because it provides superior detail which is helpful when planning surgery
- Left heart catheterisation is also done preoperatively to measure left ventricular end diastolic pressure, which helps to grade severity and to assess the coronary arteries in case a CABG may also be warranted

## Management

Asymptomatic patients with mild to moderate disease are treated conservatively and monitored in the clinic. The role of medical therapy

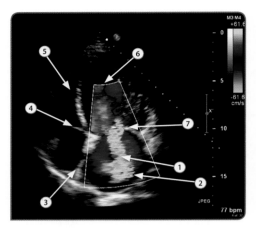

**Figure 7.9** Transthoracic echocardiogram demonstrating a central, broad jet of mitral regurgitation ① flowing into a dilated left atrium ②. Colour is generated by Doppler echo; red and blue signals indicate flow towards and away from the probe (at the top of the image) respectively according to the scale at the top right of the image. ③, right atrium; ④, tricuspid valve; ⑤, right ventricle; ⑥, left ventricle, ⑦ mitral valve.

is limited in primary mitral regurgitation but is key in functional mitral regurgitation.

## Medication

Angiotensin-converting enzyme inhibitors, beta-blockers, diuretics and mineralocorticoid antagonists may reduce mitral regurgitation by optimising left ventricular geometry in patients with secondary regurgitation and a failing, dilated left ventricle. Antianginal therapy and revascularisation with percutaneous coronary intervention or CABG are considered if ischaemia is a contributory cause.

Medical therapy has no significant role in the management of primary mitral regurgitation. However, antihypertensive therapies may improve left ventricular ejection fraction by reducing cardiac afterload. Anticoagulation should be considered if atrial fibrillation coexists.

## Surgery

Both mitral valve repair and mitral valve replacement are options. Repair (in appropriate cases) is now considered superior to replacement; it is associated with improved long-term outcome and reduced reoperation rates.

A mechanical mitral valve prosthesis is shown in **Figure 7.10.**

Deciding when to intervene can be difficult. However, it is essential for the intervention to take place before the development of left ventricular dysfunction and pulmonary arterial hypertension. Surgery is considered for symptomatic patients with severe mitral regurgitation and for asymptomatic patients with deteriorating left ventricular dimensions, pulmonary pressures or left ventricular function.

## Percutaneous therapy

Two percutaneous techniques have been developed to improve secondary (functional) mitral regurgitation. The first involves clipping the two mitral valve leaflets together at their midpoint. The second delivers an annular valve ring via the coronary sinus. Both techniques require further support from the results of prospective trials before they are used routinely.

## Prognosis

In severe mitral regurgitation, the prognosis becomes poor when the left ventricular dimensions start deteriorating. Survival falls to one third at 5 years. Comorbidities also influence prognosis; e.g. heart failure in secondary mitral regurgitation.

# Mitral valve prolapse

Mitral valve prolapse occurs if one or both mitral valve leaflets prolapse back into the left atrium, beyond the line of the mitral valve annulus. A prolapsing mitral valve is often called a Barlow's valve after John Barlow, the cardiologist who first described the condition. It is the most prevalent valvular abnormality, estimated to affect up to 5% of the general population, although this figure depends on precisely how prolapse is defined.

Mitral valve prolapse is frequently associated with mitral regurgitation which is usually mild but may progress to moderate or severe. Mitral valve prolapse without mitral regurgitation is considered a benign condition.

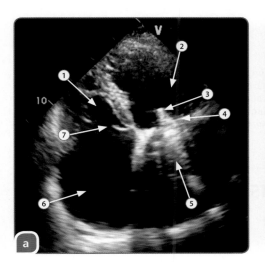
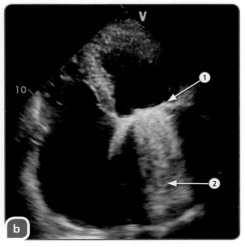

**Figure 7.10** Mechanical mitral valve replacement. (a) during diastole; the disc is tilted forwards in the open position. ① Right ventricle; ② left ventricle; ③ mechanical tilting disc; ④ main body of the prosthetic valve; ⑤ acoustic shadow cast over the dilated left atrium by the valve; ⑥ dilated right atrium; ⑦ tricuspid valve. (b) During systole; pressure changes cause the disc to tilt back closing the valve. ① prosthetic valve; ② acoustic shadow.

## Clinical features

Some patients with mitral valve prolapse experience atypical chest pain, palpitations and anxiety.

A characteristic mid-systolic click is heard as the mitral valve leaflet and apparatus tense in systole (like a yacht's spinnaker filling with wind). This is followed by a late systolic murmur if mitral regurgitation is present. In the absence of mitral regurgitation, the mid-systolic click is often the only clinical sign.

## Management

Asymptomatic patients without mitral regurgitation can be reassured and monitored every 3-5 years with clinical evaluation and echocardiography. Mitral regurgitation and arrhythmia are managed as described on pages 272 and 211. **Figure 7.11** demonstrates mitral valve prolapse causing mitral regurgitation.

## Medication

Beta-blockers, particularly propranolol, are useful for patients with palpitations, atypical chest pain and anxiety.

## Surgery

Indications for surgery are similar to those for mitral regurgitation without prolapse (see page 272). Whenever possible, mitral valve repair is preferred to mitral valve replacement.

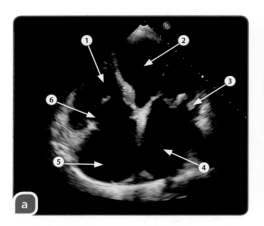 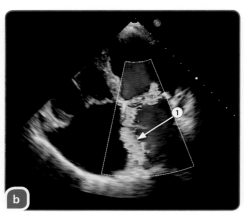

**Figure 7.11** Mitral valve prolapse causing mitral regurgitation. (a) The posterior mitral valve leaflet is prolapsing back into the left atrium during systole. ①, right ventricle; ②, left ventricle; ③,posterior mitral valve leaflet; ④, dilated left atrium; ⑤, dilated right atrium; ⑥, tricuspid valve. (b) Colour Doppler signal in the same patient showing a large jet of mitral regurgitation ① flowing into the left atrium. The jet is directed anteriorly and follows the contours of the atrial septum.

# Right-sided valve disease

Right-sided valve disease strains the right side of the heart. This leads to systemic venous hypertension, peripheral oedema and elevated jugular venous pressure. Ultimately, the right ventricle begins to fail.

## Tricuspid valve disease

Tricuspid stenosis is rare. It is most commonly rheumatic or congenital in origin. If rheumatic, it almost always coexists with mitral stenosis.

A more common problem is tricuspid regurgitation, in which blood leaks back into the right atrium during systole. Tricuspid regurgitation is usually functional, i.e. secondary to right ventricular dilatation. Causes of right ventricular dilatation include left sided heart disease (ventricular and valvular), pulmonary vascular disease, pulmonary valve disease and left to right shunts. Tricuspid regurgitation may also occur secondary to infective endocarditis, connective tissue disease, tumour, rheumatic heart disease or a congenital abnormality.

# Clinical features

Fatigue and dependent oedema are symptoms of tricuspid stenosis and tricuspid regurgitation.

Signs of tricuspid stenosis include:

- elevated jugular venous pressure (with prominent a wave)
- dependent oedema
- hepatomegaly
- low-pitched rumbling murmur (similar to that of mitral stenosis) over the lower left sternal edge

Signs of tricuspid regurgitation include:

- elevated jugular venous pressure (giant V waves)
- dependent oedema
- pulsatile hepatomegaly
- pansystolic murmur at the lower left sternal edge (louder with inspiration)
- cachexia
- jaundice (indicating hepatic congestion)
- irregularly irregular pulse secondary to atrial fibrillation (caused by atrial stretch)

# Management

Tricuspid stenosis rarely requires intervention but when it does, percutaneous valvuloplasty or surgery to repair or replace the valve are available. Tricuspid regurgitation is usually managed symptomatically with medication because most cases occur secondary to an underlying ventricular abnormality which cannot be corrected with surgery. Most cases of tricuspid regurgitation are managed symptomatically with medical therapy.

## Medication

Diuretic therapy and mineralocorticoid antagonists may improve symptoms of peripheral oedema and hepatic congestion by offloading fluid volume and reducing right heart preload.

## Surgery

Surgical repair or replacement is appropriate in only a minority of cases of severe tricuspid valve disease without dilatation of the annulus. A bioprosthetic valve is used, because the risk of valve thrombosis is increased (due to low, right-sided pressures).Functional tricuspid regurgitation can be improved with tricuspid valve annuloplasty, where annular dilatation is corrected with a prosthetic ring. This is usually considered when patients undergo cardiac surgery for another reason.

> **Tricuspid regurgitation is common and is associated with clear clinical signs,** especially prominent V waves (see page 109) in the jugular venous pressure and peripheral oedema. Therefore it is popular in medical examinations.

# Pulmonary valve disease

There are two types of pulmonary valve disease:

- Pulmonary regurgitation which is usually acquired
- Pulmonary stenosis which is usually congenital and diagnosed in childhood

Pulmonary regurgitation is more common than pulmonary stenosis. The condition occurs secondary to pulmonary arterial hypertension. Less commonly, it occurs secondary to infective endocarditis or connective tissue disease. It causes symptoms and signs of right ventricular failure. An early diastolic decrescendo murmur, analogous to aortic regurgitation, is best heard at the 3rd to 4th left intercostal space, loudest on inspiration. Treatment should be targeted at the underlying cause e.g. pulmonary hypertension. Diuretic treatment is required if the right ventricle fails. In selected, severe cases, valve replacement is performed.

Pulmonary stenosis may occur above, below, or at the level of the valve itself. The condition may be asymptomatic but symptoms develop if the right ventricle begins to fail. Clinical signs include an ejection systolic murmur in the area of the pulmonary valve. Balloon valvuloplasty, surgical valvotomy or valve replacement are options in carefully selected severe cases.

# Rheumatic heart disease

Rheumatic heart disease is a chronic inflammatory condition affecting the cardiac valves. It is the gravest complication of rheumatic fever.

Rheumatic heart disease affects an estimated 15 million children and adults across the world. In high-income countries, the prevalence of rheumatic heart disease has declined in line with the decrease in the incidence of rheumatic fever. However, the condition remains a leading cause of valvular heart disease and is still the leading cause of mitral stenosis globally. In low- and middle-income countries, rheumatic heart disease remains a major problem.

## Rheumatic fever

Rheumatic fever is an autoimmune inflammatory condition that affects multiple organ systems. It complicates < 0.5% of cases of streptococcal throat infection. The causal organism is *Streptococcus pyogenes,* a group A β-haemolytic streptococcus. Antibodies targeting an antigen in the bacterial cell wall (anti-M antibodies) cross-react with proteins in the heart and other organs, causing the disease's acute sequelae (see **Table 7.9**). The chronic sequelae of rheumatic fever, however, are limited to the heart.

About 85% of cases of rheumatic fever occur in school-aged children. Modern healthcare systems, easy access to antibiotics and improved social conditions have resulted in a decline in rheumatic fever in high-income countries to < 1 case per 100,000. The incidence in low- and middle-income countries is variable but can be over 100 times higher.

## Clinical features

### Acute phase

Rheumatic fever develops 2–5 weeks after the precipitating event: a streptococcal sore throat. The clinical features of rheumatic fever are variable and are divided into minor and major criteria, according to the modified Jones criteria (**Table 7.9**).

Diagnosis requires evidence of group A β-haemolytic streptococcal infection (throat culture, antigen test or rising antibody level) and two major or one major and two minor criteria.

Arthritis and carditis are the most commonly seen major criteria. Fever and increased inflammatory markers are the most commonly seen minor criteria. In the heart, rheumatic fever disrupts:

- the endocardium, which causes valve disruption

| Modified Jones criteria for diagnosis of rheumatic fever | |
|---|---|
| Major criteria | Minor criteria |
| Polyarthritis | Fever |
| Chorea | Arthralgia |
| Subcutaneous nodules | Increased inflammatory markers or white cell count |
| Erythema marginatum | Electrocardiographic evidence of heart block |
| Carditis | Previous rheumatic fever |

**Table 7.9** Diagnostic criteria for rheumatic fever: the modified Jones criteria

- the myocardium, which causes heart failure and arrhythmia
- the pericardium, which causes chest pain and pericardial effusion

## Chronic phase: long term cardiac sequelae

Rheumatic heart disease occurs decades later as a result of chronic inflammation and progressive fibrosis (**Figure 7.7**). Inflammation and fibrosis are induced by the autoimmune reaction and damage the endomyocardial lining on the valve leaflets or apparatus, causing valvular heart disease.

Mitral stenosis is the most common consequence. Aortic stenosis and tricuspid stenosis also occur, but when they do, the mitral valve is almost always coaffected. Occasionally, acute carditis permanently damages the myocardium, causing chronic heart failure.

## Management

Patients are usually treated in hospital, where close cardiac monitoring is available. Rheumatic fever has no cure. The aims of therapy are to eradicate the bacteria, reduce the inflammatory reaction and minimise long-term damage to the heart.

### Medication

Antibiotics such as penicillin or a macrolide (or cephalosporin, if the patient is allergic to other antibiotics) are used:

- acutely if there is evidence of active infection
- chronically, usually by parenteral injections, to eradicate infection and prevent recurrence for ≥ 5 years after the occurrence of rheumatic fever or until the age of 18 years (whichever is later)

Some advocate longer-term chronic therapy with monthly long-acting penicillin. Nonsteroidal anti-inflammatory drugs are used to reduce the inflammatory reaction. Corticosteroids are used in the acute phase if evidence of myocarditis is detected.

### Prognosis

About half of cases of rheumatic fever progress to rheumatic heart disease. This figure approaches 90% if carditis is a feature of the initial illness but is reduced by appropriate early therapy.

# Infective endocarditis

Infective endocarditis is an inflammation of the endocardium caused by infection. As part of the inflammatory reaction microbes, inflammatory cells, fibrin and platelets clump together to form vegetations (**Figure 7.14**) which threaten the integrity and function of the endocardium, valves and subvalve apparatus.

Without prompt diagnosis and early aggressive treatment, infective endocarditis rapidly results in valvular incompetence, cardiac failure, embolic complications and death.

## Epidemiology

The incidence of endocarditis in the general population varies between studies but is estimated at 6 cases per 100,000 patient-years.

However, the incidence is higher for at-risk groups, which include:

- intravenous drug users
- people with pre-existing valve disease
- those who have had prosthetic valve surgery
- men (male to female ratio, 2:1)
- people with poor dental health

## Aetiology

Causative organisms, and the approximate proportion of cases they account for, include the following species:

- oral (previously called viridans) streptococci (50%)
- staphylococci (25%)

- enterococci (10%)
- the HACEK organisms (*Haemophilus, Aggregatibacter (Actinobacillus), Cardiobacterium, Eikenella* and *Kingella*), a group of slow-growing, Gram-negative, commensal bacteria (10%)

> **Intravenous drug use is usually associated with right-sided infective endocarditis.** This is because the injected venous blood returns to the right heart.

*Staphylococcus aureus* causes a particularly aggressive endocarditis. Coagulase-negative staphylococci are common in prosthetic valve endocarditis. Very rarely, fungi cause infective endocarditis.

Blood cultures are negative in about 1 in 10 cases. This may be because the causative organism is difficult to culture (e.g. the HACEK organisms), samples were acquired during antibiotic therapy or even because there is no organism (in cases of non infective endocarditis).

Non-infective (marantic) endocarditis may occasionally occur with inflammatory, autoimmune or malignant conditions such as systemic lupus erythematosus and adenocarcinoma. Treatment is targeted at the underlying cause but anticoagulation may also be appropriate.

> **Permanent pacemaker leads may act as a focus for infection.** They are foreign bodies inserted into the right heart chambers.

Any alteration to the structure or function of a native valve increases the risk of endocarditis. Such alterations include valvular stenosis or incompetence, congenital heart disease, hypertrophic cardiomyopathy, previous surgery and previous endocarditis.

Events that cause a transient bacteraemia also predispose to endocarditis. These include poor dental hygiene (or dental surgery), surgery, instrumentation or intravenous drug use. Immunosuppressive conditions or therapies and diabetes mellitus also increase the risk.

## Clinical features

Endocarditis may present insidiously or acutely (with rapidly evolving, florid clinical signs). An insidious course is typical of streptococci, and an acute course is typical of staphylococci. Symptoms of infection include (**Figure 7.12**):

- fever
- night sweats
- weight loss
- lethargy
- anorexia

Symptoms consistent with heart failure indicate advanced, complicated disease with valve destruction.

Clinical signs of endocarditis include:

- tachycardia
- pyrexia
- a new or evolving murmur
- signs of valve dysfunction
- immune complex deposition
- embolic phenomena
- signs of cardiac failure in advanced disease

Clubbing, anaemia and splenomegaly may occur with chronic infection. **Figure 7.13** shows some subtle clinical signs in a patient with bacterial endocarditis.

> **In infective endocarditis, vegetations may embolise to cause infarction in any organ.** The lungs, brain, kidney or bowel may be affected. Embolisation is a marker of poor prognosis and recurs in half of cases. Systemic emboli indicate left-sided disease. Right-sided vegetations embolise to the pulmonary circulation.

## Diagnostic approach

Many of the signs and symptoms of infective endocarditis are non-specific. Therefore diagnosis requires a high index of suspicion, with heavy reliance on a combination of clinical features and serological, microbiological and echocardiographic findings.

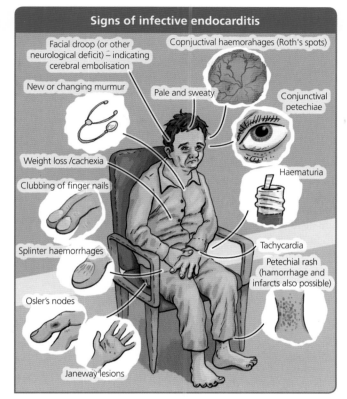

**Figure 7.12** Signs of infective endocarditis.

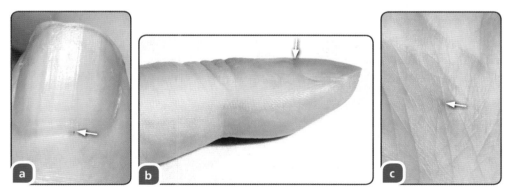

**Figure 7.13** Subtle clinical signs in the hand of a woman with bacterial endocarditis. (a) Small splinter haemorrhage in the nail bed. (b) Early clubbing, with loss of the normal nail bed angle. (c) A Janeway lesion on the palm.

Formal diagnosis is made according to the modified Duke criteria which separate the features of infective endocarditis into major and minor criteria (**Table 7.11**).

- Infective endocarditis is definitively diagnosed if two major criteria or one major criterion and three minor criteria, or five minor criteria are met
- Infective endocarditis is possible if either one major and one minor criteria or three minor criteria are met

Many autoimmune diseases can cause rashes, lumps and bumps similar to those of infective endocarditis. Antibody–antigen complexes deposit in the microcirculation in a similar way to the emboli of infective endocarditis. Signs of autoimmune deposits are shown in **Table 7.10**.

## Investigations

At least three paired blood culture specimens (aerobic and anaerobic) of > 10 mL are taken at least 30 min apart from different anatomical sites. Specimens should be taken before antibiotics are started in order to maximise the chance of a diagnostic result, but this should not delay treatment when it is needed urgently. Serum is sent (and saved) for immunological analysis, especially in culture-negative cases.

Inflammatory markers (C-reactive protein and erythrocyte sedimentation rate) and white cell count are increased in patients with

| Extra-cardiac autoimmune and vascular involvement in infective endocarditis | |
|---|---|
| Cutaneous | Petechial rash |
| | Osler's nodes (tender erythematous nodules on the palms or soles) |
| | Janeway lesions (non-tender erythematous macules on the palms and soles) |
| | Splinter haemorrhages (under the nail or nail bed) |
| Ophthalmic | Roth's spots (retinal haemorrhages with pale centre) |
| | Conjunctival haemorrhages |
| Renal (glomerulonephritis) | Haematuria |
| | Proteinurea |
| | Other signs of renal impairment |
| Rheumatological | Asymmetric arthritis |
| Haematological | Splenomegaly |
| | Pallor (anaemia) |

**Table 7.10** Signs of extra-cardiac autoimmune and vascular involvement in infective endocarditis

| Modified Duke criteria for diagnosing infective endocarditis | |
|---|---|
| Major criteria | Minor criteria |
| Two positive blood cultures for a typical microorganism or Persistently positive cultures, with a consistent organism | Fever: > 38.0°C |
| Imaging evidence of endocardial infection, such as: ■ oscillating vegetation on a valve ■ abscess ■ new prosthetic valve dehiscence or ■ new valvular regurgitation (not worsening or changing of pre-existing murmur) | Predisposing condition: Predisposing cardiac disease or intravenous drug use |
| | Vascular phenomena – septic infarction, arterial emboli, mycotic aneurysm, haemorrhage, Janeway lesions |
| | Immunological phenomena – see Table 7.10 |
| | Microbiological (or serological) – results consistent with endocarditis but do not meet a major criterion |
| | Echocardiographic findings – results consistent with endocarditis but do not meet a major criterion |

**Table 7.11** A summary of the modified Duke criteria. Diagnosis requires two major criteria or one major criterion and three minor criteria or five minor criteria. Endocarditis is possible if either one major and one minor criteria or three minor criteria are met

infective endocarditis. Full blood count, urea and electrolytes, and liver function tests may reflect anaemia or distant organ involvement. Serum albumin is frequently decreased.

Transthoracic echocardiography and, if necessary, transoesophageal echocardiography are done to identify evidence of infection (**Figure 7.14**).

Aortic valve endocarditis may cause an aortic root abscess, which may interfere with atrioventricular node conduction. Therefore all patients with aortic valve endocarditis need regular ECGs to monitor the PR interval.

## Management

All confirmed cases of infective endocarditis are managed by a specialist team of cardiologists, with regular support from cardiac surgeons, infectious disease specialists and microbiologists. All endocarditis patients also undergo a dental assessment.

### Medication

Early use of intravenous antibiotic therapy is required for all cases of endocarditis. The therapy is chosen to correspond with the cultured organism's antibiotic sensitivities, whenever possible. When there is no microbiological diagnosis, empiric therapy should cover likely organisms.

The choice of antibiotic, dose, and length of the course are guided by microbiological advice and the individual patient's response to treatment. A typical treatment period is 6 weeks, including at least 4 weeks of intravenous therapy.

### Surgery

All cases of infective endocarditis are discussed regularly with the surgical team. Surgery is a life-saving intervention in some cases.

Ideally, infection should be eradicated fully before surgical intervention. Operating on actively infected, friable tissue is more difficult, and the risk of recurrent infection is increased. However, these disadvantages must be weighed against other factors which warrant early surgery, such as ensuing cardiac failure, prosthetic valve endocarditis, uncontrolled sepsis, the presence of aggressive organisms (e.g. *Staph. aureus),* embolic phenomena and large vegetations.

### Monitoring

It is essential to monitor the patient's response to treatment. Patients receive regular clinical assessment, echocardiography, electrocardiography, blood cultures and measurement of inflammatory markers. Decreasing concentrations of C-reactive protein are a particularly encouraging sign reflecting successful treatment.

### Prognosis

Without antibiotic therapy, infective endocarditis is fatal. Even with modern antibiotic

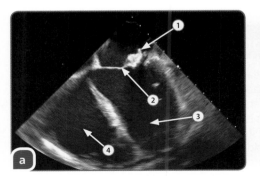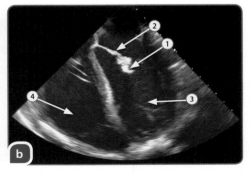

**Figure 7.14** Bacterial endocarditis affecting the mitral valve. (a) Transoesophageal echocardiogram in systole: the anterior mitral valve leaflet ② has a vegetation ① attached at its tip; ③ left ventricle; ④ right ventricle. (b) The same study but in diastole with the mitral valve open. The vegetation; ① has moved with the valve leaflet ②. ③ left ventricle; ④ right ventricle.

regimens, death occurs in about 20% of patients with infective endocarditis. Aggressive or uncontrolled infections, large vegetations and cardiac failure are all associated with a poor prognosis. The prognosis for right-sided disease is slightly better than for left because systemic embolisation is absent and tricuspid valve dysfunction is better tolerated than left-sided valve dysfunction.

## Infective endocarditis prophylaxis

Certain patient groups are considered at increased risk of developing infective endocarditis. These include those with:

- valve replacement, or repair with prosthetic material (high risk)
- previous infective endocarditis (high risk)
- certain structural congenital cardiac diseases (high risk)
- acquired valvular heart disease
- hypertrophic cardiomyopathy

Certain procedures are considered at risk of inducing bacteraemia thus increasing the risk of endocarditis. These include:

- any procedure involving an infected site or a site suspected to be infected (high risk)
- dental procedures (high risk)
- upper and lower gastrointestinal tract procedures
- genitourinary tract procedures
- upper and lower respiratory tract procedures (including ear, nose and throat)

All at-risk patients should be educated about the importance of good oral hygiene, regular dental review and the risks of non-medical procedures such as tattooing and body piercing. They should also be educated about the symptoms of endocarditis and when to seek medical help. Healthcare professionals should understand the need for stringent aseptic technique during venous catheterisation and invasive procedures.

Traditionally, at-risk patients were routinely offered antibiotic therapy prior to at-risk procedures in order to reduce the risk of developing endocarditis. However, there is controversy about the effectiveness of antibiotic prophylaxis in terms of benefit versus risk. Increasingly, antibiotic prophylaxis is restricted to the higher risk patients undergoing the higher risk procedures. Further research is needed to fully elucidate precisely which patient groups undergoing which procedures warrant antibiotic prophylaxis. To ensure the correct patients receive antibiotic prophylaxis healthcare professionals should:

- be aware of which patients are at increased risk of endocarditis
- be aware of which procedures increase the risk of endocarditis
- follow up-to-date locally applied guidelines
- discuss the risks and benefits of antibiotic prophylaxis with their patients
- consult a specialist in any case where there is doubt regarding the appropriateness of antibiotic prophylaxis.

## Answers to starter questions

1. The only definitive treatment for valve disease is structural intervention, such as surgical repair or valve replacement. Newer approaches involve transcatheter valve insertion where a replacement valve is delivered to the area of disease mounted on a balloon catheter (similar to a stent). This approach is less invasive and has shown promise, especially in the context of treating aortic stenosis. Drug therapy can improve symptoms and in cases of functional mitral or tricuspid regurgitation (see pages 270 and 274) can improve valve function by influencing ventricular morphology and volume.

2. There are many complications of valve replacement surgery including valve failure, infection (i.e. prosthetic valve endocarditis) and dehiscence. Mechanical valves require lifelong anticoagulation to avoid valve thrombosis and this increases bleeding risk. Bioprosthetic valves do not require anticoagulation beyond the first 3 months but are more susceptible to structural deterioration and therefore less durable.

**Answers** *continued*

3.  The main factors to consider involve durability and anticoagulation. Mechanical valves are more durable than biological valves and usually last for 20 years or more but also require lifelong anticoagulation. Biological valves do not require anticoagulation beyond the first 3 months but usually only last 10–15 years before needing re-do surgery. Younger patients therefore tend to opt for mechanical valves while older patients often opt for a biological valve, especially if they are not expected to outlive their valve.

4.  Left heart catheter studies can be used to further investigate valve disease but also allows coronary angiography to be performed at the same time to identify co-existing coronary artery disease. If significant coronary disease is identified, the surgeon can repair (or replace) the diseased valve and perform a coronary artery by-pass graft (CABG) operation during the same operation. Alleviating ischaemia improves the patient's prognosis and reduces the risk of having a second operation.

5.  Valvular dysfunction places the chamber immediately proximal under strain from either increased pressure (in stenotic lesions) or volume (regurgitant lesions) load. Ultimately, this results in dysfunction of the proximal compartments. Right-sided valve disease strains the right heart and systemic veins causing right ventricular failure, raised jugular venous pressure and peripheral oedema which, in severe cases, can cause hepatic impairment. Left-sided valve disease results in left heart failure and elevated pressures in the pulmonary circulation which causes pulmonary arterial hypertension. The combination of left and right ventricular failure is called congestive cardiac failure.

6.  Transthoracic echocardiography (TTE) does not provide the same level of endocardial definition or detail as transoesophageal echocardiography (TOE), especially in mitral and prosthetic valve disease. A TOE may detect a vegetation after a 'normal' or 'inconclusive' TTE and so a TTE can be falsely reassuring. When there is a strong clinical suspicion of endocarditis, a TOE should be performed. Endocarditis is diagnosed according to the Duke criteria (see page 280). Therefore, even if the TOE is also negative for signs of infection (a major criterion), a diagnosis of endocarditis can still be made if one other major criterion and three minor criteria, or five minor criteria are met.

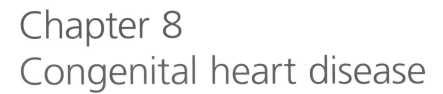

# Chapter 8
# Congenital heart disease

## Starter questions

Answers to the following questions are on page 298.

1. What are the most common congenital cardiac abnormalities?
2. Why do some cyanotic children squat to relieve their symptoms?
3. Why might a patent ductus arteriosus be lifesaving?
4. Why is using a pacemaker in a neonate problematic?
5. Why are heart defects often found alongside defects in other systems?

## Introduction

Advances in modern medicine have extended the survival into adulthood of patients with even complex congenital heart disease.

Congenital heart disease is divided into cyanotic and non-cyanotic conditions (**Table 8.1**). Patients with cyanotic congenital heart disease have inadequate oxygen saturation because of the shunting of blood from right to left and from the mixing of oxygenated and deoxygenated blood in a single chamber (e.g. a single ventricle). Patients with non-cyanotic congenital

heart disease may have less obvious symptoms. In adults, the most common cardiac congenital lesions are atrial septal defects (ASDs) and bicuspid aortic valves, both of which have a good prognosis.

Congenital heart disease encompasses a heterogeneous, diverse and complex group of conditions and patterns of disease. This chapter covers the most common congenital cardiac abnormalities; it is not an exhaustive list.

| Congenital cardiac lesions | |
|---|---|
| **Cyanotic** | **Non-cyanotic** |
| Ebstein's anomaly | Aortic stenosis |
| Hypoplastic left heart | Atrial septal defect |
| Pulmonary atresia | Atrioventricular canal (endocardial cushion defect) |
| Tetralogy of Fallot | Coarctation of the aorta |
| Total anomalous pulmonary venous return | Patent ductus arteriosus |
| Transposition of the great vessels | Pulmonic stenosis |
| Tricuspid atresia | Ventricular septal defect |
| Truncus arteriosus | |

**Table 8.1** Congenital cyanotic and non-cyanotic cardiac lesions

# Case 9 A baby with failure to thrive and laboured breathing

## Presentation

Anna Rusedski, aged 4 weeks old has been brought to see the general practitioner (GP) by her 29-year-old mother, Martha. Martha is concerned that Anna has not gained any weight since birth, appears to be working hard to breathe, and seems to cry more than other babies. She has also noticed that Anna's feet are cold.

## Initial interpretation

Anna is failing to thrive (not growing at the expected rate). There are many possible causes for this (**Table 8.2**). Martha is right to consult the GP.

## History

Anna was born at 42 weeks' gestation after a pregnancy that had progressed well and without complication. After the birth, no abnormalities were detected at a 'baby check' at the hospital. However, over the first 2–3 weeks of her life, Anna was unsettled and did not feed properly. Martha says that there is a family history of congenital heart disease on the father's side.

## Interpretation of history

The family history of congenital heart disease raises suspicion of a cardiac cause for Anna's problems. The progression of symptoms over the first 2 weeks of life also point to a cardiac condition, because this is the period over which the patent ductus arteriosus (PDA) closes.

## Examination

Anna is not cyanotic, and she appears healthy despite the lack of weight gain. However, she is using her accessory muscles to take in air and her feet are cold. Also, there is a discrepancy in blood pressure between the arms and the legs, and a harsh systolic murmur is heard on auscultation.

Palpation of the peripheral pulses reveals very weak femoral pulses and radiofemoral delay. Oxygen saturation was lower in her feet than her hands which is unusual. The chest is clear, with no signs of chest infection or pulmonary oedema. The abdomen is soft and non-tender.

**Case 9** *continued*

| Causes of failure to thrive | |
| --- | --- |
| Endogenous | Exogenous |
| Inborn errors of metabolism | Caregiver – e.g. breast milk alone not sufficient for nutrition but formula not offered |
| Physical deformity e.g. cleft palate | Caregiver purposefully limiting calorific intake |
| Food allergy e.g. milk allergy | Patient purposefully restricting own calorific intake |
| Cystic fibrosis | |
| Gastrointestinal problems e.g Coeliac disease or chronic diarrhoea | |
| Heart disease | |
| Recurrent infection | |

**Table 8.2** The main causes of failure to thrive in infants. Failure to thrive implies poor physical growth and does not necessarily mean there are associated delays in other types of development (e.g. emotional or intellectual development). Causes are usually either endogenous or exogenous as described here but of course in many cases, the two may co-exist

## Interpretation of findings

The clinical findings combined with the history indicate a diagnosis of coarctation (narrowing) of the aorta. The difference in blood pressure between the arms and the legs, the murmur, the weak femoral pulses and the radiofemoral delay are all caused by constriction of the thoracic aorta. Therefore these clinical signs are pathognomonic of coarctation.

## Investigations

Anna is urgently referred to the local children's hospital. Her electrocardiogram (ECG) is normal, but chest X-ray shows signs of pulmonary plethora. Echocardiography shows that the left ventricle is enlarged and its function impaired; the constricted aortic arch is also visible (**Figure 8.1**).

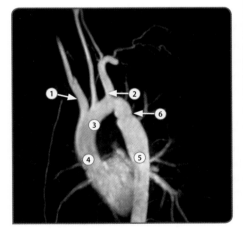

**Figure 8.1** Magnetic resonance angiogram showing coarctation of the aorta. ① Brachiocephalic artery ② left subclavian artery ③ arch of aorta ④ ascending aorta ⑤ descending aorta. ⑥ Coarctation site. Courtesy of Pankaj Garg.

## Diagnosis

The investigations confirm the diagnosis of coarctation of the aorta. Anna is started on prostagandin E1 infusion (which prevents the ductus arteriosus from closing, increasing oxygen saturation and preventing the onset of metabolic acidosis) and is transferred to the local paediatric centre, where she will undergo cardiac surgery to correct the condition.

> **Congenital heart disease affects 1% of all children globally.** In children born to affected parents, this risk increases to 2–5%.

# Atrial septal defect

An ASD is a hole in the interatrial septum between the right and left atria (**Figure 8.2**). The hole allows abnormal blood passage from the left atrium into the right atrium (**Figure 8.3**), resulting in extra flow through the right side of the heart and the pulmonary circulation.

## Types

There are two main types of ASD:

- ostium primum
- ostium secundum

## Epidemiology

Atrial septal defects account for 10% of all cases of congenital heart disease. The condition is twice as common in females than in males.

## Aetiology

The defect forms during embryonic development of the heart in the first trimester. The causes of each type of ASD are shown in **Table 8.3**.

## Pathogenesis

Left-to-right shunting of blood is normal in the womb but abnormal from birth. In the presence of an ASD, shunting continues during the first few months of life. If the increase in right-sided flow is sufficient, pressure in the pulmonary circulation increases; pulmonary hypertension occasionally results but is not usually severe.

## Clinical features

Atrial septal defects often have no clinical features. However, an ASD is sometimes part of a wider syndrome, such as Down's syndrome.

- A primum ASD sometimes presents in childhood with failure to thrive
- Patients with a secundum ASD are often asymptomatic, so the condition is often not diagnosed until adulthood

Right heart failure can complicate both types of ASD. Patients present with signs of

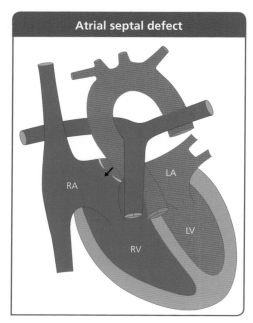

**Figure 8.2** Atrial septal defect. Arrow indicates abnormal blood flow across the atrial septal defect. LA, left atrium; LV, left ventricle; RA, right atrium; RV, right ventricle.

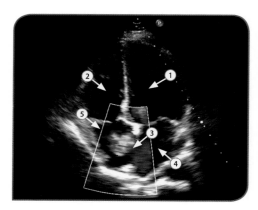

**Figure 8.3** Atrial septal defect. The (orange) colour Doppler signal demonstrates abnormal flow across the defect from left to right atrium. ① Left ventricle ② Right ventricle ③ Atrial septal defect ④ Left atrium ⑤ Right atrium.

right heart failure in middle age. Atrial fibrillation because of the resulting dilated atria also occurs.

| Types of atrial septal defect | |
|---|---|
| Type | Cause |
| Ostium primum | Incomplete fusion of the septum primum with the endocardial cushion |
| Ostium secundum | Deficiency, perforation or absence of the septum primum |

**Table 8.3** Types of atrial septal defect

Affected patients usually present with signs of right heart failure: raised jugular venous pressure, pulmonary or tricuspid murmurs, and a fixed split-second heart sound. As the disease progresses, signs of pulmonary hypertension become apparent: right ventricular heave, loud P2, and pulmonary regurgitation and tricuspid regurgitation murmurs.

## Diagnostic approach

The diagnostic approach for ASDs is shown in **Table 8.4**

In adults, the definitive diagnosis of ASD (and differentiation from patent foramen ovale) requires transoesophageal echocardiography. Transthoracic echocardiography is often not diagnostic, because of difficulties in obtaining accurate images of the interatrial septum.

## Management

Correction through surgery or with a specialised closure device is recommended in childhood to prevent the development and progression of right ventricular failure and pulmonary hypertension. Small ASDs are often left untreated. However, closure is advised once clinical signs of right heart volume loading are apparent.

## Prognosis

After closure of the defect, most patients go on to live full and active lives; their life expectancy is normal. However, the risk of atrial fibrillation remains because of the dilated atria.

| Diagnostic approach in atrial septal defect | |
|---|---|
| Diagnostic approach | Finding(s) |
| Electrocardio-graphy | Helps distinguish between primum and secundum ASDs<br><br>■ Primum ASD: right bundle branch block and left axis deviation<br>■ Secundum ASD: right bundle branch block and right axis deviation |
| Chest X-ray | Cardiac enlargement is caused by an enlarged right heart (both ventricle and atrium) |
| | Pulmonary plethora is seen in some cases |
| Echocardio-graphy | A hole between the right and left atria is often all that is required to diagnose ASD in children |
| Cardiac catheterisation | May be necessary to confirm diagnosis or assess the right-to-left shunt |

**Table 8.4** Diagnostic approach in atrial septal defect

# Ventricular septal defect

A ventricular septal defect (VSD) is a defect of the wall between the right and left ventricles of the heart (**Figure 8.4**). The condition may be congenital or acquired. An example of an acquired VSD is the type caused by necrosis of the myocardium after a large myocardial infarction.

This section discusses congenital VSDs. These account for one in five cases of congenital cardiac abnormalities.

## Epidemiology

Between 2 and 7 neonates in every 1000 have a ventricular septal defect.

## Aetiology

Congenital VSDs arise from an embryological abnormality during the formation of the heart in the first trimester. VSDs are associated with syndromes such as Fallot's tetralogy,

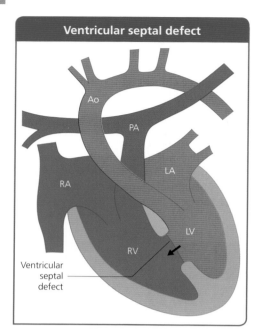

**Ventricular septal defect**

**Figure 8.4** Ventricular septal defect. Ao, aorta; LA, left atrium; LV, left ventricle; PA, pulmonary artery; RA, right atrium; RV, right ventricle. Arrow indicates abnormal blood flow across the ventricular septal defect.

which are also associated with other congenital lesions (e.g. PDA).

## Pathogenesis

The haemodynamic effects of a VSD depend on its size and the pulmonary vascular resistance.

$$\text{Pulmonary vascular resistance} = \frac{\text{(Input pressure–output pressure)}}{\text{Blood flow}}$$

Small VSDs are common. They often have no clinical features apart from a pansystolic murmur at the lower left sternal edge and apex.

Large VSDs cause left-to-right shunting of blood. This effect causes increased left ventricular volume, excess pulmonary blood flow, and decreased cardiac output. Ultimately, cardiac failure occurs.

## Clinical features

Neonates with large VSDs present with a pansystolic murmur and symptoms of heart failure: laboured and rapid breathing, feeding difficulties, failure to thrive and an enlarged liver.

Clinical signs include:

- pansystolic murmur
- laterally displaced apex beat
- right ventricular heave

If cardiac failure develops, jugular venous pressure becomes raised and peripheral and pulmonary oedema is present. Patients sometimes develop right-sided volume overload and consequent pulmonary hypertension.

## Diagnostic approach

### Electrocardiography

In small VSDs, the ECG is normal. However, in larger VSDs it often shows left or right axis deviation reflecting left and right ventricular enlargement, respectively.

### Chest X-ray

Chest X-ray is often normal when the VSD is small. However, with large VSDs biventricular enlargement and signs of cardiac failure may be visible.

### Echocardiography

Echocardiography is usually diagnostic (**Figure 8.5**).

### Cardiac catheterisation

Cardiac catheterisation is used to assess the size of the left-to-right shunt. On occasion, it is used to identify the site of the VSD, although this is rarely required.

## Management

Spontaneous closure occurs in 30–50% of cases; almost all small VSDs close spontaneously. Therefore treatment is often unnecessary.

### Medication and surgery

Medical therapy with diuretics to offload the ventricle is used as a temporary measure until either spontaneous closure or definitive surgery.

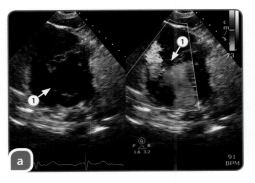 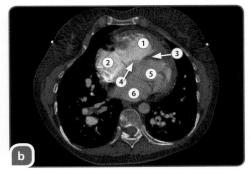

**Figure 8.5** (a) A short axis view echocardiogram of ① a large VSD with color flow across the septum (b) CT scan showing a VSD. ① Right ventricle ② right atrium ③ interventricular septum ④ VSD ⑤ left ventricle ⑥ left atrium.

Indications for surgical closure include:

- failure to thrive
- evidence of left-sided volume overload
- heart failure

The surgical mortality rate is < 2%.

## Prognosis

After spontaneous closure or successful surgical correction of an isolated lesion, patients with a VSD can expect to lead active lives. Their life expectancy is normal.

# Eisenmenger's syndrome

In Eisenmenger's syndrome, patients with an uncorrected congenital defect associated with a significant left-to-right shunt (commonly a VSD or PDA) develop fixed, irreversible pulmonary vascular disease and pulmonary hypertension. When pulmonary hypertension develops, there comes a time when the right-sided pressure becomes greater than that on the left. At this point, blood no longer shunts from left to right but flows from right to left. This reversal in blood flow causes cyanosis.

Eisenmenger's syndrome is a late sign of advanced and irreversible pulmonary haemodynamic changes. The condition affects up to 5% of patients with a VSD. Classically, patients

with Eisenmenger's syndrome become more cyanotic on exercise.

The prognosis for this group of patients is improving because of earlier detection and better treatments, and many survive into middle age.

> **The murmur associated with a VSD is a harsh and pansystolic.** It differs from those caused by mitral regurgitation and aortic stenosis, because it is audible all over the precordium and is not localised to one specific area. Always consider this in your differential diagnosis when examining patients.

# Patent ductus arteriosus

The ductus arteriosus allows blood to flow from the pulmonary circulation to the aorta during fetal life (see page 10). It usually closes spontaneously in the first month of life.

However, in cases of PDA, the ductus fails to close, resulting in a permanent connection between the descending aorta and the pulmonary artery. Postnatally, the aortic pressure is greater than the pulmonary pressure, which causes a left-to-right shunt of blood (**Figure 8.6**).

## Epidemiology

Patent ductus arteriosus accounts for 5–10% of all congenital lesions. The condition affects 0.08% of all neonates and is more common in those born prematurely.

## Clinical features

Patent ductus arteriosus is often diagnosed incidentally during routine auscultation. Babies with a large defect present with a left-to-right shunt and behave in a similar fashion to babies with a VSD.

Patients with a PDA are often asymptomatic. However, if flow across the ductus is large, patients present with signs and symptoms of cardiac failure.

A continuous, machinery-like murmur is heard in the pulmonary area. If the PDA is large, patients often have a palpable thrill in the pulmonary area and a collapsing pulse associated with a wide pulse pressure.

## Diagnostic approach

Echocardiography is the investigation of choice. Magnetic resonance imaging (MRI) of the heart also determines the anatomical defect.

> All newborn babies have a 'baby check', which includes auscultation of the heart and assessment of peripheral pulses. This examination is often the first step in the diagnosis of previously undetected congenital heart problems such as coarctation of the aorta and PDA.

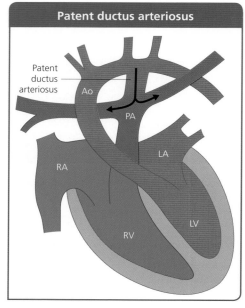

**Figure 8.6** Patent ductus arteriosus. Ao, aorta; LA, left atrium; LV, left ventricle; PA, pulmonary artery; RA, right atrium; RV, right ventricle.

## Management

Spontaneous closure may occur up to 6 months from birth. If defects are large, closure by surgery or a catheter-delivered device is usually indicated.

In the womb, prostaglandin synthesis maintains ductal patency. Therefore, if the PDA is detected in the immediate neonatal period, non-steroidal anti-inflammatory drugs such as indometacin (an inhibitor of prostaglandin synthesis) is given to try to stimulate duct closure.

## Prognosis

Patients expect to lead a normal life provided no complications develop (e.g. pulmonary hypertension or heart failure).

# Tetralogy of Fallot

Tetralogy of Fallot (**Figure 8.7**) is the commonest cyanotic congenital heart defect. As the name suggests, it comprises four different features:

- pulmonary stenosis
- VSD
- overriding of the aorta
- right ventricular hypertrophy

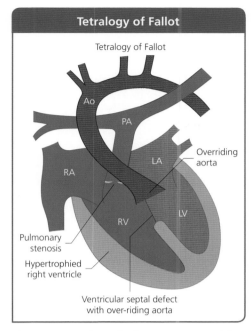

**Tetralogy of Fallot**

Tetralogy of Fallot

Ao

PA

LA

Overriding aorta

RA

LV

RV

Pulmonary stenosis

Hypertrophied right ventricle

Ventricular septal defect with over-riding aorta

**Figure 8.7** Tetralogy of Fallot. Ao, aorta; LA, left atrium; LV, left ventricle; PA, pulmonary artery; RA, right atrium; RV, right ventricle.

## Epidemiology

Tetralogy of Fallot accounts for 10% of all cases of congenital heart disease. The condition affects 3–6 neonates in every 10,000 and is more common in males than in females.

## Aetiology

During embryological development of the affected heart, the bulbus cordis fails to rotate, so the aorta is further forward and more to the right than normal (see page 7). This malalignment results in pulmonary stenosis, a VSD below the aortic valve and right ventricular hypertrophy.

The pulmonary stenosis prevents blood leaving the right ventricle, therefore deoxygenated blood leaves through the over-riding aorta into the systemic circulation. Some patients with the tetralogy of Fallot have pulmonary atresia or critical pulmonary stenosis. In such cases, the only way blood can enter the lungs is through the PDA. However, most patients have enough flow from the right ventricle to the pulmonary artery to allow oxygenation of blood.

## Pathogenesis

In addition to the classic tetralogy, other anomalies are sometimes present. These include a hypoplastic left pulmonary artery, an ASD and a right-sided aortic arch.

The large VSD means that the left and right ventricles have the same systemic pressure. However, the pulmonary stenosis causes a net right-to-left shunt, with associated cyanosis.

## Clinical features

Tetralogy of Fallot usually presents from 3 months of age. Neonates often appear normal and are not cyanosed. Infants may have clubbed fingers, but this feature is rare because of earlier diagnosis (often at birth).

Cyanosis is sometimes present and classically occurs with stress, for example during feeding or crying (feeding leads to reduced air intake and therefore stress). The tendency to become cyanosed increases with age.

There are signs of right ventricular hypertrophy: a right ventricular heave and a murmur consistent with pulmonary stenosis and a VSD (i.e. a murmur during systole). Polycythaemia (the production of too many red blood cells), also occurs.

Older patients often squat to relieve the cyanosis, because this position reduces the shunt by increasing systemic vascular resistance. However, this remedial action is now rarely seen, because of earlier diagnosis and surgical correction.

## Diagnostic approach

The ECG shows signs of right ventricular hypertrophy with right axis deviation. Chest X-ray is abnormal; the heart is often described as having a boot-like appearance (coeur en sabot; **Figure 8.8**). Echocardiography confirms the diagnosis. Cardiac MRI is used to provide more detailed morphological information.

## Management

Primary corrective surgery by 1 year of age is preferred. Until then, patients need to be treated medically.

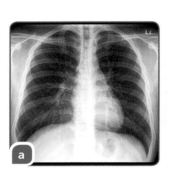
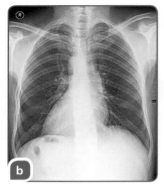
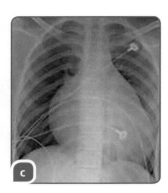

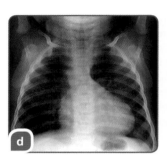
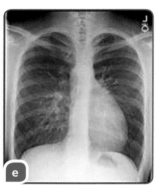

**Figure 8.8** Radiographic comparison of the major congenital heart diseases.( a) Normal. (b) Dextrocardia. (c) Ebstein's anomaly. (d) Tetralogy of Fallot. (e) Transposition of the great arteries.

**Professional patients?** Many children with congenital heart defects, and their parents, become experts in their condition and its management.

Management of congenital heart disease is a highly specialised area of medicine. Always call for help early; senior support is often required when considering treatment plans for patients who have come into hospital. Remember that regional hospitals often treat patients with congenital heart defects, so it may be necessary to seek help from outside the unit.

In patients with more severe cyanosis caused by low pulmonary blood flow,a staged operation is done. First, before 3 months of age, a Blalock–Taussig or Waterston shunt is formed. A Blalock–Taussig shunt involves the creation of a subclavian artery to pulmonary artery shunt to increase pulmonary circulation.

A Waterston shunt involves the creation of a narrow opening between the ascending aorta and the right pulmonary artery to increase pulmonary circulation. Complete correction is carried out later, when the child is 2 years old.

## Prognosis

Surgical correction confers good long-term survival (> 85% at 30 years). However, even following complete correction, children sometimes experience pulmonary regurgitation that is symptomatic later in life.

# Transposition of the great arteries

There are two types of transposition of the great arteries (TGA): complete and corrected. Only in corrected TGA is the circulation normal.

## Complete transposition of the great arteries

The aorta arises from the right ventricle, and the pulmonary artery from the left ventricle. The two circuits are completely separate. Survival in these patients depends on the presence of a shunt (an ASD, a VSD or a PDA), which allows oxygenated blood to enter the systemic circulation (**Figure 8.9**).

## Epidemiology

Transposition of the great arteries accounts for 5–7% of all congenital heart defects. The condition affects 2 or 3 neonates per 10,000. It is the commonest congenital lesion presenting with cyanosis at birth.

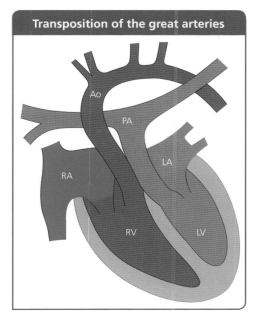

**Figure 8.9** Transposition of the great arteries. Ao, aorta; LA, left atrium; LV, left ventricle; PA, pulmonary artery; RA, right atrium; RV, right ventricle.

## Pathogenesis

Complete TGA often have an associated shunt, for example in cases of PDA or VSD. The shunt can be life-saving, but the blood flow it provides may be insufficient for survival.

## Clinical features

Complete TGA presents with cyanosis at birth. The cyanosis increases as the life-sustaining PDA closes. Without surgical correction, progressive heart failure occurs and ultimately death is inevitable.

Clinical signs include a hyperdynamic circulation. Murmurs are difficult to hear unless there is an associated shunt (an ASD or a VSD).

## Diagnostic approach

The ECG is usually abnormal, with right axis deviation and signs of right heart strain. Chest X-ray is abnormal; the heart has an 'egg on its side' appearance. An echocardiogram is diagnostic.

## Management

Several surgical strategies are available for correction of complete TGA. The commonest is definitive anatomical surgical correction.

In the neonatal period, intravenous prostaglandin infusion is used to maintain the patency of the PDA. Prostaglandin administration ensures that mixing of blood between the two circulations continues through the PDA. However, in this condition the drug's effects are limited, and a balloon atrial septostomy is required urgently. This is a life-saving measure until surgery is performed.

> **Prostaglandin maintains the patency of the PDA by causing it to dilate and remain open.** The infusion starts as soon as TGA is clinically suspected in a neonate; they are transferred to a paediatric cardiac surgical unit. for urgent atrial septostomy followed by corrective surgery.

## Prognosis

The longer the time without treatment, the higher the mortality (**Table 8.5**). Surgical correction yields excellent long-term results, with 97% survival at 25 years.

# Congenitally corrected transposition of the great arteries

In congenitally corrected TGA, the circulation is normal but the ventricles are reversed.

- The left ventricle is in the position of the right ventricle; it receives blood from the right atrium and pumps blood to the lungs
- The right ventricle takes the position and job of the left ventricle; it receives blood from the left atrium and pumps blood to the body

## Epidemiology

Like complete TGA, this condition is rare. However, the risk of congenital heart disease in the children of a mother with corrected TGA is as high as 6%.

## Pathogenesis

Congenitally corrected TGA is usually associated with other lesions. The most common of these are a VSD (80%), pulmonary stenosis (40%), aortic regurgitation and complete heart block.

## Clinical features

The symptoms of congenitally corrected TGA are:

- Systemic ventricular failure: the right ventricle (the systemic ventricle) is not designed to cope with the higher pressures in the systemic circulation
- Dizziness
- Syncope: caused by complete heart block (common)
- Arrhythmias (common)

The clinical signs often reflect the associated lesions, for example pulmonary stenosis and aortic regurgitation. Detection of such lesions in a cyanosed neonate immediately raises the suspicion of congenitally corrected TGA.

# Diagnostic approach

The ECG sometimes shows 1st, 2nd or 3rd degree heart block. Chest X-ray may show an enlarged heart, again caused by the associated lesions. Furthermore, the aorta is left-sided and resembles a duck's back.

# Management

This is a rare diagnosis and definitive management should be performed in as specialist paediatric centre. Treatment options are shown in **Table 8.6**.

## Prognosis

Prognosis is very variable. The outcome depends on the early clinical course of the patient.

| Prognosis for complete transposition of the great arteries | |
|---|---|
| Time without treatment | Mortality (%) |
| 1 week | 30 |
| 1 month | 50 |
| 1 year | 90 |

**Table 8.5** Prognosis for complete transposition of the great arteries

| Management of congenitally corrected transposition of the great arteries | |
|---|---|
| Medical therapy | Required for any heart failure that develops (see page 247) |
| Surgical treatment options | Pacemaker insertion for heart block |
| | Cardiac ablation for supraventricular tachycardias |
| | Closure of any associated ventricular septal defect or valve lesions |

**Table 8.6** Management of congenitally corrected transposition of the great arteries

# Coarctation of the aorta

Coarctation of the aorta is caused by a congenital focal narrowing of the aorta. The condition causes high blood pressure in the arteries that arise proximal to the constriction, as well as reduced blood flow distally (**Figure 8.10**).

## Epidemiology

Coarctation of the aorta accounts for 5–8% of all congenital defects in the UK.

## Aetiology

The condition arises during development of the vascular system. Infantile coarctation presents soon after birth and is caused by hypoplasia of the aortic isthmus. Coarctation also presents in adulthood. In such cases, the obstruction is usually progressive and patients present with complications such as high blood pressure.

## Pathogenesis

Associated lesions, such as bicuspid aortic valves, are common. Coarctation is also associated with PDAs and other complex cardiac lesions.

> Many other aortopathies are commonly seen in clinical practice, for example bicuspid aortic valves and Marfan's syndrome (Figure 10.6). These conditions require regular screening for aortic dilation, a common feature. Surgery is indicated if the sinus of Valsalva dilates to > 5 cm.

## Clinical features

Infantile heart failure presents with failure to thrive and cardiac failure. If the condition is undetected in infancy, the patient often presents with proximal hypertension, usually restricted to the upper body, in later life.

> In coarctation of the aorta, the anastomoses between the anterior and posterior intercostal arteries provide an alternative route for blood to travel to the lower body. These arteries dilate and may erode the lower borders of the ribs. This effect is visible on chest X-ray as rib notching.

Blood pressure differs between the left and right arms, depending on the precise location of the constriction. Femoral pulses are weak, delayed or absent when compared with the radial pulse on the same side (radiofemoral delay). A systolic murmur is usually heard under the left clavicle.

## Diagnostic approach

No specific ECG changes reflect aortic coarctation necessarily. However, left ventricular hypertrophy and right bundle branch block are seen, reflecting secondary myocardial hypertrophy. Chest X-ray is often normal

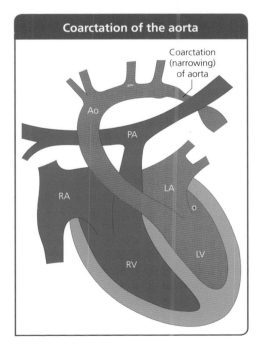

**Figure 8.10** Coarctation of the aorta. Ao, aorta; LA, left atrium; LV, left ventricle; PA, pulmonary artery; RA, right atrium; RV, right ventricle.

in infancy but as the patient ages, shows rib notching.

Echocardiography is the first choice investigation. The echocardiogram shows increased flow velocity through the coarctation and often shows the shape of the narrowing itself. Cardiac MRI or computerised tomography provides more comprehensive and detailed morphological assessment.

## Management

Management of coarctation of the aorta depends on the age of the patient (**Table 8.7**). Corrective surgery is performed in both infants and adults.

## Prognosis

All patients who have undergone surgery are followed up for life, because complications occasionally develop many years later.

These include hypertension, aneurysm formation and recurrent coarctation (which sometimes requires further surgical correction). However, once a coarctation is corrected, prognosis is good.

| **Management of coarctation of the aorta** | |
|---|---|
| Patient group | Corrective surgery |
| Infants | Insertion of a patch to widen the aorta |
| | Removal of the narrow section and completion of repair by end-to-end anastomosis (more common) |
| Adults | Conventional open aortic surgery |
| | Dilation of the constriction by balloon angioplasty or aortic stent insertion (more common) |

**Table 8.7** Management of coarctation of the aorta

---

## Answers to starter questions

1. Atrial septal defects and bicuspid aortic valves are the most common congenital cardiac lesions.

2. Children who are cyanotic because they have Fallot's tetralogy squat to relieve the cyanosis because it increases pulmonary blood flow and systemic vascular resistance reducing the right to left shunt and relieving symptoms. This usually occurs when there is infundibular pulmonary stenosis.

3. A patent ductus arteriosus is lifesaving in Fallot's tetralogy with a critical pulmonary stenosis because it allows blood to pass back into the lungs thereby increasing oxygen levels.

4. Using a pacemaker in a neonate is problematic because of the small size of the patient and because they develop and grow rapidly over the first few years of life. This means they will require repeated box changes and each procedure carries the risk of infection, pericardial effusion and pneumothorax. Pacemaker leads may also become too short as the patient grows up.

5. Congenital defects are formed during the embryological development of the fetus and it is common for more than one body system to be affected at the same time.

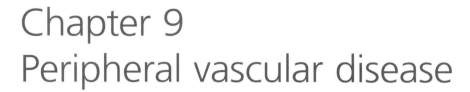

# Chapter 9
# Peripheral vascular disease

## Starter questions

Answers to the following questions are on page 323–324.

1. Why are patients with asymptomatic varicose veins no longer treated in some areas?
2. What are the pros and cons to screening for diseases such as aortic aneurysm?
3. Why would one blood vessel 'steal' blood from another?
4. Why do some young, otherwise fit and healthy, athletes develop peripheral vascular disease?
5. If a patient refuses to stop smoking, should they receive treatment for their vascular disease?
6. How can clots in the peripheral venous circulation cause blockages in the brain?

# Introduction

Peripheral vascular disease affects 15% of the population, and its incidence increases with age. It is a significant, preventable cause of:

- stroke
- limb amputation
- pulmonary embolism
- sudden death

Peripheral vascular disease encompasses various pathological processes, including stenosis, thrombosis, spasm, embolism and inflammation. These processes affect both arteries and veins, and peripheral vascular disease is divided into peripheral arterial disease and peripheral venous disease.

Peripheral arterial disease is caused by atherosclerosis. Atherosclerotic plaques narrow or occlude the arterial lumen, causing acute or chronic ischaemia in the distal tissues.

Peripheral venous disease results from mechanical failure of veins. This causes abnormal venous dilatation (varicosities), venous hypertension and pooling of blood. Stasis of blood may result in deep vein thrombosis. If a deep vein thrombus embolises, it travels through the right heart, passing from the systemic circulation into the pulmonary circulation. Here, it occludes one or more pulmonary arteries – a condition known as pulmonary embolism.

Peripheral vascular disease and the discipline of vascular surgery traditionally exclude diseases of the cerebral, coronary, pulmonary, mesenteric, renal and splenic circulations.

# Case 10   A collapse on the street

## Presentation

George Sharp, a 66-year-old retiree, is seen clutching his abdomen in pain shortly before collapsing to the ground. Luckily, an off-duty nurse is present to help him and immediately phones for an ambulance.

## Initial interpretation

Male gender and old age are risk factors for atherosclerosis and malignancy. Collapse is a result of severe pain (if the patient is conscious) or life-threatening hypotension (if they are unconscious). Possible diagnoses include:

- myocardial infarction manifesting as epigastric pain
- perforated bowel
- rupture of an abdominal aortic aneurysm

## Further history

Mr Sharp's wife says that he has been complaining of stomach ache and backache for a couple of weeks, with no particular pattern. He has not complained

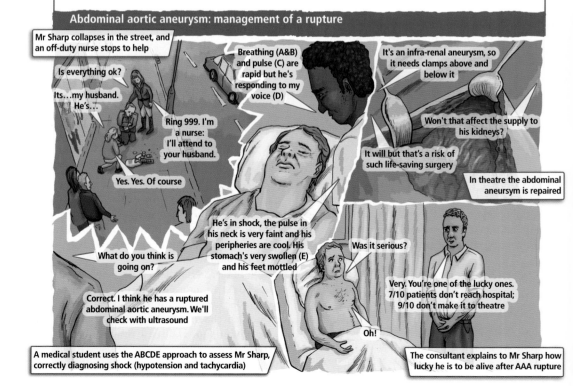

Abdominal aortic aneurysm: management of a rupture

Mr Sharp collapses in the street, and an off-duty nurse stops to help

Is everything ok?

Its…my husband. He's…

Ring 999. I'm a nurse: I'll attend to your husband.

Yes. Yes. Of course

What do you think is going on?

Correct. I think he has a ruptured abdominal aortic aneurysm. We'll check with ultrasound

A medical student uses the ABCDE approach to assess Mr Sharp, correctly diagnosing shock (hypotension and tachycardia)

Breathing (A&B) and pulse (C) are rapid but he's responding to my voice (D)

He's in shock, the pulse in his neck is very faint and his peripheries are cool. His stomach's very swollen (E) and his feet mottled

It's an infra-renal aneurysm, so it needs clamps above and below it

Won't that affect the supply to his kidneys?

It will but that's a risk of such life-saving surgery

In theatre the abdominal aneursym is repaired

Was it serious?

Very. You're one of the lucky ones. 7/10 patients don't reach hospital; 9/10 don't make it to theatre

Oh!

The consultant explains to Mr Sharp how lucky he is to be alive after AAA rupture

of breathlessness, dizziness, chest pain, weight loss or a change in bowel habit. He suffers from high blood pressure and high cholesterol.

He had a mini stroke (transient ischaemic attack) last year, but Mrs Sharp cannot remember what medication her husband is taking. His father died suddenly in his sixties, but his mother died of 'old age' in her eighties.

## Examination

The nurse examines Mr Sharp at the roadside, using the ABCDE approach for assessment of the critically ill patient.

- Airway: the patient is groaning and confused but maintaining his own airway
- Breathing: respiratory rate is 38 breaths/ min, chest expansion is symmetrical, and there is no dullness or hyper-resonance
- Circulation: carotid pulse rate is 140 beats/min and capillary refill time is 5 s
- Disability: the patient responds to voice only
- Exposure: his stomach is distended and pulsatile, and his lower legs appear mottled

## Interpretation of findings

Abdominal pain radiating to the back indicates intra-abdominal, usally retroperitoneal, pathology. Without breathlessness or an angina-like chest pain, a diagnosis of ischaemic heart disease is unlikely. There is no weight loss or any change in bowel pattern to suggest intestinal malignancy.

If atherosclerosis is present in one anatomical region (e.g. the carotid artery), it is likely in other areas (e.g. the abdominal aorta). Mr Sharp's transient ischaemic attack could have arisen from atherosclerotic disease of the carotid artery, making abdominal aortic aneurysm more likely.

It is also possible that his father died from a ruptured abdominal aortic aneurysm.

The combination of hypotension and tachycardia suggests shock. Mr Sharp's confusion and the mottling of his legs indicate reduced perfusion of the brain and lower limbs, respectively. His distended, pulsatile abdomen is likely to be the result of a ruptured abdominal aortic aneurysm.

> **In emergency or prehospital settings, systolic blood pressure can be estimated without the use of a sphygmomanometer.** Remember that the further away an artery is from the heart, the higher the blood pressure must be to reach that point. Therefore, the carotid artery becomes palpable with a blood pressure of > 60 mmHg, the femoral artery palpable with a blood pressure of > 70 mmHg and the radial artery palpable with a blood pressure of > 80 mmHg.

## Investigations

Mr Sharp is taken by ambulance to the local emergency department. On the way, paramedics measure his blood pressure, blood glucose and temperature; they also record an electrocardiogram (**Table 9.1**).

On arrival, the paramedics hand over the case to a medical student and the emergency department registrar, who perform a further rapid assessment and a focused

| Results of investigations after the collapse | |
|---|---|
| Investigation | Result |
| Blood pressure | 68/50 mmHg |
| Blood glucose | 5.5 mmol/L |
| Temperature | 36.5°C |
| Electrocardiogram | Sinus tachycardia |

**Table 9.1** Results of investigations for the man found collapsed on the street

**Case 10** *continued*

ultrasound examination. This is used to assess for the three most common forms of shock: heart failure, pericardial tamponade and ruptured abdominal aortic aneurysm. Ultrasound visualises a 10-cm abdominal aortic aneurysm.

> **A ruptured abdominal aortic aneurysm is a clinical diagnosis.** The diagnosis is based on the triad of abdominal pain, shock and a pulsatile mass in the abdomen.

## Diagnosis

The normal blood sugar and temperature rule out hypoglycaemia or sepsis as a working diagnosis. However, Mr Sharp's low blood pressure, tachycardia and confusion are signs of haemorrhagic shock resulting from a ruptured abdominal aortic aneurysm. This diagnosis is also supported by his recent abdominal pain, history of vasculopathy and pulsatile abdominal mass.

He undergoes life-saving emergency surgery to repair the aneurysm.

# Case 11 Painful, cold left foot

## Presentation

Ms Newton, a 56-year-old shopkeeper, presents to her local emergency department complaining of a painful and cold left foot (**Figure 9.1**).

## Initial interpretation

Foot pain is common; causes include gout, plantar fasciitis and ligament sprain. However, coolness suggests a problem with the blood supply. Constant perfusion of warm blood maintains normal tissue temperature and respiration. It is important to establish:

- rapidity and time of onset

- whether or not the condition is worsening
- associated symptoms, such as numbness and radiation

## History

The pain has been increasing for a couple of days. It was not preceded by trauma, and has no focal tender point. The pain is worse when Ms Newton lies in bed, causing her to hang her foot out. She is a lifelong smoker but has no other significant medical history of note and takes no medications. Her parents are both in their eighties and are well.

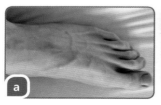 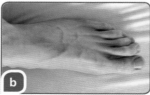 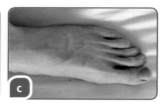

**Figure 9.1** (a) Cold, painful, pale and pulseless acutely ischaemic foot before reperfusion therapy. (b) Immediate return of colour with associated reactive hyperaemia (see page 68) following reperfusion. (c) Normal colour of the foot the following day.

**Case 11** *continued*

The symptoms of acute limb ischaemia are known as the six P's.

- Pain
- Pulseless
- Pallor
- Perishingly cold
- Paraesthesia
- Paralysis

## Interpretation of history

Lack of trauma from the history or focal tenderness on examination means that the pain is unlikely to originate from the musculoskeletal system. Night pain is common in lower limb ischaemia, because gravity cannot facilitate blood flow to the feet when the patient is horizontal in bed. This problem is remedied when the foot is below the level of the heart, a position commonly achieved by dangling the foot out of bed.

## Examination

Other than a blood pressure of 155/95 mmHg, Ms Newton's cardiovascular, respiratory and abdominal systems are all normal. She is afebrile and has normal oxygen saturation and blood glucose.

Her left foot is pale and pulseless, with a delayed capillary refill time of 10 s. The most distal palpable pulse are her femoral arteries. She has difficulty both dorsiflexing and plantar flexing her foot actively, and it is painful when done passively.

## Interpretation of findings

Delayed capillary refill time indicates impaired blood supply and suggests a problem with either the heart or the arteries. The normal cardiovascular, respiratory and abdominal examination help exclude diagnoses such as aortic dissection or ruptured aortic aneurysm, which do not cause ischaemia in a single limb in isolation. The normal oxygen saturation, blood sugar and temperature rule out hypoxia, hyperglycaemia or hypothermia/sepsis as con-

tributing factors. Furthermore, the normal blood pressure and singularly affected limb eliminates any form of shock, such as cardiogenic or septic shock, and heart failure as the cause. All limbs would be affected if this was the case.

A unilateral pulseless and cold foot confirms an arterial aetiology. The left femoral artery is palpable in the left groin indicating that the problem is distal to this. The presence of a motor deficit indicates that tissue viability is threatened. Urgent revascularisation is needed.

## Investigations

An electrocardiogram and blood tests (including full blood count and renal and liver function tests) are performed; all are normal. The normal electrocardiogram rules out a thrombus, formed due to atrial fibrillation, causing acute limb ischaemia and the normal blood tests are an important pre-operative baseline as blood loss and significant organ injury may follow any life-saving operation.

The ankle–brachial pressure index (ABPI) is < 0.5 (75 mmHg/155 mmHg) in the left foot demonstrating that the blood pressure perfusing the legs is significantly lower than the arms (it should be the same). There is only a faint very Doppler ultrasound signal present in the distal femoral artery. This further supports the working diagnosis of acute limb ischaemia.

## Diagnosis

The diagnosis is acute lower limb ischaemia, as indicated by the unilateral painful, cold and pulseless foot. The foot pain at rest and delayed capillary refill show that the ischaemia is severe enough to threaten tissue viability (see **Table 9.2**). The difficulty in moving the foot means that urgent revascularisation is required.

Ms Newton's condition is likely to be the result of peripheral arterial disease, accelerated by cigarette smoking and untreated hypertension.

# Abdominal aortic aneurysm

Abdominal aortic aneurysm is a focal dilatation of the abdominal aorta (**Figure 9.2**). The aneurysm is most commonly located below the kidneys (i.e. infrarenal), and this may, or may not, involve the iliac arteries. Abdominal aortic aneurysm is defined as a diameter > 50% larger than normal. The normal abdominal aortic diameter is around 2 cm (corrected for age, sex and body size). Therefore, a diameter >3 cm would indicate an aneurysm.

## Epidemiology

Abdominal aortic aneurysms are present in 10% of men and 2% of women worldwide, most commonly in people aged 65–75 years. The condition occurs most frequently in Caucasians and is less common in other ethnic groups. It is one of the leading causes of death in the UK and the USA.

More than half of patients whose abdominal aortic aneurysm ruptures die before reaching hospital, most without ever knowing they had the disease.

## Aetiology

Risk factors are the same as for atherosclerosis: smoking, hypertension, hypercholesterolaemia, old age and male gender. In less than 5% of cases, the abdominal aortic aneurysm is caused by a disease of collagen architecture (such as Marfan's syndrome; see page 336), mycotic emboli from infective endocarditis (see page 277) or in rare cases syphilis.

> Patients with multiple risk factors for atherosclerosis, or signs of the condition, are sometimes referred to as **vasculopaths or arteriopaths**.

## Prevention

Early diagnosis and treatment of risk factors help prevent progression of abdominal aortic aneurysm. Ultrasound screening allows early diagnosis, monitoring of expansion and early intervention before rupture, but it does not prevent disease. In the UK, abdominal ultrasound is used to screen all men over 65; the aim is to intervene prior to rupture, reducing the number of deaths from this disease.

## Pathogenesis

Degradation and structural failure of collagen and elastin in the tunica media of the aorta (see page 57) causes a focal weakening of the wall. This leads to progressive aortic dilatation, causing further weakening, the start of a viscious circle. The risk of rupture increases as the size of the abdominal aortic aneurysm increases (**Figure 9.3**).

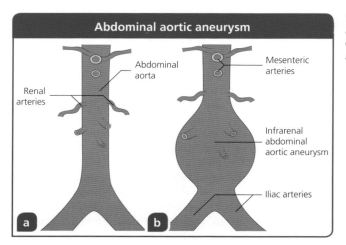

**Abdominal aortic aneurysm**

Renal arteries

Abdominal aorta

Mesenteric arteries

Infrarenal abdominal aortic aneurysm

Iliac arteries

a    b

**Figure 9.2** Saccular swelling of an abdominal aortic aneurysm. (a) Normal aorta. (b) Aorta with abdominal aneurysm.

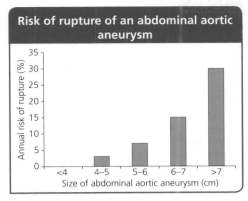

**Risk of rupture of an abdominal aortic aneurysm**

(y-axis) Annual risk of rupture (%)
(x-axis) Size of abdominal aortic aneurysm (cm): <4, 4–5, 5–6, 6–7, >7

**Figure 9.3** Annual risk of rupture of an abdominal aortic aneurysm. The risk increases with the size of the aneurysm. Data from Brewster DC, et al. J Vasc Surg 2003; 37:1106–117.

> **Aneurysms affecting both the thoracic aorta and the abdominal aorta are called thoracoabdominal aneurysms.** Unlike abdominal aortic aneurysms, 20% are caused by aortic dissections, and their surgical management is riskier and more complex.

## Clinical features

Abdominal aortic aneurysms are asymptomatic until they expand significantly (by > 5 cm) or rupture. Symptoms include:

- back, flank, abdominal or groin pain
- compression of the femoral nerves, causing paraesthesia of the anterior thigh and quadriceps weakness
- embolic phenomena leading to acute lower limb ischaemia
- a pulsatile sensation or mass in the stomach

Clinical examination misses abdominal aortic aneurysm in half of cases. Therefore if suspicion is high, patients are referred for further investigation.

## Diagnostic approach

Abdominal ultrasound (see page 133) is quick, cheap, non-invasive and does not expose the patient to ionising radiation. This makes it an ideal screening tool. However, its use is limited by body habitus and overlying bowel gas.

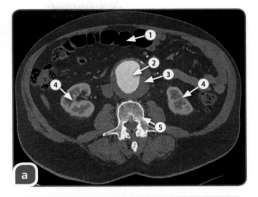

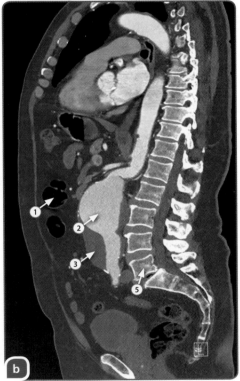

**Figure 9.4** Computerised tomography scan showing an abdominal aortic aneurysm. (a) Transverse plane. (b) Sagittal plane. ①, Overlying bowel gas; ②, aortic lumen; ③, clot (within the aneurysm); ④, kidney; ⑤, spine.

Computerised tomography (CT) demonstrates the precise anatomy, location and involvement of other vessels (e.g. renal iliac arteries) and identifies presence of thrombus. It is useful in planning therapy such as surgery or stenting (**Figure 9.4**).

Many emergency departments now have physicians trained to use ultrasound when patients present with suspected abdominal aortic aneurysm It is used at the patient's bedside in order for a quick diagnosis. One in a hundred cases are diagnosed incidentally. For example, a magnetic resonance imaging scan for a patient presenting with radicular neck pain may reveal an abdominal aortic aneurysm in addition to disc pathology.

Differential diagnoses are shown in **Table 9.2.**

## Management

In all patients with abdominal aortic aneurysm, risk factors should be managed appropriately. Smoking cessation, and treatment of hypertension and hypercholesterolaemia, are the mainstay of conservative treatment. Whilst medication cannot halt or reverse the condition, aggressive treatment of risk factors slows progression.

Patients requiring elective surgical repair of their aneurysm are increasingly being assessed using cardiopulmonary exercise testing, so that clinical decisions are based on physiological fitness and not chronological age. This helps avoid procedures in those simply not fit enough to withstand and recover from a physiological insult such as open abdominal aortic aneurysm repair.

## Watchful waiting

Watchful waiting is the monitoring of a condition at regular intervals until the threshold for intervention is reached. For patients with an abdominal aortic aneurysm of < 5.5 cm, watchful waiting is indicated because the risk of repair exceeds that of rupture. Follow-up ultrasound scans are required once or twice a year, depending on the whether the aneurysm is < 4.0 cm or < 5.5 cm respectively. This is to monitor the rate of progression of the aneursym, with intervention being reserved for patients with aneurysms > 5.5 cm.

| Differential diagnosis of abdominal aortic aneurysm | | | | |
|---|---|---|---|---|
| Differential diagnosis | Site of pain | Associated symptoms | Risk factor(s) | Abdominal examination findings |
| Abdominal aortic aneurysm | Back | Variable | Hypertension Smoking | Pulsatile mass |
| Oesophageal varices | None | Haematemesis and melaena | Chronic liver disease | Chronic liver disease |
| Gastric ulcer | Epigastric | Haematemesis and melaena | Aspirin or NSAID use | Epigastric tenderness |
| Bowel obstruction | Central | Nausea and vomiting | Cancer surgery Hernia | Tinkling bowel sounds |
| Appendicitis | Right lower quadrant | Fever Rigors | Not applicable | Tender right iliac fossa |
| Kidney stones | Right or left flank | Urgency Haematuria | Dehydration Hot climate | Tender renal angle |
| Gallstones | Right upper quadrant | Nausea and vomiting | Obesity Poor diet | Tender right hypochondrium |

NSAID, non-steroidal anti-inflammatory drug.

**Table 9.2** Differential diagnosis of abdominal aortic aneurysm from other intra-abdominal pathology

> There is controversy over abdominal aortic aneurysm screening: who, when and how often to screen, as well as which test to use. This is because although abdominal aortic aneurysm is common, many patients will die with, and not from, their disease.

## Elective endovascular aneurysm repair

Patients with an unruptured abdominal aortic aneurysm are referred for an elective endovascular aneurysm repair if they are at higher risk and unsuitable for surgery. This procedure involves insertion of a Teflon-covered stent (**Figures 9.5** and **9.6**) to seal the aneurysm from the native aorta, preventing further growth and rupture.

The complication rate for elective endovascular aneurysm repair is 15%. Complications include arterial dissection, ischaemic colitis, leakage, contrast nephropathy and device failure.

The procedure is popular with patients, because it requires only about 2 days in hospi-

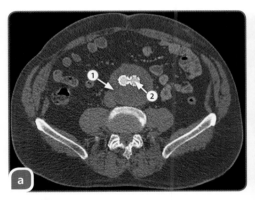
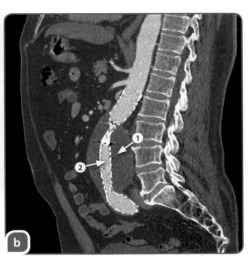

**Figure 9.5** Computerised tomography scan showing stenting of an abdominal aortic aneurysm. (a) Transverse plane. (b) Sagittal plane. (1) abdominal aortic aneurysm; (2) the stent in place. The individual stent struts are visible

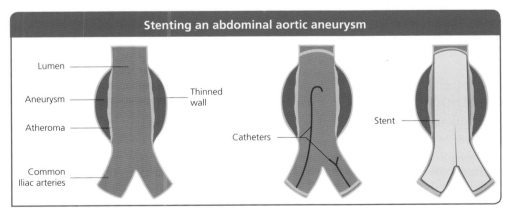

**Stenting an abdominal aortic aneurysm**

Lumen

Aneurysm

Atheroma

Thinned wall

Catheters

Stent

Common Iliac arteries

**Figure 9.6** Stenting an abdominal aortic aneurysm. The catheters are inserted using a minmially invasive technique into both femoral arteries. Under X-ray guidance, a wire, with a collapsed covered stent, is positioned above and below the aneurysm and then deployed into the abdominal aortic aneurysm.

tal, and the recovery period is short. However, more studies are needed to evaluate long-term survival rates.

## Open abdominal aortic aneurysm repair

For all patients with a ruptured abdominal aortic aneurysm, open surgery is indicated. Most patients are referred for elective repair.

Open surgery requires direct access to the aneurysm through an abdominal approach. A clamp is placed both proximal and distal to the aneurysm, and the aneurysmal segment is then removed and replaced by a conduit graft (**Figure 9.7**).

The mortality rate for open surgery approaches 10%, and the complication rate is up to 30%. Complications include acute kidney injury, myocardial infarction and lower limb paralysis.

## Complications

Rupture of the aneurysm is the most feared complication of abdominal aortic aneurysms. Rupture can lead to sudden death, infection and thromboembolic phenomena, leading to acute ischaemia of the lower limbs.

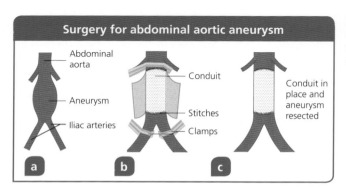

**Surgery for abdominal aortic aneurysm**

Abdominal aorta

Aneurysm

Iliac arteries

Conduit

Stitches

Clamps

Conduit in place and aneurysm resected

a       b       c

**Figure 9.7** Surgery for abdominal aortic aneurysm. (a) Before surgery. (b) During surgery. (c) After surgery.

# Aortic dissection

An aortic dissection is a tear in the intimal lining of the aorta. The condition is most common in those aged 50–65 years and in African-Caribbean people, and it is twice as common in men than in women. The mortality rate is 30%.

## Aetiology

Aortic dissection can be congenital, acquired or iatrogenic.

■ Congenital causes are connective tissue disorders such as Marfan's syndrome, and in those with other aortopathy such as bicuspid aortic valve and coarctation of the aorta
■ Acquired aortic dissection results from hypertension (in > 70% of cases), pregnancy

(due to increased stress and hormones such as relaxin and progesterone leading to cystic medial necrosis), atherosclerosis and aortic aneurysm
■ Iatrogenic aortic dissection develops during surgery for aortic and mitral valve replacement, coronary artery bypass grafting and percutaneous cardiac catheter placement

## Prevention

Early diagnosis and treatment of risk factors such as hypertension is key to the prevention of cystic medial necrosis of the aortic wall leading to aortic dissection. Regular screening of people who are at increased risk, including those with Marfan's disease or those with known dilated aorta, is also important. Transthoracic echocardiography is used to detect, measure and monitor dilation of the aortic arch so that early intervention can be performed before dissection occurs.

## Pathogenesis

Aortic dissection starts with a tear in the tunica intima, allowing blood to enter the medial layer, 'splitting' the two layers apart. As the split extends, a false lumen is created between the tunica intima and the media (see page 57).

Cystic medial necrosis plays a role in the initial tear of the arterial wall. Degradation of the connective tissue fibres, such as collagen, elastin and smooth muscle makes the aorta more susceptible to shearing stress, leading ultimately to a tear.

Two systems are used to classify aortic dissection: the DeBakey (types I–III) and the Stanford (types A and B) (**Figure 9.8**). DeBakey classification type I dissections originate in the ascending aorta and extend to at least the aortic arch; type

II dissections involve the ascending aorta only. Type III dissections begin in the descending aorta usually just distal to the left subclavian artery. Stanford classification type A dissections involve the ascending aorta whereas type B dissections do not.

## Clinical features

In > 90% of cases, there is a sudden, severe, tearing-like pain. It is usually retrosternal, because the dissection extends proximally to involve the aortic sinus and thus occlude the coronary arteries. Radiation of pain into the neck suggests propagation of the dissection to involve the aortic arch. Radiation of pain into the back suggests the dissection has continued to involve the descending aorta.

Other ways in which aortic dissection may present include:

- stroke
- syncope
- heart failure
- mesenteric ischaemia
- renal and liver injury

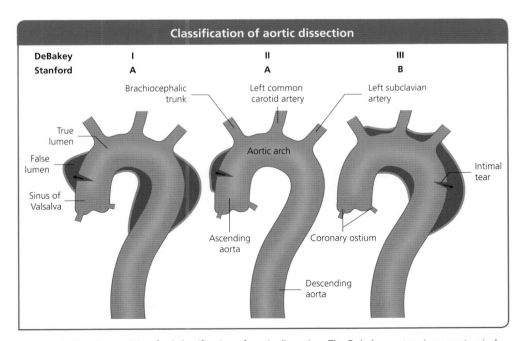

**Figure 9.8** DeBakey and Stanford classification of aortic dissection. The Debakey system is an anatomical description of the origin and extent of the dissection. The Stanford system is based on whether the dissection extends to the descending aorta or not.

A difference in blood pressure of > 20 mmHg between the left and right arms suggests the presence of an aortic dissection. Aortic dissection leads to aortic regurgitation if a proximal tear extends into the sinus of Valsalva to cause acute aortic valve insufficiency. This is indicated by a diastolic murmur, a wide pulse pressure and other signs (see page 266) such as breathlessness and chest pain.

## Diagnostic approach

Differential diagnoses for aortic dissection include:

- myocardial infarction
- pulmonary embolism
- myocarditis
- musculoskeletal back pain

The diagnosis of aortic dissection is challenging, because of the wide variety of ways in which it presents. Unlike many diagnoses, even if a good history and examination suggest the presence of aortic dissection, immediate imaging is required to confirm.

## Investigations

Blood tests showing increased cardiac enzymes indicate cardiac ischaemia. Increased urea or creatinine suggests renal injury, due to either hypoperfusion or dissection of the renal arteries.

Electrocardiography shows typical ST elevation in only a minority of patients, e.g. those with coronary involvement.

### Imaging

Computerised tomography is the gold standard test for diagnosing aortic dissection. It may also exclude other diagnoses, such as pulmonary embolism. CT allows detailed study of the anatomy of the aorta, and it is used to determine the type of aortic dissection, its location and any complications (**Figure 9.9**). However, aortic regurgitation cannot be assessed by CT. It is also not ideal in the unstable patient, because of the difficulty in monitoring their vital signs during scanning. Early discussion with cardiothoracic surgeons and anaesthetists is essential.

Chest X-ray shows widening of the medias-

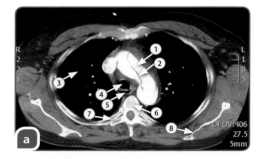

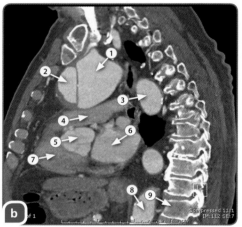

**Figure 9.9** Thoracic computerised tomography scans. (a) Aortic dissection in the transverse plane, with a flap in the aortic arch (the tennis ball sign). ①, aortic arch; ②, intimal flap; ③, lung; ④, trachea; ⑤, oesophagus; ⑥, thoracic vertebra; ⑦, rib; ⑧, scapula. (b) Ascending aortic dissection. ①, false lumen; ②, true lumen; ③, aortic arch; ④, main pulmonary artery; ⑤, aortic valve; ⑥, left atrium; ⑦, right ventricle; ⑧, descending aorta; ⑨, spine.

tinum (> 8 cm in the anteroposterior view) in two thirds of clinical cases.

Transthoracic echocardiography allows assessment of aortic regurgitation (see page 266), but only detects the intimal dissection flap (the tear in the aortic intima) in cases where the proximal ascending aorta is affected (**Figure 9.10**).

## Management

Regular blood pressure monitoring and reduction of blood pressure (aiming for systolic < 120 mmHg) are essential to reduce the risk of further dissection propagation.

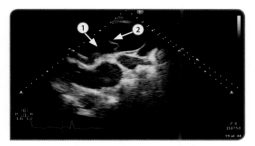

**Figure 9.10** Transoesophageal echocardiogram showing Stanford type A dissection (the tennis ball sign). ①, ascending aorta; ②, intimal flap.

Management depends on whether the dissection is proximal or distal and uncomplicated.

■ Proximal dissections involving the ascending aorta are managed surgically: the affected region is resected and replaced with a conduit graft, the aortic valve may need replacing and coronary arteries bypassed if they have become compromised by the dissection

■ Distal and uncomplicated aortic dissections are managed medically

All patients with aortic dissection need long-term follow-up, medication to control blood pressure, and in some cases, annual imaging of the dissection to monitor progression.

> **Dr DeBakey proposed a classification system for aortic dissections and developed a surgical procedure for their treatment.** At 97, he was the oldest patient ever to undergo the operation that bears his name.

## Complications

These include:

■ aortic regurgitation
■ myocardial infarction
■ stroke
■ regional ischaemia
■ pleural or pericardial effusion

# Carotid artery disease

Carotid artery disease is a narrowing of the carotid arteries, typically as a consequence of atherosclerosis. It affects around 5% of the population, is twice as common in men than in women, and is three times as common in the over 70s than in younger people.

Prompt diagnosis and early intervention to reduce risk factors for atherosclerosis provide the best prevention.

## Pathogenesis

When an atherosclerotic plaque ruptures, the resulting thrombus (clot) can either occlude the carotid artery or travel in pieces (emboli) to the smaller arteries of the brain.

■ A large occlusion, sometimes of the carotid artery itself, causes a cerebrovascular accident
■ Transient occlusion of a small cerebral vessel causes a transient ischaemic attack

## Clinical features

Patients present after a complication, such as a cerebrovascular accident (stroke) or transient ischaemic attack. Rarely, carotid artery disease is detected incidentally, for example when a carotid bruit is heard on examination of the neck.

## Diagnostic approach

Ultrasound is used to make a diagnosis of carotid artery disease. Narrowing of the arteries is detected, with reduced blood flow distally. The finding is considered significant if >75% of the lumen is narrowed (**Figure 9.11**).

## Management

The aims of management are to stabilise the existing atherosclerosis, reduce the risk of thrombosis and control blood pressure.

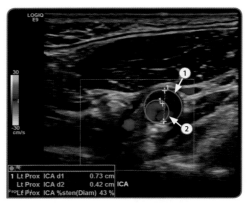

**Figure 9.11** Carotid Doppler ultrasound showing 43% narrowing as a consequence of atherosclerosis of the carotid artery. (1) Occluded carotid artery lumen with no blood flow (0.73 cm total diameter). (2) Patent carotid artery lumen with colour demonstrating blood flow (0.42 cm diameter).

## Medication

All patients require lifelong aspirin to lower the risk of thrombosis. They also need statins to stabilise the atherosclerotic plaque and slow its progression.

## Surgery

Surgical or radiological interventions are warranted in patients who have experienced symptoms (e.g. transient ischaemic attack or stroke) and whose arteries have 70–99% stenosis. This approach is used because with < 70% stenosis, the risks of intervention outweigh the benefits, and arteries that are 100% stenosed cannot be reopened.

> **Statin medications do not just reduce low-density lipoprotein cholesterol and inflammation.** These drugs also stabilise atherosclerotic plaques, thus reducing the risk of rupture and subsequent thrombosis.

Procedures include carotid endarterectomy, in which the carotid artery is clamped proximally and distally to the narrowing, opened for removal of the atherosclerotic plaque, and then closed. Complications include bleeding and stroke in 5% of patients.

Stenting is an alternative to carotid endarterectomy in patients with multiple comorbidities, for whom surgery is considered too high risk.

# Acute limb ischaemia

Acute limb ischaemia is the sudden loss of blood supply to a limb. The condition affects 0.1% people per year worldwide. Its incidence increases with age but is unaffected by gender or ethnicity.

Outcome is improved by early diagnosis and treatment of atherosclerosis risk factors and use of anti-coagulant medication to prevent thrombus formation or embolisation in patients with atrial fibrillation or mural thrombus (see page 229).

## Aetiology

The major cause of acute limb ischaemia, accounting for > 80% of cases, is atherosclerosis. An atherosclerotic plaque ruptures and a thrombus forms, leading to complete occlusion of the lumen of the lower limb artery.

About 15% of cases arise through thromboembolism. Most emboli originate from the left atrial appendage, as a result of atrial fibrillation (see page 229). Trauma and thrombosis within a surgical graft may also cause thromboembolism.

## Clinical features

An acutely ischaemic limb is painful, pulseless, pale and cold (**Table 9.3**). In severe cases, paraesthesia and loss of power ensue. There are different categories of acute limb ischaemia which require varying levels of treatment (**Table 9.4**).

## Diagnostic approach

Blood tests are generally unhelpful for diagnosis, but they are done to obtain baseline

## Clinical features of acute limb ischaemia

| Feature | Embolic cause | Thrombotic cause |
|---|---|---|
| Occlusion severity | Total | Subtotal |
| Onset | Minutes/hours | Days/weeks |
| Site(s) | Sometimes multiple | Single |
| Preceding claudication | No | Yes |
| Arterial palpation | Soft, tender | Hard |
| Bruits | No | Yes |
| Contralateral pulses | Yes | Weak or absent |

**Table 9.3** Clinical features of embolic and thrombotic acute limb ischaemia

values for reference when monitoring the patient.

Palpating peripheral pulses provides useful information: the occlusion will be distal to the most peripheral palpable pulse. For example, if the femoral pulse is palpable, but not the popliteal, the occlusion is between the two.

Ultrasound and CT are used to visualise the anatomy and locate the occlusion.

## Management

The aim of management is to return blood flow to the affected limb as quickly as possible. This is achieved pharmacologically or surgically, depending on what therapy is available locally.

## Medication

Patients are commenced immediately on intravenous heparin to prevent clot propagation. If the clot is embolic in origin, long-term oral anticoagulation is used to reduce the risk of clot recurrence, especially in the context of atrial fibrillation (see page 146).

Intra-arterial catheter delivered thrombolysis (e.g. streptokinase or tissue plasminogen activator) is used to break down the clot and restore the blood flow.

## Embolectomy

In this procedure, the embolus is removed either percutaneously with catheter-based techniques, or by open surgery.

## Bypass surgery

If other treatments are unsuccessful or not feasible, an urgent bypass of the blockage is performed. A harvested vein or artificial conduit, typically made from Teflon, is used to connect a point proximal to the occlusion (e.g. the abdominal aorta) to a point distal to it (e.g. the popliteal artery). As a result of the procedure, blood supply bypasses the affected area.

> **Calciphylaxis is a rare but serious disease typically seen in patients with end-stage renal failure.** It is a syndrome comprising vascular calcification, thrombosis and skin necrosis.
>
> Calciphylaxis can mimic acute limb ischaemia. However, patients with calciphylaxis have diffuse ischaemia and necrosis of the skin.

## Categories and treatment of acute limb ischaemia

| Feature or treatment | Viable | Threatened | Non-viable |
|---|---|---|---|
| Pain | Mild | Severe | Variable |
| Capillary refill | Normal | Delayed | Absent |
| Motor deficit | None | Partial | Complete |
| Sensory deficit | None | Partial | Complete |
| Arterial Doppler signal | Audible | Inaudible | Inaudible |
| Treatment | Urgent work-up | Revascularisation | Amputation |

Adapted from the Society of Vascular Surgery–International Society for Cardiovascular Surgery Clinical Categories of acute lower limb ischaemia. 1997.

**Table 9.4** Clinical categories and treatment of acute limb ischaemia

## Complications

The possible complications of acute limb ischaemia are:

- irreversible tissue ischaemia requiring debridement
- gangrene requiring amputation
- compartment syndrome, where the ischaemic tissue swells within a fascial component, leading to further ischaemia requiring fasciotomy

# Chronic limb ischaemia

Chronic limb ischaemia is the gradual loss of blood supply to the lower limbs. It affects 1 in 10 people worldwide; the risk increases with age and the condition affects different genders and ethnicities equally. Risk factors include those for atherosclerosis (see page 181).

> Patients with peripheral arterial disease are at high risk of developing and dying from ischaemic heart disease or cerebrovascular disease. Therefore these conditions must also be identified and managed optimally.

## Pathogenesis

Atherosclerosis develops in the arteries supplying the legs thus limiting blood flow. The flow-limiting stenosis means that the blood supply to tissues cannot be met at times of increased oxygen demand, such as during exercise. This failure results in tissue ischaemia, which manifests as pain and causes the patient to stop their activity.

## Clinical features

Patients present with calf, leg or buttock pain on walking, called claudication, which settles on resting. Claudication can be thought of as angina of the legs.

As the condition progresses, the patient starts to develop pain at rest, arterial ulcers (**Table 9.6**) and even gangrene. On examination, the pulses are impalpable, the skin appears pale or dusky and hair loss becomes apparent (**Figure 9.12**).

## Diagnostic approach

The Fontaine classification is used to stratify patient's symptoms. Increasing pain (duration, frequency, intensity) indicates increasing severity of disease (**Table 9.5**).

> Neurogenic claudication can mimic peripheral vascular disease. However, the former refers to lumbar spinal stenosis leading to entrapment of the spinal roots as they near the spinal cord. This condition can cause cramping and weakness in the legs.

## Investigations

Ankle–brachial pressure index (see page 117) is used to diagnose, and assess the severity of, peripheral vascular disease. It is the ratio of ankle systolic blood pressure to brachial systolic blood pressure:

ABPI = ankle systolic blood pressure/brachial systolic blood pressure

| Fontaine classification | |
|---|---|
| Stage | Symptom |
| I | Asymptomatic |
| IIa | Intermittent claudication at >200 m |
| IIb | Intermittent claudication at <200 m |
| III | Resting limb pain |
| IV | Limb necrosis or gangrene |

**Table 9.5** The Fontaine classification for chronic limb ischaemia

| Features of venous and arterial ulcers | | |
|---|---|---|
| Feature | Venous ulcers | Arterial ulcer |
| Medical history | Deep vein thrombosis | Hypertension |
| | Varicose veins | Smoking |
| | Thrombophlebitis | Hypercholesterolaemia |
| Position | Medial malleolus | Lateral malleolus |
| | | Pressure areas |
| Pain | Throbbing | Claudication |
| | Improved by elevation of limb | Improved by gravity (worse when elevated) |
| Ulcer | Shallow and sloughy | Punched-out, deep and irregular |
| | Heavy exudate | Little exudate |
| Lower limb | Oedematous | Delayed capillary refill time |
| | Haemosiderin deposition | Pulses absent |

**Table 9.6** Features of venous and arterial ulcers

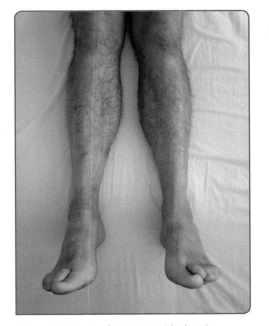

**Figure 9.12** Legs of a patient with chronic peripheral arterial disease, with loss of hair distally and pale peripheries.

| Ankle-brachial pressure index and symptoms of chronic limb ischaemia | |
|---|---|
| Symptoms | Ankle-brachial pressure index |
| Symptom free | 0.95–1.0 |
| Intermittent claudication | 0.5–0.95 |
| Resting pain | 0.3–0.5 |
| Ulceration and gangrene | <0.2 |

**Table 9.7** Ankle-brachial pressure index and symptoms of chronic limb ischaemia

pressure lower than brachial blood pressure) indicates a problem. **Table 9.7** shows the correlation between ABPI and symptom severity.

Ultrasound scanning is the investigation of choice to confirm an occlusion because it demonstrates blood flow, even in the absence of pulses. It also assesses the location, severity and extent of atherosclerotic disease causing chronic occlusion.

These two blood pressures are normally equal, which gives an ABPI of 1. Atherosclerosis in the lower limbs reduces blood pressure in the lower limbs, but it is unusual to develop atherosclerosis in the arm, so its blood pressure is preserved. Therefore a value of < 0.9 (ankle blood

**Peripheral arterial disease affecting the arms or hands is rare.** It can be caused by inflammatory disorders such as Tayakasu's arteritis (a disorder affecting the large arteries) or thromboangiitis obliterans, also known as Buerger's disease (which affects the small arteries).

## Management

The aims of medical management are to treat atherosclerosis risk factors and stabilise existing plaque. Percutaneous and surgical intervention are indicated when symptoms become disabling or if critical limb ischaemia develops.

The key elements of conservative management are:

- risk factor modification and plaque stabilisation; smoking cessation; good diabetic control and antiplatelet and lipid-lowering therapy
- encouragement of regular exercise, which not only increases high-density lipoprotein cholesterol but also improves cardiorespiratory fitness and muscular endurance, which reduces symptoms
- regular attendance at the foot clinic and chiropody appointments for the early detection of signs of peripheral arterial disease in diabetic patients

### Endovascular techniques

These techniques, which include angioplasty and stenting, are used to reopen relatively short segments of disease in an occluded artery; 90% remain open at 1 year. However, there is a small risk (around 2%) of complications which include acute thrombosis, arterial rupture and distal embolisation.

### Resection and bypass grafting

Surgical options include resection of non-viable tissue and bypass grafting. Either a vein or an artificial conduit is used to bridge the blockage.

### Complications

Consequences of chronic ischaemia include arterial ulcers, disabling symptoms and ultimately gangrene which may necessitate amputation of the limb.

# Deep vein thrombosis

Deep vein thrombosis is the formation of a blood clot in a deep vein of a lower limb. It is a common condition: 1 in 20 people develop deep vein thrombosis during their lifetime. The risk is increased by male gender, white ethnicity and increasing age.

## Prevention

Prevention of deep vein thrombosis is mostly through avoidance of blood stasis. During prolonged periods of immobility, for example on long haul flights, venous stasis is avoided by moving the legs regularly and drinking plenty of (non-alcoholic) fluids.

All patients admitted to hospital require assessment of their risk of deep vein thrombosis and bleeding. If the risk is high, they are given subcutaneous low-molecular-weight heparin (LMWH). Patients undergoing elective surgery are given compressive stockings to stop venous stasis perioperatively.

## Pathogenesis

Virchow's triad summarises the three key factors that contribute to the development of thrombosis. It is helpful when considering the possible risk factors for deep vein thrombosis (**Table 9.8** and **Figure 9.13**).

## Clinical features

Half of all cases are asymptomatic. Symptomatic patients present with a painful, warm, swollen and erythematous (red) lower limb. Differential diagnoses include a ruptured Baker's cyst, trauma and cellulitis.

## Diagnostic approach

The Wells score is a useful diagnostic aid used in patients presenting with an acutely swollen lower limb to assess the likelihood of a deep venous thrombosis; therefore, a decision on the most appropriate diagnostic test is made (**Table 9.9** and **9.10**).

## Risk factors for deep vein thrombosis

| Factor | Examples |
|---|---|
| Hypercoagulability | Pregnancy |
| | Malignancy |
| | Infection/inflammation |
| | Inherited thrombophilia |
| | Smoking |
| Blood stasis | Immobility |
| | Compression |
| | Varicose veins |
| | Plaster cast |
| | Crush injury |
| Endothelial damage | Trauma |
| | Surgery |

**Table 9.8** Risk factors for deep vein thrombosis according to Virchow's triad

## Wells score for risk of deep vein thrombosis

| Criterion | Score |
|---|---|
| Active cancer | +1 |
| Unilateral calf swelling ≥ 3 cm | +1 |
| Unilateral swollen veins | +1 |
| Unilateral pitting oedema | +1 |
| Previous deep vein thrombosis | +1 |
| Swelling of entire leg | +1 |
| Deep venous localised tenderness | +1 |
| Paralysis, paresis or recent cast | +1 |
| Recently bedridden or has undergone major surgery | +1 |
| Another diagnosis at least as likely | −2 |

**Table 9.9** The Wells clinical prediction score for risk of deep vein thrombosis

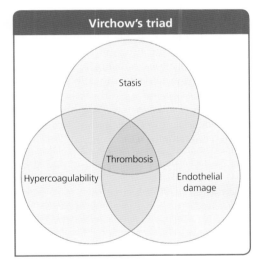

**Figure 9.13** Virchow's triad.

## Likelihood of deep vein thrombosis and recommended investigations

| Wells score | Likelihood of deep vein thrombosis (%) | Recommended investigation |
|---|---|---|
| ≥ 2 (high) | 50 | Ultrasound scan |
| 1–2 (moderate) | 20 | D-dimer test |
| < 1 (low) | 5 | |

**Table 9.10** Wells score, likelihood of deep vein thrombosis and recommended investigations

## Investigations

D-dimer is a by-product of fibrinolysis, therefore an increased blood concentration suggests activation of the coagulation system and thrombosis. A raised D-dimer indicates a higher likelihood of deep vein thrombosis. D-dimer does not indicate the location or underlying cause of the clot. There are many other causes of raised D-dimer including trauma, recent surgery, liver or kidney disease, infection, malignancy and pregnancy.

> **D-dimer is very sensitive, but poorly specific, for detecting DVT.** Therefore, if the D-dimer is elevated there may be a DVT, but if the D-dimer is below the reference range DVT is very unlikely

Patients should undergo a venous ultrasound examination if deep vein thrombosis is suspected; if there is a high likelihood of deep vein thrombosis according to the Wells score (**Table 9.10**) or if the D-dimer is elevated along with a low or moderate likelihood of deep vein thrombosis. Ultrasound has high diagnostic accuracy for diagnosing or excluding clotting in the lower limb (**Figure 9.14**).

## Management

With or without treatment, over time the venous lumen becomes recanalised and venous blood flow is restored. Therefore the aim of treatment is to prevent clot propagation or recurrence. Patients are given LMWH while receiving loading doses of warfarin, until their international normalised ratio (INR) is within acceptable limits, after which the LMWH is stopped.

The INR is the patient's prothrombin time divided by the reference range (normal) prothrombin time, then raised to the power of the international sensitivity index. This value standardises the test across different analytical systems and reagents used worldwide.

Once the INR has been stabilised, patients are maintained on warfarin for 3–6 months.

If a patient has difficulty with repeated blood samples due to poor venous access for phlebotomy, has an unstable INR, bleeding or poor concordance with warfarin, they are prescribed a novel oral anticoagulant (see page 147) or

remain on LMWH. These drugs do not require regular monitoring of their anticoagulant effect and do not effect the INR.

If a patient has recurrent deep vein thrombosis or is unable to take warfarin or LMWH because of the risk of bleeding, they may be suitable for insertion of an inferior vena cava filter. Clots collect in the filter, which prevents dangerous embolisation, for example to the lungs.

> **The international normalised ratio, like prothrombin time, is a measure of the extrinsic pathway of coagulation.** It is a measure of factors I, II, V, VII and X.
>
> A normal INR is about 1. However, for a patient with deep vein thrombosis, the optimal INR is medicated so that it is between 2 and 3, meaning that the blood takes 2–3 times longer to clot than normal.

## Complications

If a deep vein thrombus embolises it may travel through the lungs and lodge in the pulmonary arteries causing a pulmonary embolus. Alternatively, the affected lower limb may develop post-thrombotic syndrome: chronic pain, swelling and heaviness. Venous ulcers are another common complication (**Table 9.6**).

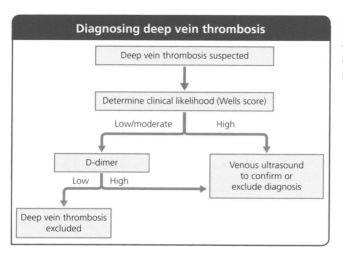

**Figure 9.14** A suggested scheme for diagnosing or excluding deep vein thrombosis which combines clinical probability scoring and imaging.

# Varicose veins

Varicose veins are a result of chronic insufficiency of the one-way venous valves, allowing retrograde blood flow, blood pooling and engorgement of the veins. The condition is common, affecting 40% of women and 20% of men worldwide. It is more common in western, ageing, obese and inactive populations.

## Aetiology

Some risk factors cannot be modified, but others can.

- Non-modifiable: genetic factors (as yet unknown) and ageing
- Modifiable: prolonged standing, obesity, chronic abdominal straining (constipation) and pregnancy

These risk factors either compromise the structural integrity of the veins or cause venous hypertension. Ultimately, this causes valve incompetence which results in the condition of venous insufficiency. This leads to venous dilatation, blood pooling and reduced venous return from the veins of the lower limbs (**Figure 9.15**).

## Clinical features

Patients complain of aching and heavy legs, swelling during the day and the appearance of telangiectasia (small, red and spidery veins; **Figure 9.16**). Other symptoms include varicose eczema (dryness and pruitis of overlying skin), leg cramps and delayed healing of minor injuries.

## Diagnostic approach

The diagnosis of varicose veins is based on the findings of the history and examination. Doppler ultrasound is the gold standard test for diagnosing varicose veins and assessing venous anatomy and truncal reflux (back flow of blood through a main superficial vein).

## Management

Patients with asymptomatic varicose veins can be reassured. Patients should be referred to a vascular service if symptomatic or if they have associated skin changes (pigmentation or varicose eczema), superficial vein thrombosis, (hard, tender veins) or venous ulceration. Referred patients should undergo investigation with Doppler ultrasound.

Interventional options include endothermal ablation, endovenous laser treatment and ultrasound-guided sclerotherapy. If these are unsuitable, surgical removal ('stripping') is advised. Conservative strategies include weight loss, exercise, compression stockings and avoidance of standing for long periods.

Varicose veins are largely benign but some cases become complicated by venous ulcers (**Table 9.6**), deep vein thrombosis, pain and tenderness or superficial thrombophlebitis.

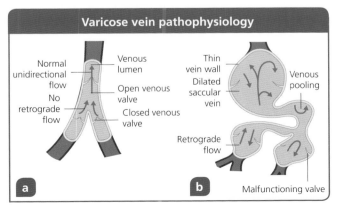

**Figure 9.15** Varicose vein pathophysiology. (a) Normal vein. (b) Varicose vein.

### Varicose vein pathophysiology

Normal unidirectional flow · No retrograde flow · Venous lumen · Open venous valve · Closed venous valve · Thin vein wall · Dilated saccular vein · Retrograde flow · Venous pooling · Malfunctioning valve

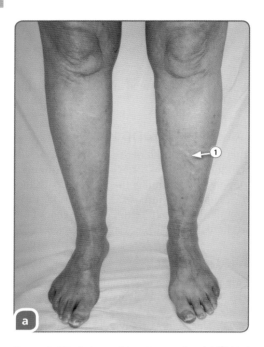
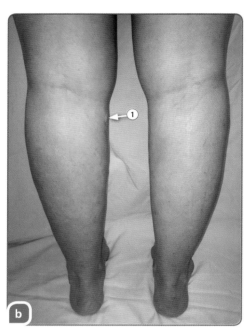

**Figure 9.16** Patient with varicose veins. (a) ① Varicose veins demonstrated on the left leg on the anterior tibial border. (b) ① Varicose veins demonstrated on the left leg, at the medial border of the calf.

# Superficial thrombophlebitis

Thrombophlebitis is the presence of clot (thrombo) and venous (phleb-) inflammation (-itis), typically in the superficial tissues of the lower limb.

Superficial thrombophlebitis affects around 5% of the population worldwide. It is more common in women, in the elderly and in patients with varicose veins.

## Clinical features

Patients typically present with pain, erythema and swelling in the affected limb, and a palpable cord-like vein.

## Diagnostic approach

Diagnosis is clinical unless symptoms or signs are detected above the knee. In these cases, ultrasound is needed to rule out deep vein thrombosis.

## Management

Elevation, compression, warmth and non-steroidal anti-inflammatory drugs are effective in reducing symptoms and preventing propagation of the clot.

## Complications

These include extension into deep vein thrombosis, venous ulcers (**Table 9.6**) and persistence of the thrombosed vein as a nodule.

# Raynaud's phenomenon

Raynaud's phenomenon is when blood flow to an area of the body is compromised secondary to excessive transient vasoconstriction (vasospasm) in response to the cold or emotional stress. It usually affects the peripheries, i.e. the fingers, toes and other appendages, although other areas can also be affected.

The phenomenon is subdivided into idiopathic primary Raynaud's disease and secondary Raynaud's syndrome (vasospasm in the context of another disease; see **Table 9.11**). Primary Raynaud's disease affects 10% of the population worldwide and typically occurs in the second or third decade.

| Conditions that cause or mimic secondary Raynaud's phenomenon | |
| --- | --- |
| Causes | Conditions |
| Autoimmune | Systemic sclerosis |
| | Lupus |
| | Rheumatoid arthritis |
| Infectious | Hepatitis B and C |
| | *Mycoplasma* infection |
| Malignant | Lymphoma |
| | Leukaemia |
| | Myeloma |
| Environmental | Vibration injury |
| | Frostbite |
| Endocrine | Acromegaly |
| | Diabetes |
| | Hypothyroidism |
| Haematological | Polycythaemia |
| | Paroxysmal nocturnal haemoglobinuria |
| Drug-related | Oral contraceptive pill use |
| | Beta-blocker use |
| Mimic | Thromboembolic disease |
| | Thoracic outlet syndrome |

**Table 9.11** Conditions that cause or mimic secondary Raynaud's phenomenon

## Pathogenesis

Primary Raynaud's disease is a benign vasospasm which usually involves the small digital arteries supplying the fingers. This leads to transient reduction in blood flow to the fingers, which results in pain, discolouration and cold digits. Secondary Raynaud's phenomenon is a combination of endothelial dysfunction, structural microvascular changes and increased platelet aggregation causing transient arterial occlusion.

## Clinical features

The precise cause of attacks is unknown, but exposure to cold, smoking and caffeine are well recognised triggers. During an attack, the affected digits change colour from white to blue to red, before returning to their normal colour. The colour change is in this order, reflecting the underlying pathophysiology.

- White/pale: as a result of vasospasm of the artery reducing local blood flow
- Blue: caused by cyanosis, with a marked drop in blood oxygen saturation
- Red: as a result of reactive hyperaemia following vaso-relaxation and restoration of blood flow

## Diagnostic approach

The diagnosis is clinical in primary Raynaud's disease following examination of the hands, e.g. during an attack. Attacks typically occur bilaterally in response to a trigger and in the absence of any discernible cause.

Conditions that cause or mimic Raynaud's phenomenon are shown in **Table 9.11.** If there is suspicion of a secondary cause, such as lupus, this possibility must be investigated appropriately, for example by referral to the rheumatology department for further examination and antinuclear antibody titres.

## Management

Primary Raynaud's disease is treated with smoking cessation, avoidance of triggers by keeping peripheries warm and vasodilating drugs (e.g. calcium channel blockers). In more severe cases, alpha-adrenergic blockers (e.g. prazosin), ACE inhibitors, angiotensin receptor blockers, topical nitrates, phodiesterase inhibitors (e.g. sildenafil) and prostaglandins (iloprost) can be used.

In secondary Raynaud's phenomenon, treatment focuses on the underlying disease, in addition to the use of calcium channel blockers to control symptoms.

## Complications

In extreme cases, arterial ulcers (**Table 9.6**) and gangrene occur.

# Subclavian or axillary vein thrombosis

Subclavian or axillary vein thrombosis is a rare condition in which a clot develops in the veins of a proximal upper limb. It is also known as effort thrombosis or Paget–von Schrötter disease, and accounts for 1% of all cases of venous thrombosis.

## Pathogenesis

The disease typically occurs in the dominant upper limb because of repeated and sustained overhead activity, such as painting. It also occurs in malignancy, after radiotherapy or in the presence of thrombophilia (e.g. protein C or S deficiency; see **Table 9.12**) or long-term indwelling central venous catheters.

Venous return from the upper limb is restricted, when the arms are positioned overhead, because of compression of veins by:

- soft tissue (e.g. anterior scalene)
- bony tissue (e.g. 1st rib)
- endothelial damage (e.g. repetitive motion or cannulation)
- hypercoagulable states (e.g. dehydration)

## Clinical features

The arm feels heavy, swollen and weak and appears cyanotic, with distended superficial veins.

If thrombophilia is suspected, blood samples are taken for screening.

| Causes of emboli | | | | |
|---|---|---|---|---|
| Embolus | Cause | Example | Population at risk | Manifestation |
| Air | Gas bubbles | Decompression sickness | Deep sea divers | Joint pain, rashes and death |
| Infection | Mycotic | Infective endocarditis | Patients with valvular disease and requiring surgery | Stigmata of endocarditis, e.g. splinter haemorrhages |
| Fat | Bone marrow | Hip replacement | Patients with long bone fractures | Dyspnoea, hypotension and death |
| Amniotic | Amniotic fluid | During delivery | Women whose baby requires instrumental delivery | Dyspnoea, confusion and rash |
| Tumour | Haematogenous spread | During growth | Patients with solid malignant tumours | Depends on the location, grade and type of tumour |

**Table 9.12** The different causes of emboli

> **Thrombophilia means 'to like clotting'.**
> It refers to an increased tendency to
> form blood clots; synonymous terms are
> hypercoagulability and prothrombotic
> state. Thrombophilia is inherited (e.g.
> protein C deficiency) or acquired (e.g.
> antiphospholipid syndrome).

## Diagnostic approach

Ultrasound may reveal the clot, unless it is
obscured by the clavicle or sternum. Therefore if suspicion is high, an alternative imaging modality is used, such as CT.

## Management

Management of subclavian or axillary vein
thrombosis is the same as that for deep vein
thrombosis: use of subcutaneous LMWH and
warfarin until the INR is in the therapeutic
range (normally 2–3), followed by discontin-
uation of LMWH and continuation of warfarin for 3–6 months. Novel oral anticoagulants
(see page 147) are becoming a useful alternative to warfarin. Some thrombophillic conditions require anticoagulation indefinitely in
order to reduce the long-term risk of thromboembolic disease.

> **In the initial warfarin loading phase,
> there can be paradoxical and transient
> prothrombotic tendency.** This is because
> it inhibits anticoagulant factors protein C
> and S more than the procoagulant
> factors II, VII, IX and X. This is why patients
> continue to receive subcutaneous LMWH,
> alongside warfarin, for 5 days and until
> the INR ≥2 for at least 24 h.

## Complications

These include pulmonary embolism, post-
thrombotic syndrome and recurrent thrombosis.

## Answers to starter questions

1. Routine surgery for all cases of varicose veins has been reduced in some areas
   to rationalise treatment and reduce healthcare costs. Many patients remain
   asymptomatic where the condition presents a purely cosmetic problem; these
   patients can be given advice and reassurance. Within the UK National Health Service
   for example, interventional treatment is reserved for symptomatic patients with
   ultrasound-confirmed varicose veins and Doppler evidence of truncal reflux. Of course,
   asymptomatic patients may still seek surgery within the private healthcare sector, but
   this may require separate insurance or additional personal cost.

2. The problem with screening for any disease is that the screening test result might be
   falsely reassuring (false negative result) or may result in excess cost, risk and anxiety of
   unnecessarily investigating those without disease (false positive results). Equally, the
   significant costs of implementing a screening program should be justified by improved
   clinical outcomes. The World Health Organisation criteria (based upon the original
   Wilson and Junger criteria) set out 10 principles that a screening program should meet.

3. One artery may 'steal' blood from another in the presence of altered haemodynamics.
   For example, vertebral-subclavian steal syndrome occurs when there is a proximal
   subclavian artery stenosis prior to the origin of the vertebral artery. Increased
   resistance to blood flow through the stenosis means that, under certain circumstances,
   blood supply to the distal subclavian artery is preferentially supplied by 'stolen'
   retrograde flow from the adjoining vertebral artery. This is triggered by exercise
   of the affected upper limb (increased demand for flow). When it occurs, vertebral
   artery blood flow becomes sacrificed and symptoms of cerebral hypoperfusion occur
   including visual disturbance, dizziness, syncope and pre-syncope.

**Answers** *continued*

4.  External iliac artery endofibrosis is a rare condition that can affect cyclists and triathletes. Fibrotic scar tissue develops around the external iliac artery due to the adoption of aerodynamic postures whilst at maximal exertion. This leads to strain and kinking of the artery until a progressive build-up of scar tissue occludes it causing symptomatic claudication, but only at peak exertion.

5.  This is an extremely contentious issue. While smoking is the single biggest modifiable risk factor for vascular disease and by stopping (not reducing) an individual is taking responsibility for their own health, patients who do not stop should not be considered less worthy of treatment. They may find it hard to stop, as they have few other pleasures in their life. Indeed, they may even feel that being told to stop is an infringement of their civil liberties. Sportsmen with osteoarthritis, alcoholics with liver disease and cocaine users with myocardial infarctions are all similar examples of what some might regard as self-inflicted diseases. A clinician's place is not to judge the patient but to provide the best possible advice and treatment in all circumstances.

6.  An embolised clot can travel from the systemic veins (right heart) into the systemic arteries system (left heart) if there is a 'hole in the heart' such as a patent foramen ovale or atrial septal defect (see page 288). This is called a paradoxical embolism, where a venous thrombosis, rather than embolising to the lungs within the pulmonary arteries (the natural path), traverses the atria from right to left leading to a cerebrovascular accident. There needs to be a transient right-left shunting of blood across the atrial septum (normally left atrial pressure exceeds right atrial pressure). This occurs in right ventricular failure, positive-pressure ventilation, pulmonary hypertension and during valsalva-like manoeuvers (forced expiration against a closed glottis) such as sneezing and difficult urination and defecation. There remains some controversy regarding the most appropriate indications for patent foramen ovale closure procedures.

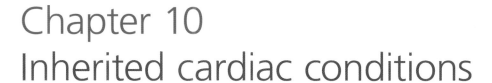

# Chapter 10
# Inherited cardiac conditions

## Starter questions

Answers to the following questions are on page 339.

1. Do all patients with hypertrophic cardiomyopathy have symptoms?
2. What investigations are required to diagnose hypertrophic cardiomyopathy?
3. Why is diagnosing hypertrophic cardiomyopathy more difficult in Afro-Caribbean populations?
4. Why do athletes often have abnormal ECGs and echocardiograms?
5. Why do patients with Marfan syndrome have a higher mortality than the general population?

# Introduction

Inherited cardiac conditions are diseases with a known genetic basis that affect the heart. They are usually multisystem conditions. However, this chapter focuses on their cardiovascular effects.

It is important to remember that, as genetic diseases, these conditions have implications not only for the person with the disease but also for the whole family. Diagnosis of an inherited cardiac condition in one person leads to screening of family members. Thus screening often results in the diagnosis of potentially life-threatening conditions in persons who are otherwise well.

Ideally, patients with an inherited cardiac condition are treated by a cardiologist with a special interest in this group of diseases.

# Case 12 Cardiac arrest in a football player

## Presentation

James Smith is 18 years old and has been playing football for Ecclesall United for one season. During an important cup tie, James collapsed on the pitch. The club physician found that James was in ventricular fibrillation, started cardiopulmonary resuscitation and restored a cardiac output with electrical direct current cardioversion. James's condition was stabilised, and he was transferred to the local hospital for ongoing care.

## Initial interpretation

Cardiac arrest in a young athlete is an uncommon event. Differential diagnoses to consider are:

- myocardial ischaemia
- an arrhythmia, such as Brugada's syndrome or long QT
- cardiomyopathy

Electrolyte abnormalities and other non-cardiac causes are also considered but are less likely.

## History

James had been fit and well up to the time of his cardiac arrest. He had never complained of any cardiac symptoms and had never lost consciousness before. He says that his mum and dad are well and have no medical problems. However, his mum reports that James's uncle died of a heart problem in his early twenties.

## Interpretation of history

Patients who suffer cardiac arrest are at risk of a further event. Therefore all possible steps must be taken to establish the underlying cause. In the absence of any chest pain, and in such a young person, a myocardial infarction is unlikely. The family history of sudden cardiac death raises suspicion of an inherited cardiac condition.

## Examination

James is pale and clearly shaken by his experience. His condition was stabilised in the accident and emergency department using an ABCDE approach. This is the standard approach used to assess acutely ill patients: Airway, Breathing, Circulation, Disability, Exposure (see page 349). He is now maintaining his own airway and breathing for himself, with good oxygen saturation.

His blood pressure, 130/70 mmHg, is good. His heart rate is normal at 68 beats/min. On auscultation of his precordium, a harsh systolic murmur is heard at the lower left sternal edge. His lung fields are clear.

## Interpretation of findings

James is now maintaining his own airway and is haemodynamically stable. The harsh systolic murmur may represent: a valvular problem, e.g. aortic stenosis, mitral regurgitation or tricuspid regurgitation; the presence of a ventricular septal defect; or an obstruction in the left ventricular outflow tract. His chest is clear indicating there is no evidence of pulmonary oedema.

## Investigations

Chest X-ray and all standard blood test results are normal. However, the electrocardiogram (ECG) is abnormal. It shows large voltage complexes throughout the precordial leads, as well as T-wave inversion in leads V4–V6 (**Figure 10.1**). The QT interval is normal.

An echocardiogram shows asymmetrical left ventricular hypertrophy. There is also evidence of left ventricular outflow tract obstruction (**Figure 10.2**).

**Case 12** *continued*

### Electrocardiogram showing left ventricular hypertropy

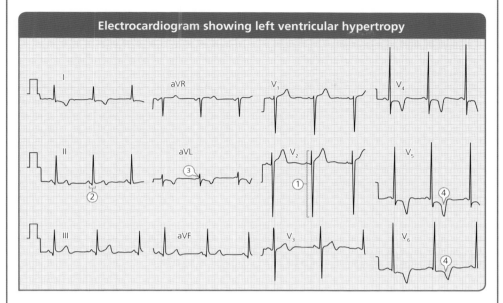

**Figure 10.1** An electrocardiogram showing left ventricular hypertrophy. ① Large amplitude QRS complexes. ② Slight widening of the QRS complex. ③ Delayed intrinsicoid deflection. ④ T wave inversion ('strain pattern').

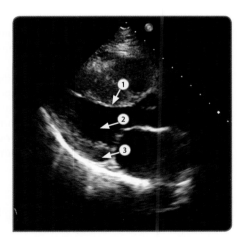

**Figure 10.2** An echocardiogram showing left ventricular hypertrophy. ① The interventricular septum and ③ posterior wall of the septum are both > 12 mm thick. ② left ventricle.

## Diagnosis

The electrocardiographic changes are consistent with left ventricular hypertrophy. This diagnosis is confirmed by the asymmetrical left ventricular hypertrophy and left ventricular outflow tract obstruction shown by the echocardiogram. It is this obstruction of the left ventricular outflow tract that is responsible for the murmur heard on auscultation.

The diagnosis is hypertrophic cardiomyopathy (HCM). James is referred to a cardiologist with a special interest in inherited conditions for ongoing investigation and care.

**Case 12** *continued*

Patients with HCM are often symptomatic because of left ventricular outflow tract obstruction. The obstruction is caused by both the hypertrophy of the ventricular wall and the abnormal systolic anterior motion of the mitral valve (see page 327).

Because James has presented with a cardiac arrest, he requires an implantable cardioverter defibrillator as secondary prevention. This intervention does not prevent recurrent arrhythmia, but it does provide early defibrillation and reduce the risk of sudden death.

Members of James's family require clinical and genetic screening to determine whether they are also affected. If possible, a copy of his uncle's post mortem report should be obtained to try to establish whether he too had HCM.

# Inherited cardiomyopathies

Cardiomyopathies are diseases of the heart muscle. The European Society of Cardiology defines cardiomyopathy as 'a myocardial disorder in which the heart muscle is structurally and functionally abnormal, in the absence of coronary artery disease, hypertension, valvular disease and congenital heart disease sufficient to cause the observed myocardial abnormality'.

Cardiomyopathies are described according to the shape of the ventricles: hypertrophied or dilated. They are often classified as primary or secondary.

■ Primary cardiomyopathies are confined to heart muscle
■ In secondary cardiomyopathies, the cardiac involvement is part of a wider, more generalised clinical syndrome

A syndrome is a collection of symptoms, signs and other clinical features that commonly coexist. Many chromosomal and inherited diseases have syndromic features.

## Hypertrophic cardiomyopathy

Hypertrophic cardiomyopathy is the abnormal hypertrophy of the left or (less commonly) the right ventricular myocardium, with no apparent haemodynamic or systemic cause.

## Epidemiology and aetiology

Hypertrophic cardiomyopathy affects about 1 in 500 adults and typically presents in adolescence.

The condition shows autosomal dominant inheritance with incomplete penetrance and variable expression. Hundreds of genetic mutations are associated with HCM, but more than half affect genes that code sarcomeric proteins with a structural role, such as myosin, actin and troponin.

In genetic terminology, **incomplete penetrance** means that a disease trait is not expressed in some people who carry the defective allele. **Variable expression** means that people with the same genetic abnormality (genotype) express the clinical trait to differing degrees.

## Pathogenesis

Hypertrophic cardiomyopathy is characterised by myocyte hypertrophy and extracellular fibrosis.

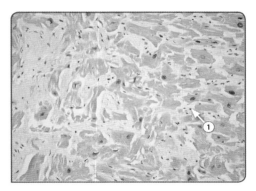

**Figure 10.3** Microscopic appearance of hypertrophic cardiomyopathy. There is profound myocyte disarray and prominent background fibrosis ①. The cardiac myocytes are clearly disorganised and non-linear in architecture. The pale pink matrix is fibrous tissue.

- Microscopically, the normal, ordered myocytic arrangement is lost, and is replaced by a chaotic cellular arrangement (**Figure 10.3**); the small intramural coronary arteries become fibrotic and narrowed
- Macroscopically, the hypertrophy usually affects the ventricular septum in an asymmetrical fashion; less commonly, a concentric pattern is seen

The hypertrophy usually affects the free left ventricular wall. Right ventricular hypertrophy is sometimes present but does not usually occur in isolation.

## Clinical features

Hypertrophic cardiomyopathy commonly presents as an incidental finding secondary to abnormalities seen on an ECG done for a separate reason.

- Chest pain is common; it is caused by the increased oxygen demand of the hypertrophied muscle and the narrowed intramural arteries
- Patients occasionally present with shortness of breath, palpitations and syncope (caused by atrial and ventricular arrhythmias)
- Diastolic dysfunction (see page 241) is common (myocardial fibrosis and stiffening)

- One in 10 patients develop left ventricular systolic dysfunction

Clinical signs may be absent, but patients with left ventricular outflow tract obstruction often have an ejection systolic murmur. Patients sometimes have a jerky central pulse.

## Diagnostic approach

Electrocardiographic changes such as left ventricular hypertrophy, left axis deviation and repolarisation abnormalities often precede echocardiographic changes. On an echocardiogram, left ventricular hypertrophy is usually asymmetrical.

A maximal ventricular wall thickness of > 15 mm is required to diagnose HCM. About a third of patients have obstruction of the left ventricular outflow tract. The obstruction results from the combination of hypertrophy and systolic displacement of the mitral valve.

Systolic displacement of the mitral valve, referred to as systolic anterior motion, occurs when the mitral valve is 'sucked' up towards the septum secondary to the high-velocity jet of blood flowing around the hypertrophied segment (the venturi effect). Systolic anterior motion results in mitral valve regurgitation and contributes to the physical obstruction of the left ventricular outflow tract in late systole.

Cardiac magnetic resonance imaging (MRI) is used to detect early disease. The technique is also used to help characterise established cases of HCM.

### Family screening

All first-degree family members of the affected patient are counselled appropriately and screened for the disease. Screening includes:

- an ECG
- clinical assessment
- an echocardiogram
- genetic testing for known genetic mutations

The absence of any recognised genetic mutation does not exclude the diagnosis of HCM. Screening is usually repeated before a diagnosis is be confidently excluded, especially in those first screened as young children.

## Management

No other intervention apart from insertion of an implantable cardioverter defibrillator in appropriately selected patients (see **Table 10.1** for assessment of risk) changes prognosis or prolongs life. Therefore symptom management is the primary aim in this condition.

In HCM, susceptibility to sudden cardiac death varies but peaks during adolescence and early adulthood; it is caused by ventricular arrhythmias. The factors listed in **Table 10.1** are assessed regularly to determine risk for each patient with HCM. Sudden cardiac death is associated with competitive and contact sports, so all patients should avoid these activities.

### Medication

Drug treatment includes beta-blockers, which suppress supraventricular arrhythmias, reduce heart rate and reduce left ventricular filling pressures. Verapamil is an option if beta-blockers are contraindicated.

Disopyramide is often added if a left ventricular outflow tract obstruction persists and the patient is symptomatic after medical therapy.

| Risk assessment for sudden cardiac death | |
|---|---|
| Major risk factor | Investigation or detection |
| Family history of sudden cardiac death | Pedigree analysis |
| Unexplained syncope (one or more episodes in the preceding 12 months) | History |
| Ventricular arrhythmias | 24-h electrocardiographic monitoring to detect non-sustained ventricular tachycardia |
| Maximal left ventricular wall thickness > 30 mm | Echocardiography or magnetic resonance imaging |
| Abnormal blood pressure response to exercise | Blood pressure does not increase by 20–30 mmHg from baseline during an exercise tolerance test (because of abnormal autonomic response) |

**Table 10.1** Assessment of risk of sudden cardiac death in patients with hypertrophic cardiomyopathy

Left ventricular systolic impairment arising from HCM is treated in the same way as left ventricular systolic impairment resulting from other causes (see page 247). Anticoagulation is considered if atrial fibrillation develops.

### Surgery

If symptomatic left ventricular outflow tract obstruction persists, debulking of the hypertrophied myocardium by surgical myomectomy or alcohol septal ablation is considered.

### Prognosis

Prognosis of patients with HCM is good. It is important that the risk of sudden cardiac death is repeatedly assessed and an implantable defibrillator implanted if required.

# Dilated cardiomyopathy

Dilated cardiomyopathy (DCM) is characterised by:

- impaired ventricular function
- ventricular chamber dilatation
- normal or reduced ventricular wall thickness
- absence of a secondary cause

Secondary causes include coronary, valvular or congenital heart disease; hypertension; and any other haemodynamic abnormality. These conditions are excluded before a diagnosis of DCM is made.

## Types

Dilated cardiomyopathy has many different causes (**Table 10.2**). Most patients have idiopathic DCM; its cause is unknown. About a third of patients in this group have a familial (i.e. genetic) form of the condition.

**Excessive alcohol consumption is one of the commoner causes of DCM.** The problem of alcohol-related DCM is increasing, especially in younger adults. The physiological response to alcohol varies between individuals, which is why not all heavy drinkers develop a DCM. Alcohol-related DCM is one of the few potentially reversible forms of heart failure. Patients are strongly advised to completely abstain from alcohol.

| Causes of dilated cardiomyopathy | |
|---|---|
| Type | Definition or example(s) |
| Familial | One or more family member affected, or family history of sudden cardiac death at < 35 years of age |
| Drug-induced | Anthracycline or doxorubicin |
| Toxins | Alcohol and anabolic steroids |
| Endocrine disorders | Hypo- or hyperthyroidism, phaeochromocytoma and Cushing's syndrome |
| Post-partum | Develops during the last month of pregnancy or first 5 months after delivery |
| Tachycardia-induced | Persistent atrial or ventricular tachycardias can cause a dilated cardiomyopathy that is usually reversible once the tachycardia is controlled |
| Idiopathic | No other identifiable cause |
| Inflammatory | Sarcoidosis or vasculitis |
| Infections | Viral or bacterial |
| Storage disorders | Haemochromatosis |

**Table 10.2** Common causes of dilated cardiomyopathy

## Epidemiology and aetiology

Many different genetic mutations have been discovered;

- 90% are inherited in an autosomal dominant fashion, for example mutations of the *lamin* A/C and *SCN5A* genes (this gene encodes the sodium channel)
- 5% are X-linked, for example Duchenne's and Becker's muscular dystrophy

The incidence and prevalence of familial DCM in the general population is unknown, but it is estimated to affect 0.05%. It is the commonest cause of heart failure in the young but typically presents in middle age.

## Clinical features

Patients present with the symptoms and signs of heart failure (see page 243). Shortness of breath, chest pain, oedema and fatigue are common. Cardiac enlargement often results in a laterally displaced apex beat, a 3rd or 4th heart sound and often a pansystolic murmur (secondary to functional tricuspid or mitral regurgitation; see pages 271 and 274).

## Diagnostic approach

Chest X-ray shows an enlarged cardiac shadow (**Figure 10.4**). Echocardiography is used to confirm and quantify the degree of ventricular dilatation and impairment.

The ECG is normal or show evidence of conduction defects such as bundle branch block. Conduction abnormalities arise sec-

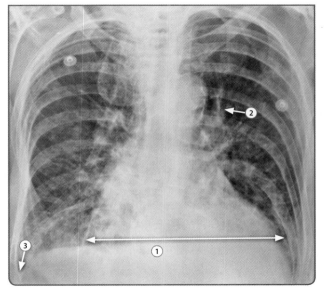

**Figure 10.4** Chest X-ray showing interstitial oedema. ①, cardiomegaly; ②, upper lobe blood diversion; ③, loss of clarity of perihilar vessels and blunting of costophrenic recesses, indicating small effusions.

ondary to progressive disease or to specific disease genotypes that cause particular electrophysiological abnormalities (e.g. lamin A/C mutations and myotonic dystrophy). Ambulatory ECG monitoring is required to exclude or identify arrhythmia.

Cardiac MRI is used to help distinguish between the different causes of DCM.

## Management

### Medication

The mainstay of management of DCM is conventional heart failure treatment with diuretics, angiotensin-converting enzyme (ACE) inhibitors and beta-blockers (see pages 152 and 158).

### Device therapy

Pacemaker implantation is warranted if the patient has a coexisting electrical conduction disorder.

Cardiac resynchronisation therapy (CRT) is indicated for patients with DCM. The indications mirror those for conventional systolic heart failure. Insertion of an implantable cardioverter defibrillator is indicated for primary and secondary prevention of sudden cardiac death in DCM. Therefore a CRT defibrillator is usually the device of choice.

## Prognosis

Heart failure is usually a progressive disease and patients have periods of stability followed by periods of exacerbations of fluid overload. The prognosis is variable and depends upon the cause of the DCM, but in all cases appropriate medication prolongs life.

## Family screening

Family screening is required for first-degree relatives of patients with seemingly idiopathic DCM, especially in those with a positive family history of the disease.

**Dilated cardiomyopathy presents in the same way as severe left ventricular impairment and heart failure.** The conditions are treated in the same way: with diuretics, ACE inhibitors, beta-blockers and spironolactone. However, for DCM careful clinical assessment is necessary to identify cases in which a familial cause is possible, because of the implications for other family members.

# Arrhythmogenic right ventricular cardiomyopathy

Arrhythmogenic right ventricular cardiomyopathy is an inherited cardiomyopathy that predominantly affects the right side of the heart. The condition is characterised by fibrofatty replacement of the right ventricular myocardium and is associated with myocyte loss.

## Epidemiology and aetiology

Arrhythmogenic right ventricular cardiomyopathy is estimated to affect about 1 in 5000 people.

The genetic basis of the condition is poorly understood. However, it is associated with mutations of several genes, including desmoplakin (*DSP)* and desmoglein-2 (*DSG2*).

## Clinical features

Patients present with ventricular arrhythmias, cardiac failure and sudden cardiac death. The last of these often occurs in younger persons.

## Diagnostic approach

All patients require echocardiography and cardiac MRI.

Diagnosis is often difficult. Therefore patients in whom arrhythmogenic right ventricular cardiomyopathy is suspected are referred to a cardiologist for further assessment. Diagnosis is made by:

■ history

- echocardiography
- cardiac MRI
- ECG
- cardiac biopsy (occasionally)

Internationally accepted criteria for diagnosis comprise a series of historical, structural, histological and electrophysiological abnormalities (see **Table 10.3**).

## Management

Medical therapy is used to treat the signs and symptoms of heart failure. Antiarrhythmic drugs such as beta-blockers and amiodarone are commonly used to suppress atrial and ventricular arrhythmias.

The following patients are considered for insertion of an implantable cardioverter defibrillator:

- those assessed to be at high risk of sudden cardiac death (for example, with evidence of ventricular tachycardia)
- those with previous cardiac arrest

| Criteria for arrhythmogenic right ventricular cardiomyopathy | |
|---|---|
| Category | Criterion |
| Historical | Family history of arrhythmogenic right ventricular cardiomyopathy or sudden cardiac death |
| Structural | Abnormal right ventricular appearance or movement |
| Histological | Fibrofatty myocytic replacement |
| Electrophysiological abnormalities | Non-sustained ventricular tachycardia and abnormal repolarisation |

**Table 10.3** Criteria for diagnosis of arrhythmogenic right ventricular cardiomyopathy

High-risk features include wide QRS complexes on ECG, a family history of sudden cardiac death, syncope and poor right ventricular function.

# Other cardiomyopathies

There are other less common cardiomyopathies which present in clinically distinct ways.

## Restrictive cardiomyopathy

Restrictive cardiomyopathy is the least common of all the cardiomyopathies. The condition is characterised by endocardial fibrosis and increased stiffness of the heart muscle. Consequently, small changes in volume within the ventricles result in large increases in ventricular pressures.

This type of cardiomyopathy is idiopathic in some cases. In others, it is associated with storage disorders (e.g. haemochromatosis and Fabry's disease) or infiltrative disease (e.g. amyloidosis, scleroderma and carcinoid).

Clinical presentation is one of congestive cardiac failure. Investigations include ECG, echocardiography and cardiac catheterisation.

The results show characteristic haemodynamic features.

The aims of treatment are to:

- treat the heart failure
- suppress arrhythmias
- halt disease progression by treating the cause, if possible

Restrictive cardiomyopathy carries a particularly poor prognosis.

## Takotsubo cardiomyopathy

Takotsubo cardiomyopathy is also known as stress-induced cardiomyopathy or broken heart syndrome. Patients present with chest pain, shortness of breath and an ECG that is consistent with acute myocardial ischaemia.

Diagnosis is made by cardiac catheterisation, which shows normal coronary arteries but left ventricular apical ballooning during systole.

Treatment is mainly supportive. Heart failure is treated until a good left ventricular recovery is made.

Prognosis is good, and many patients recover fully. Takotsubo cardiomyopathy is commoner in women and does recur in up to 10% of patients. Be aware that until coronary angiography, the condition presents with features identical to acute myocardial infarction.

> **Takotsubo cardiomyopathy is so-called because of the angiographic appearance of the ballooning left ventricle and contracted left ventricular base.** These resemble a Japanese octopus trap (a 'takotsubo').
>
> The condition is also known as broken heart syndrome, because it can be triggered by acute, severe physical or emotional stress, such as that experienced after a sudden bereavement or end to a romantic relationship.

# Inherited arrhythmias

There are different kinds of inherited arrythmias. They are caused by abnormalities in the ion channel genes. They often present with symptoms of syncope or dizziness and are important to diagnose and manage as they can also present with sudden cardiac death.

## Brugada's syndrome

Brugada's syndrome is an inherited channelopathy that occasionally presents with sudden cardiac death. Patients are often referred because a family member has been diagnosed with the condition or has died from it. They are often asymptomatic.

## Aetiology

The syndrome shows autosomal dominant inheritance. Mutations of the gene encoding the sodium channel (*SCN5A)* occur in up to a fifth of cases.

## Clinical features

Patients are often asymptomatic but also present with palpitations or syncope. The disease rarely presents with sudden cardiac death.

## Diagnostic approach

Diagnosis is confirmed by the combination of a characteristic ECG and another feature of the condition, for example:

- documented polymorphic ventricular tachycardia or fibrillation
- a family history of sudden cardiac death
- inducible ventricular tachycardia in electrophysiological studies
- family members with Brugada's syndrome–type ECGs or syncope

The ECG has several characteristic features, typically the combination of ST elevation with right bundle branch block in leads V1–3 (**Figure 10.5**).

## Management

The only effective treatment in preventing sudden cardiac death is insertion of an implantable cardioverter defibrillator. Patients should avoid drugs that have been shown to induce Brugada's syndrome, such as certain antiarrhythmic, psychotropic and anaesthetic agents. A list of drugs is available from the internet. This can be printed off and handed to patients.

First degree family members should be screened for the condition and screening cascaded forward as appropriate.

## Long QT syndrome

### Types

Long QT syndrome is a recognised cause of sudden cardiac death. It is disorder of myocyte ion channels.

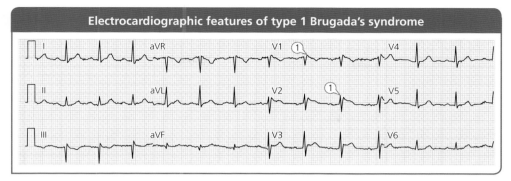

**Figure 10.5** A 12-lead electrocardiogram showing the classic changes seen in type 1 Brugada's syndrome. Note the coved ST elevation in leads V1 and V2 ①.

The condition is congenital or acquired and has several subtypes. Long QT types 1–10 have been identified; the commonest are types 1–3.

## Aetiology

Multiple mutations cause long QT syndrome (see **Table 10.4**).

## Clinical features

The condition is often asymptomatic but rarely presents with sudden cardiac death or palpitations and syncope. Syncope and sudden cardiac death are caused by either ventricular fibrillation or polymorphic ventricular tachycardia (torsades de pointes) (see pages 226 and 257).

These arrhythmias have recognised stimuli, such as swimming in long QT syndrome type 1 and loud noises in long QT syndrome type 2.

## Diagnostic approach

Diagnosis is based on an abnormally prolonged corrected QT interval on the ECG. An exercise ECG or a signal-averaged ECG, a Holter monitor QT interval assessment, and occasionally an adrenaline challenge are also useful in selected cases. All immediate family members are screened.

Diagnosis is often difficult. Not uncommonly, patients are first diagnosed with epilepsy. Schwartz's criteria can be used, and a suitably specialised cardiologist should determine the diagnosis.

| Mutations that cause long QT syndrome | |
| --- | --- |
| Long QT syndrome type | Details |
| 1 | Accounts for a third of cases |
| | Caused by a mutation in the *KCNQ1* gene, which encodes the slow potassium rectifier channel |
| | May have autosomal dominant or autosomal recessive inheritance |
| 2 | Accounts for a quarter of cases |
| | Caused by a mutation in the *KCNH2* gene, which encodes the rapid delayed potassium rectifier channel |
| 3 | Caused by a mutation in the *SCN5A* gene, which encodes the sodium channel |
| | Has autosomal dominant inheritance |
| 4–10 | Much less common than types 1–3 |

**Table 10.4** Mutations that cause long QT syndrome

> **In long QT syndrome, triggering events differ by genotype.** In long QT syndrome type 1, events are usually preceded by exercise, commonly swimming because of a vagotonic response to cold water. In type 2, events may follow exposure to auditory stimuli or emotion. In type 3, events most commonly occur during sleep ('dead-in-bed syndrome').

## Management

Lifestyle modifications include avoiding competitive sports, swimming alone and loud noises. Patients are advised to avoid QT-prolonging drugs.

Long QT syndrome is treated primarily with beta-blockers. Insertion of an implantable cardioverter defibrillator is considered for all patients with recurrent syncope or documented ventricular tachycardia, as well as survivors of a cardiac arrest.

# Other inherited cardiac conditions

Other conditions with a genetic basis and that affect the heart are described here.

## Marfan's syndrome

Marfan's syndrome is a multisystem connective tissue disease that predominantly affects the eyes, the cardiovascular system and the musculoskeletal system.

## Epidemiology and aetiology

This inherited cardiac condition is estimated to affect 2–3 people in 10,000.

Marfan's syndrome is inherited in an autosomal dominant fashion. Most patients have a mutation of a gene encoding fibrillin. About a quarter of cases arise spontaneously (no family history) from a new mutation.

## Clinical features

Marfan's syndrome has characteristic clinical features (**Figure 10.6**).

- Musculoskeletal features include a tall and thin physique, with long arms and fingers, a high arched palate with overcrowded dentition, and striae of the skin
- Cardiac features include dilatation, dissection or rupture of the aorta; patients may also have valvular involvement with aortic regurgitation or mitral valve prolapse
- Ophthalmic features include lens subluxation and myopia

## Diagnostic approach

Diagnosis is based on the international criteria known as the Ghent nosology. These are

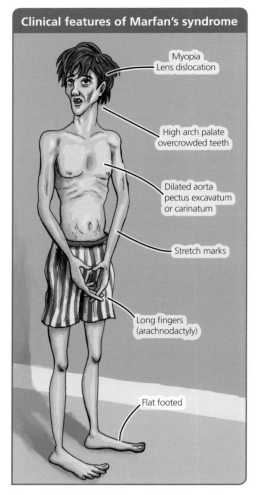

**Clinical features of Marfan's syndrome**

Myopia
Lens dislocation

High arch palate
overcrowded teeth

Dilated aorta
pectus excavatum
or carinatum

Stretch marks

Long fingers
(arachnodactyly)

Flat footed

**Figure 10.6** Clinical features of Marfan's syndrome.

divided into major and minor criteria and combine family history with various clinical features.

# Investigations

Patients are assessed at least annually, because some features may develop over years and are not apparent at first presentation. Each affected system should be managed by an appropriate specialist (an ophthalmologist, a cardiologist, etc.).

The focus of cardiovascular management is assessment and surveillance of the thoracic aorta with echocardiography and cardiac MRI. This is because aortic dissection or rupture is the gravest complication of Marfan's syndrome, and is predicted by increasing aortic dimensions.

# Management

Beta-blockers are given if any evidence of aortic dilatation is detected. Hypertension is managed aggressively. Angiotensin II receptor blockers are given to even normotensive patients, because there is some evidence that their use reduces aortic dilatation. Aortic root surgery is considered when the diameter of the aortic root is > 4.5 cm at the level of the sinus of Valsalva.

> **The diagnosis of any condition with a genetic basis has implications for the whole family.** Patients should be referred to a specialist inherited cardiac conditions service and a full family pedigree documented. Post-mortem studies may be necessary to confirm causes of death and thus help establish the inheritance of a condition.
>
> Once a genetic basis has been established, patients are referred to a clinical geneticist for screening of the index case (the patient with the condition) and members of their family.

# Familial hypercholesterolaemia

Familial hypercholesterolaemia is an inherited condition that leads to accumulation of low-density lipoprotein (LDL) cholesterol. This increases the incidence of premature atherosclerosis. However, the risk is dramatically reduced if the condition is identified and treated.

# Epidemiology and aetiology

Familial hypercholesterolaemia is an autosomal dominant condition. Many different associated mutations have been identified. Most of these mutations affect the *LDLR* gene, which encodes the LDL receptor.

Heterozygous patients have a change in one copy of the *LDLR* gene. The prevalence of heterozygous familial hypercholesterolaemia in the general population is about 1 in 500. If the condition is left untreated, about 50% of men and 30% of women have clinical coronary heart disease by the age of 50.

Patients with the homozygous form of the disease have a change in both copies of the *LDLR* gene, which leads to a more serious condition. Homozygous familial hypercholesterolaemia affects one in a million people, and is therefore much rarer then the heterozygous form. Homozygous familial hypercholesterolaemia often presents in childhood with the sequelae of atherosclerosis.

# Clinical features

Patients present with premature atherosclerosis, most commonly coronary heart disease. with either myocardial infarction or symptoms of angina. Other people present with alternative manifestations of atherosclerosis, such as stroke and peripheral vascular disease.

# Diagnostic approach

Familial hypercholesterolaemia is diagnosed according to the Simon Broome criteria (**Table 10.5**). The diagnosis is either definite or possible, depending on the presence of tendon xanthomas (**Figure 10.7**), family history of myocardial infarction, and serum cholesterol concentrations in affected family members.

| Criteria for diagnosis of familial hypercholesterolaemia | |
|---|---|
| Definite familial hypercholesterolaemia | Possible familial hypercholesterolaemia |
| Adult | Adult |
| Cholesterol > 7.5 mmol/L<br>OR<br>LDL cholesterol > 4.9 mmol/L | Cholesterol > 7.5 mmol/L<br>OR<br>LDL cholesterol > 4.9 mmol/L |
| Child (age < 16 years) | Child (age < 16 years) |
| Cholesterol > 6.7 mmol/L<br>OR<br>LDL cholesterol > 4 mmol/L | Cholesterol > 6.7 mmol/L<br>OR<br>LDL cholesterol > 4 mmol/L |
| AND | AND |
| Tendon xanthomas in the patient, or a first- or second-degree relative<br>OR<br>DNA evidence of a known mutation associated with family history | A family history of myocardial infarction (< 60 years in a first-degree relative; < 50 years in a second-degree relative)<br>OR<br>A family history of increased total cholesterol (> 7.5 mmol/L in a first- or second-degree adult relative; > 6.7 mmol/L in a child or sibling younger than 16 years) |
| LDL, low-density lipoprotein. | |

**Table 10.5** The Simon Broome criteria for diagnosis of definite and possible familial hypercholesterolaemia

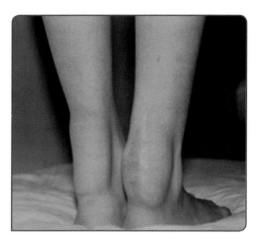

**Figure 10.7** Tendon xanthoma in familial hypercholesterolaemia; note the obvious thickening of the Achilles tendon.

and LDL cholesterol is 50% of baseline values. All patients need to make lifestyle modifications, which include smoking cessation, weight loss and switching to a low-fat diet.

> Patients with hypothyroidism should have their thyroid biochemistry corrected before starting lipid-lowering medication. Normalisation of thyroid function may be enough to treat the lipid abnormality.

Patients with the heterozygous form of familial hypercholesterolaemia require intense lipid-lowering therapy with statins as first-line therapy. If lipid concentrations remain above the targets, a second agent (usually ezetimibe) is recommended.

## Management

Patients are referred to a specialist lipid clinic. The target reduction in serum total cholesterol

## Answers to starter questions

1. Patients are often asymptomatic. When they do complain of symptoms it is usually of chest pain, shortness of breath and palpitations.

2. Hypertrophic cardiomyopathy is diagnosed by the characteristic ECG changes (specifically increased precordial voltages and non specific ST- and T-wave abnormalities) and echocardiographic findings showing thick muscle of the left ventricular wall.

3. Afro-Caribbeans tend to have thicker left ventricular walls and therefore larger voltage complexes on ECG traces than Caucasian populations. These changes can mimic hypertrophic cardiomyopathy making its diagnosis less clear.

4. Athlete's heart is a non-pathological condition that develops with aerobic exercise and training, and presents with bradycardia, cardiomegaly and ventricular hypertrophy. As such, their ECGs often look abnormal with evidence of left ventricular hypertrophy and a slow heart rate. It can be difficult to diagnose but should always be considered in asymptomatic patients who do a lot of exercise (more than 1 hour of aerobic exercise a day).

5. Patients with Marfan's syndrome have a higher chance of aortic dissection or rupture because of weakness of the vessel walls. Cardiovascular management is focused on the assessment, and surveillance of the thoracic aorta with echocardiography and CMR since aortic dissection or rupture can be predicted by rising aortic dimensions.

# Chapter 11
# Pericardial disease and tumours

## Starter questions

Answers to the following questions are on page 347.

1. Why is pressure more important than volume in pericardial effusion?
2. How can you tell a pericardial rub from a pleural rub or cardiac murmur?

## Introduction

Pericarditis is inflammation of the fluid sac surrounding the heart. Its presentation can mimic acute coronary syndromes but it is managed differently. Sometimes, pericarditis causes a pericardial effusion, which must be treated to prevent cardiac tamponade developing (a clinical emergency). Pericardial effusions also develop because of other conditions which must be recognised and treated.

Cardiac tumors are rare and primary cardiac tumours even rarer. Therefore, they usually represent metastatic disease from a tumour located elsewhere. If a cardiac tumor is the first manifestation of disease, an alternative primary tumor should always be looked for.

# Case 13 Chest pain at work

## Presentation

Andrew Coles is a 25-year-old builder. He smokes 20 cigarettes a day, but is otherwise well with no medical history of note. He has been suffering from what he describes as a cold. While mixing concrete at work, he developed a sharp central chest pain. His colleagues were worried and called for an ambulance.

## Initial interpretation

Andrew is complaining of chest pain and a cardiac cause must be considered. He is a smoker but has no other risk factors for premature heart disease at this point.

## History

Andrew's pain developed over the course 30 minutes and was sharp. He had never had anything similar before. There is no family history of heart problems. He has no associated symptoms but says the pain was worse when the ambulance crew laid him on the trolley or when he takes a deep breath. The pain eases when he sits back up. Although the pain developed while working, he has not noticed a relationship between the pain and exertion. No risk factors for thromboembolic disease are identified.

## Interpretation of history

Differential diagnoses of chest pain include acute coronary syndrome, pulmonary embolus and aortic dissection. Other possibilities include acute pericarditis or musculoskeletal chest pain. Neither his age nor the nature of the pain are classic presentations of an acute coronary syndrome; it is not exacerbated by exertion but is by deep inspiration and lying flat. The pain is pleuritic in nature. He has also experienced a recent coryzal (likely viral) illness. This is in keeping with the pain of pericarditis. Musculoskeletal chest pain should be considered because he has a manual job with a lot of lifting.

## Examination

His pulse is 100 bpm and blood pressure is 120/80 mmHg. His heart sounds are normal, with no added sounds and his chest is clear to auscultation. There is no peripheral oedema. The pain is not reproduced on palpation of the chest wall.

## Interpretation of Findings

Examination findings are largely normal, but this can be the case in all of the possible diagnoses. That palpation of the chest wall did not reproduce the pain makes musculoskeletal pain unlikely.

## Investigations

Andrew's ECG demonstrates widespread concave ST elevation (**Figure 11.1**). His chest X-ray is normal. His blood tests show raised inflammatory markers and a mildly elevated white cell count (**Table 11.1**). His haemoglobin, platelets, and renal, liver and thyroid function are all normal, as is the initial troponin (cardiac enzyme) assay.

## Interpretation of Investigations

Andrew's investigations indicate an active inflammatory process and demonstrate the classic ECG signs of pericarditis, in the absence of any radiographical evidence of lung disease. The inflammation has involved the adjacent epicardium, because there is concave ST-segment elevation, tall T waves and PR-segment depression on the ECG.

**Case 6** *continued*

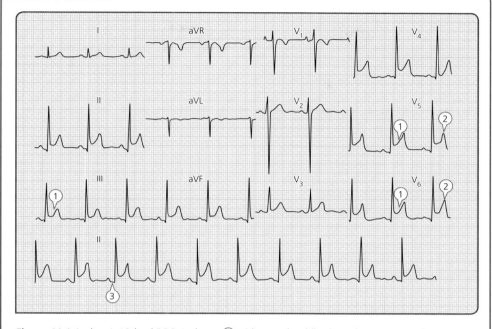

**Figure 11.1** Andrew's 12-lead ECG. It shows ① widespread saddle-shaped ST segment elevation; ② tall T waves; ③ PR segment depression.

| Andrew's blood test results | |
|---|---|
| Test | Result (normal) |
| White cell count (WCC) | 13.2 x10⁹/L (4–11 x10⁹/L) |
| Erythrocyte sedimentation rate (ESR) | 55 mm/h (< 15 mm/h) |
| C-reactive protein (CRP) | 70 mg/L (<5 mg/L) |

**Table 11.1** Andrew's blood test results

## Diagnosis

In an otherwise healthy young man with pleuritic chest pain, a recent coryzal illness, raised inflammatory markers, with typical ECG changes, the diagnosis is acute pericarditis. Andrew requires an echocardiogram to investigate for pericardial effusion, which can be caused by pericarditis.

# Acute pericarditis

Pericarditis is inflammation of the pericardium. It accounts for 5% of all acute chest pain admissions. The cause often remains unknown (idiopathic), although in many cases it occurs several weeks after a preceding viral infection (**Table 11.2**).

## Pathogenesis

Inflammation of the pericardial sac causes the parietal and visceral pericardial layers to rub together with increased friction. This causes pain and sometimes a pericardial

| Causes of pericarditis | |
|---|---|
| Cause | Example |
| Trauma | Seatbelt injury |
| Uremia | Renal failure |
| Myocardial Infarction | Dressler's syndrome |
| Other infections | Viral, e.g. Epstein–Barr virus, CMV, HIV, coxsackie virus |
| | Bacterial, e.g. TB, rheumatic fever |
| | Fungal |
| Rheumatoid arthritis and other autoimmune disorders and radiation | Rheumatoid arthritis, systemic lupus erythematosus |
| Surgical | Post coronary artery bypass graft surgery |

**Table 11.2** Causes of acute pericarditis. These can be remembered using the mnemonic TUMORS. Metastatic cancer is also a cause of pericarditis (paraneoplastic phenomenon)

effusion. If the inflammation affects the adjacent myocardium it causes myocarditis, (myo-pericarditis) or pan-carditis (epi-myo-endocarditis, e.g. in rheumatic fever). Involvement of the myocardium causes ECG abnormalities, elevation of cardiac enzymes and in some cases, significant impairment of systolic function and heart failure.

> **Pericarditis causes acute chest pain, ECG changes and a rise in cardiac enzymes (troponin).** It is therefore, often mistaken for acute coronary syndrome.

## Clinical features

The principle complaint is chest pain which is pleuritic in nature. It is typically a 'sharp', 'stabbing' or 'burning' sensation exacerbated by lying flat and by taking deep breaths, and eased by sitting upright (due to how the heart lies inside the pericardial sac). Patients are tachypnoeic, taking shallow, rapid breaths to avoid painful deep breaths. A pericardial rub may be heard (lower left sternal edge). Significant myocarditis presents with the signs and symptoms of heart failure.

## Diagnosis

Diagnosis is based on the clinical history and examination. Investigations include:

- Blood tests: Inflammatory markers (CRP, ESR and white cell count) are elevated, and cardiac enzymes (e.g. troponin) rise if there is myocardial involvement
- ECG: abnormalities if the myocardium is involved, including concave 'saddle-shaped' ST segment elevation, tall T waves and PR-segment depression (if the atrial myocardium is affected). ST-segment elevation is concave and not constrained to arterial territories
- Chest X-ray: an enlarged, globular cardiac silhouette indicates a pericardial effusion
- Echocardiography: is performed in all cases to exclude effusion and assess myocardial systolic function

## Management

Idiopathic pericarditis is managed with reassurance, analgesia, non-steroidal anti-inflammatory drugs (NSAIDs, e.g. colchicine or aspirin) and rest. Management of secondary pericarditis focusses on treating the underlying cause, e.g. uraemia (in renal failure) requires dialysis and tuberculosis requires antimicrobials.

Pericarditis with effusion may require drainage (pericardiocentesis). There are two indications for aspiration: therapeutic (to relieve cardiac tamponade) and diagnostic (to analyse the composition of the fluid). Patients with myocarditis require a cardiac MRI to assess the degree of myocardial involvement, and may require heart failure therapy and long-term follow up.

## Prognosis

Idiopathic pericarditis can recur and is treated with colchine. Prognosis is determined by whether a significant effusion develops and the degree of myocardial involvement, and in the long-term by whether scarring and fibrosis develop. Myocardial scarring causes chronic impairment of systolic function and heart failure. Scarring of the pericardial sac is a cause of constrictive pericarditis which occurs years later and impairs cardiac diastolic function.

# Pericardial effusion

Pericardial effusion is the collection of fluid between the visceral and parietal pericardial layers. It is an uncommon condition with multiple causes (**Table 11.3**). At its worse, it presents with cardiac tamponade, which is life-threatening and requires emergency drainage (see page 358). The haemodynamic consequences are related to the volume of accumulated fluid, the speed at which it collects and the pressure inside the pericardial space. The pericardium can stretch to accommodate large volume effusions if this occurs over a long period of time whereas a low-volume effusion can cause cardiac tamponade if it accumulates quickly.

> Pericardial effusion should be considered in patients who become acutely unwell with low blood pressure following an invasive cardiac procedure.

## Clinical features

Patients are asymptomatic with small, or chronic, effusions but have dyspnoea or chest pain if the effusion is large. Patients present in extremis or following cardiac arrest if there is tamponade. Clinical signs include a combination of elevated jugular venous pressure, hypotension, impalpable apex beat, tachycardia and tachypnoea. Pulsus paradoxus (abnormal reduction in pulse volume on inspiration) and Kussmaul's sign (abnormal rise in JVP with inspiration) may also be found.

ECG signs include small complexes due to the effusion impeding the conduction of electrical signals. Electrical alternans occurs where the electrical cardiac axis frequently changes (alternates) as the heart swings freely, to-and-fro, within the pericardial cavity in a large effusion. Chest X-rays show an enlarged and globular cardiac silhouette. Diagnosis is confirmed with echocardiography (**Figure 11.2**).

## Management

Management depends on the cause and the degree to which function is compromised. Tamponade requires emergency drainage. It is not unusual to drain more than 2L from a large effusion. If small and the patient is not compromised then diuretic therapy is given. Effusions treated conservatively are monitored with serial echocardiography until they resolve.

| Causes of pericardial effusion |
| --- |
| Acute pericarditis |
| Idiopathic |
| Myocardial infarction |
| Trauma |
| Post cardiac surgery or intervention (e.g. CABG, EP or PCI procedure) |
| Aortic dissection |
| Malignancy |
| Renal failure (uraemic effusion) |
| Infection: <br> ■ viral (e.g. coxsackievirus, echovirus, cytomegalovirus, HIV) <br> ■ bacterial (e.g. tuberculosis) |
| Autoimmune disease (e.g. rheumatoid arthritis, systemic lupus erythematosus) |

**Table 11.3** Causes of pericardial effusion

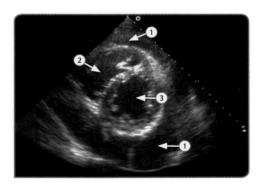

**Figure 11.2** Echocardiogram showing. ① a rim of fluid around the heart in the pericardial space. The image is a short axis (cross section) view of the heart hence the left ventricle; ③ appears doughnut shaped; ② right ventricle.

# Cardiac tumours

All cardiac tumors are rare and are either benign or malignant. Benign tumours, (e.g. myxoma, rhabdomyomas, lipomas, fibromas) have local effects and rarely spread or recur once removed. They are generally not life-threatening. Malignant tumours (e.g. rhabdomyosarcomas, angiosarcomas, myxosarcomas, fibrosarcomas, leiomyosarcomas) are four times rarer. They spread to other sites and may recur after removal.

Secondary tumours are found distant from their origin (i.e. have metastasised) and are malignant, with a very poor prognosis. Malignant cancer in the heart is almost always a metastasis from another site.

Echocardiography, CT and MRI scanning are used to diagnose cardiac tumours. Management depends on the extent of the cardiac involvement, tumour type, the degree of invasiveness, the stage of malignancy and the patient's health. Treatment of primary malignant or secondary disease is usually palliative, as resection generally fails and postoperative mortality is high.

## Cardiac myxoma

Cardiac myxomas are slow-growing, fibrous tumours which occur in all cardiac chambers but most commonly in the left atrium. They affect 1 in 5000 adults, 75% of which are women, and take years to cause symptoms.

Asymptomatic cardiac myxoma is usually discovered incidentally during echocardiography and causes weight loss, malaise, fever and night sweats. A murmur is evident if tumour interferes with valve function. A 'diastolic plop' occurs if a semi-mobile tumour prolapses through the mitral valve annulus during diastole.

> **Myxoma is often mistaken for endocarditis** because of the combination of an intracardiac mass and fever.

Diagnosis is made by echocardiography which shows a mobile, pedunculated mass attached to the myocardium, most commonly arising from the left-side of the interatrial septum (**Figure 11.3**). A transoesophageal echo is used to define the size and site of the tumor. Myxomas are removed surgically and rarely recur.

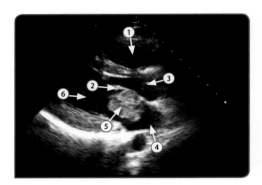

**Figure 11.3** Echocardiogram showing a ⑤ left atrial myxoma. The mitral valve ② is open during diastole and the myxoma has moved towards the left ventricle ⑥. ① Right ventricle ③ aortic valve ④ left atrium.

# Answers to starter questions

1. The most dangerous complication of a pericardial effusion is cardiac tamponade, when the cardiac chambers become compressed under the pressure exerted by the surrounding pericardial fluid. If an effusion accumulates slowly, the pericardial sac adapts and stretches, so even in large volume effusions the pericardial pressure won't rise high enough to cause tamponade. If fluid accumulates quickly the pressure rises quick enough to cause tamponade, even with low-volume effusions.

2. A rub sounds like a crunch or a creak. Pericardial rubs are timed with the cardiac cycle (with the pulse when examining) whereas pleural rubs occur when the patient takes a breath following the ventilatory pattern. Cardiac murmurs are also timed to the cardiac cycle but are more of a 'whoosh' than a crunch or creak.

# Chapter 12
# Cardiac emergencies

## Introduction

Cardiovascular disease accounts for 40% of all deaths and hospital admissions worldwide. Cardiac emergencies are potentially life-threatening, so they must be recognised and treated promptly. Cardiac emergencies typically present with chest pain, collapse, dyspnoea or palpitations.

Medical emergencies are approached using the 'safe ABCDE' scheme which prioritises the key assessment and management steps.

The assessor should only proceed to the next step when they are confident that the current step is satisfied.

- Safe: check it is safe to approach and assess the patient
- A: airway and oxygenation
- B: breathing and ventilation
- C: circulation and management of shock
- D: disability, i.e. level of consciousness
- E: exposure and examination

# Case 14 Collapse, no breathing and no pulse

## Presentation

A 60-year-old man is brought to the emergency department after being found unresponsive in his taxi, without a pulse.

## Initial interpretation

The patient appears to have suffered a cardiac arrest, because he has no pulse and is unconscious. Therefore cardiopulmonary resuscitation is started immediately to maintain perfusion to the vital organs.

## History and examination

A collapsed patient should be assessed for cardiac arrest and CPR commenced immediately. A medical history can be gained from the patient, a friend or family member afterwards.

The primary ABCDE survey reveals:

- Airway: his airway is patent but unprotected
- Breathing: there are no signs of breathing

## Case 14 continued

### Ventricular fibrillation: diagnosis and management

Hello? Can you hear me

He is not breathing and there is no pulse. He is in cardiac arrest. Start CPR

In the resuscitation area of the emergency department, CPR is performed and he is defibrillated into sinus rhythm

What do you think of the rhythm?

Looks like coarse VF; it's broad and completely irregular

Ok. I'll do compressions, you look after the airway. We'll need to phone him in

That's right. What's the next step

Defibrillation

Two paramedics on their break are asked to check a taxi driver found slumped in his cab

Why are we taking him to intensive care?

Can you see the tight narrowing in the LAD?

So therapeutic hypothermia can be used to reduce...

Of course. But he'll also need secondary prevention including anti-platelet medication to stop further thrombosis

Errr... yes. Are you going to re-open with balloon angioplasty and a stent?

...metabolic activity of his brain and other tissue?

Precisely!

Primary PCI to re-opens a blocked coronary artery

After resuscitation, defibrillation and primary PCI, he now has a good cardiac output. 24 hours of cooling aims to minimise cerebral damage.

- Circulation: the patient has no pulse and therefore no recordable blood pressure, therefore CPR is commenced
- Disability: his Glasgow coma scale score is 3 out of a maximum of 15 (the lowest possible)
- Exposure: no external signs of trauma are evident

Medical staff attach defibrillator pads to the patient's chest. These also act as ECG monitoring leads which demonstrate he is in ventricular fibrillation (**Figure 12.1**).

## Immediate intervention

The patient undergoes cardiopulmonary resuscitation. His airway is opened using a jaw thrust manoeuvre and is protected with airway adjuncts.

> **Most hospitals have a 'crash' team who respond to emergencies, including cardiac arrest.** The team is typically led by a medical registrar, an anaesthetic registrar or both.

### Rhythm strip showing ventricular fibrillation

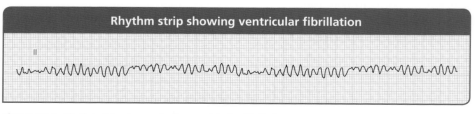

**Figure 12.1** Rhythm strip demonstrating ventricular fibrillation.

**Case 14** *continued*

The patient is ventilated using a bag valve mask. The ratio of chest compressions to ventilations is 30:2.

His heart rhythm (VF) is identified as shockable according to the advanced life support guidelines (**Figure 12.4**). He is therefore defibrillated and this restores sinus rhythm.

During cardiopulmonary resuscitation, reversible causes of cardiac arrest are sought and corrected. (for which a collateral history is useful)

# Case 15 Collapse, chest pain and tachycardia

## Presentation

A 75-year-old woman is found collapsed while visiting her husband in hospital. The crash team is called. On their arrival, she has roused but has a pulse rate of 160 beats/min while palpating her carotid artery.

## Initial interpretation

The patient has a tachyarrhythmia and has experienced a syncopal episode. The concern is that the syncope has resulted from arrhythmia causing cerebral hypoperfusion.

## History and examination

There is no background information and therefore no history available.

Examination follows the ABCDE approach.

- Airway: the airway is patent
- Breathing: the patient is breathing with a respiratory rate of 20 breaths/min; there is good air entry bilaterally, and no added sounds are audible on chest auscultation
- Circulation: her heart sounds are difficult to auscultate, and her pulse rhythm is irregularly irregular at 160 beats/min; capillary refill time is 3.5 s and her brachial blood pressure is 80/40 mmHg
- Disability: the patient's Glasgow Coma Scale score is 15 (out of 15), her blood glucose is 7 mmol/L and her temperature is 37°C
- Exposure: there are no abnormal findings on examination

The ECG rhythm strip (**Figure 12.2**) shows an irregularly irregular narrow complex tachycardia.

## Immediate intervention

The patient has a narrow complex tachycardia, specifically atrial fibrillation with rapid ventricular respone and has adverse features (syncope and hypotension). According to advanced life support guidelines (**Figure 12.7**), this patient requires

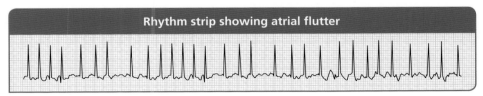

Rhythm strip showing atrial flutter

**Figure 12.2** ECG rhythm strip showing atrial fibrillation with vast ventricular response.

**Case 15** *continued*

direct current cardioversion with appropriate anticoagulant therapy. The aim of this treatment is to cardiovert the heart back into sinus rhythm. She should the be monitored until stable.

# Cardiac arrest

A cardiac arrest is when there is no effective blood circulation, secondary to cessation of cardiac output. It occurs in 4 in every 100,000 people in the general population and in 4 in every 1000 hospital in-patients. Only 10% of these survive to discharge.

Cardiac arrest has various causes (**Table 12.1**). Around two-thirds of cardiac arrests arise secondary to a heart disorder, usually ischaemic heart disease. Other cardiac causes include heart failure, cardiomyopathy and congenital and inherited disorders. Common non-cardiac causes include lung disease (hypoxia), pulmonary embolus (thromboembolism), haemorrhage (hypotension), metabolic abnormalities (hyper- and hypokalaemia) and multiorgan failure.

Cardiac arrest is diagnosed in an unconscious patient, with no palpable pulse and no respiratory effort. It is subdivided into shockable and non-shockable according to the cardiac rhythm (**Figure 12.3**). Shockable rhythms are:

- Ventricular tachycardia: regular broad complex tachycardia (> 100 beats/min)
- Ventricular fibrillation: irregular and chaotic rhythm, rate and amplitude (> 200 beats/min)

| Reversible causes of cardiac arrest | |
|---|---|
| Four H's | Four T's |
| Hypoxia | Thromboembolism (coronary or pulmonary) |
| Hypothermia | Tension pneumothorax |
| Hypotension | Tamponade (cardiac) |
| Hyper- or hypokalaemia | Toxins |

**Table 12.1** The eight reversible causes of cardiac arrest: four H's and four T's

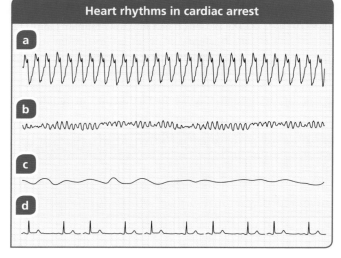

**Figure 12.3** ECG rhythm strips showing the four heart rhythms found in cardiac arrest. (a) Ventricular tachycardia. (b) Ventricular fibrillation. (c) Asystole. (d) Pulseless electrical activity.

Non-shockable rhythms do not respond to defibrillation:

- Asystole: no rhythm, rate or complexes
- Pulseless electrical activity: any rhythm compatible with life but without a pulse (also known as electromechanical dissociation, EMD)

The only treatment for cardiac arrest is cardiopulmonary resuscitation and prompt defibrillation where appropriate. This must be started immediately, because every 1-min delay decreases the likelihood of survival by 10%.

Cardiopulmonary resuscitation is performed using a ratio of 30 chest compressions (at a depth of 6 cm and a rate of 100 per min) to 2 rescue breaths (10 per min). During resuscitation, possible reversible causes for the cardiac arrest must be assessed and treated (**Table 12.1**). Drugs such as adrenaline (epinephrine) and amiodarone are used according to **Figure 12.4**.

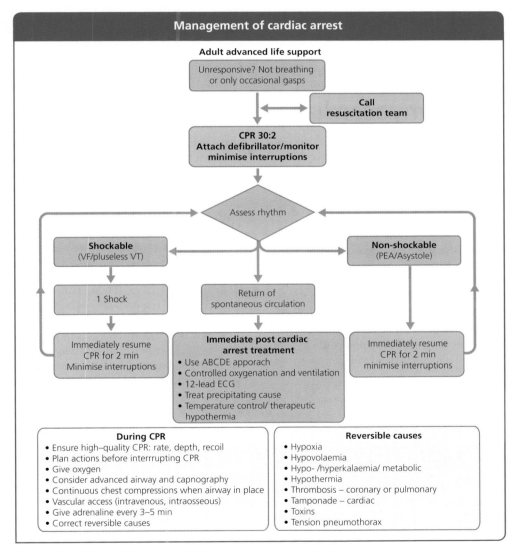

**Figure 12.4** Advanced life support guidelines for the management of a cardiac arrest. CPR, cardiopulmonary resuscitation; ECG, electrocardiogram; PEA, pulseless electrical activity; VF, ventricular fibrillation; VT, ventricular tachycardia. Reproduced with the kind permission of the Resuscitation Council (UK).

In patients with a shockable rhythm, early defibrillation to restore sinus rhythm and cardiac output is crucial (**Figure 12.5**). Automated external defibrillators are provided in some public buildings such as airports and shopping centres. They are also carried by paramedics and hospital crash teams.

Once spontaneous circulation has returned, patients are transferred to an appropriate location, for example an intensive care unit. Once stable, further investigations, such as coronary angiography, may be necessary.

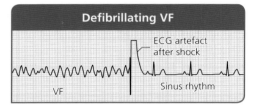

**Defibrillating VF**

ECG artefact after shock

VF

Sinus rhythm

**Figure 12.5** Successful defibrillation from ventricular fibrillation to sinus rhythm.

It is essential to check that cardiopulmonary resuscitation is appropriate for the individual patient. Before starting, check that there is not a 'Do not attempt cardiopulmonary resuscitation' order in their notes.

# Acute myocardial infarction

Acute myocardial infarction is caused by rupture of an atherosclerotic plaque in a coronary artery, leading to the formation of a thrombus that occludes the arterial lumen (see page 185).

In the acute stages, patients typically experience:

■ central chest discomfort or pain (a tight, constricting or heavy sensation), which may radiate to the jaw, neck, shoulders or arms
■ dyspnoea
■ sweating
■ nausea and vomiting

Presentations vary; some patients have no symptoms while others experience severe pain. Most present with two or more of these symptoms.

All patients require oral aspirin 300 mg to reduce thrombus formation, glyceryl trinitrate given sublingually as a spray or tablet to dilate the coronary arteries, and possibly intravenous morphine to control pain. Only patients who are hypoxic (saturation < 94%) are given oxygen. The management of patients with acute myocardial infarction can be remembered with the acronym MONA (**Table 12.2**).

A 12-lead ECG is used to diagnose myocardial infarction: ST segment elevation indicates ST elevation myocardial infarction (STEMI) and its absence indicates non–ST elevation myocardial infarction (NSTEMI) (**Figure 12.6**). Cardiac enzymes such as troponin are elevated in both conditions.

Patients with STEMI require urgent reperfusion by primary percutaneous intervention; angioplasty and stenting are used to reopen the blocked coronary artery (see page 185). If this is not available, the patient should receive thrombolytic therapy.

| Inital management of acute myocardial infarction | | | |
|---|---|---|---|
| Initial letter | Medication | Action | Example |
| M | Morphine | Analgesia | 2.5–5 mg intravenously |
| O | Oxygen | Reverses hypoxia | 100%, 15 L, high flow |
| N | Nitrates | Dilates coronary arteries | Two puffs glyceryl trinitrate sublingually |
| A | Antiplatelet drugs | Reduces thrombosis | 300 mg orally (chewed or crushed) |

**Table 12.2** The MONA acronym for the initial management of acute myocardial infarction

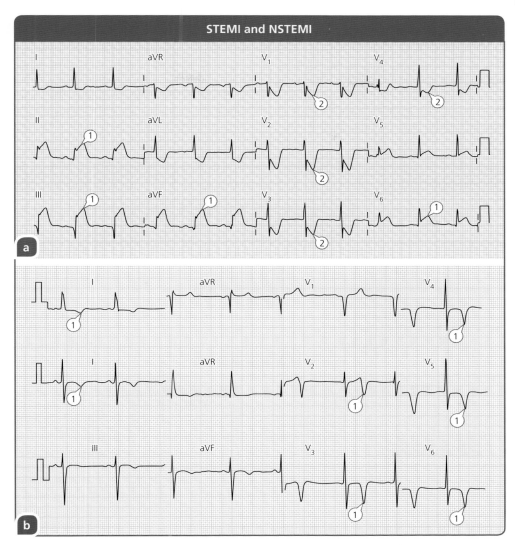

**Figure 12.6** 12-lead ECGs demonstrating typical acute STEMI and NSTEMI changes. (a) ST elevation myocardial infarction with ST segment elevation ① in leads II, III, aVF (inferior leads) and in V6 (indicating lateral territory involvement). There is reciprocal ST depression ② in V1-4. (b) Non–ST elevation myocardial infarction with deep T wave inversion ① in V2-6 and in leads I and II.

> **Not all patients with acute myocardial infarction experience chest pain.**
> Patients with diabetic neuropathy may have an acute myocardial infarction without chest pain. Furthermore, not all chest pain is cardiac in origin; it may, for example, be musculoskeletal.

Patients with NSTEMI undergo urgent percutaneous intervention only if their pain and ischaemia do not settle with medical therapy.

After percutaneous intervention, patients need cardiac monitoring on the coronary care unit.

Patients can develop acute heart failure (see page 249), cardiogenic shock, cardiac arrest (see page 352), tachyarrhythmia or bradyarrhythmia (see page 360).

# Narrow complex tachycardia

Patients with narrow complex tachycardias have a heart rate > 100 beats/min and a normal QRS duration (< 0.12 s). (see page 223). They are an emergency if adverse signs are present (**Figure 12.7** and **Table 12.3**), in which case direct current cardioversion (DCCV) is required.

DCCV is extremely uncomfortable and unless the patient is already unconscious, it should only be performed under a general

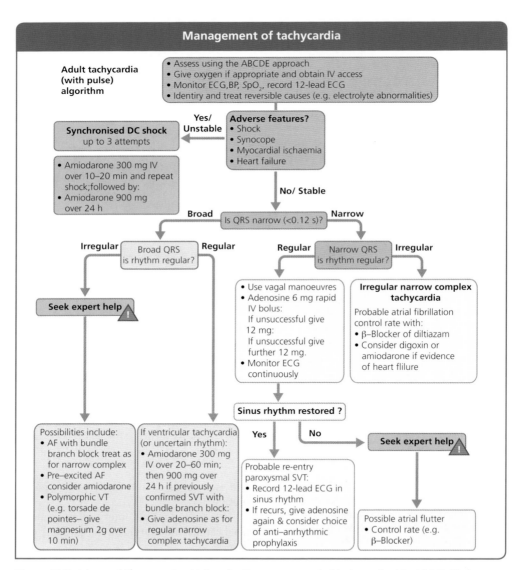

**Figure 12.7** Advanced life support guidelines for the management of tachycardia. AF, atrial fibrillation; BP, blood pressure; DC, direct current; ECG, electrocardiogram; IV, intravenous; SpO$_2$, oxygen saturation; SVT, supraventricular tachycardia; VT, ventricular tachycardia. Reproduced with the kind permission of the Resuscitation Council (UK).

| Adverse features in patients with tachycardia | | | |
|---|---|---|---|
| Adverse feature | Definition | Presentation | Meaning |
| Shock | Systolic blood pressure < 90 mmHg | Pallor and sweating | Reduced cardiac output |
| Syncope | Loss of consciousness | Loss of consciousness | Reduced cerebral perfusion |
| Heart failure | Raised jugular venous pressure and pulmonary oedema | Breathlessness | Reduced cardiac output |
| Myocardial ischaemia | Ischaemic electrocardiographic changes | Chest pain | Reduced coronary perfusion |
| Heart rate extremes | Heart rate > 150 beats/min | Palpitations , pre-syncope and syncope | Reduced diastolic filing |

**Table 12.3** Adverse features in patients with tachycardia

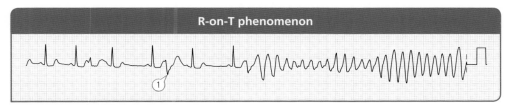

**R-on-T phenomenon**

**Figure 12.8** Rhythm strip showing the R-on-T phenomenon. An ectopic beat coincides with the T wave ① converting sinus rhythm into polymorphic ventricular tachycardia.

anaesthetic or heavy sedation. In the absence of overt adverse signs, acute management uses vagal stimulating manoeuvres and/or intravenous adenosine (to transiently block the atrioventricular node) to restore sinus rhythm. If these are unsuccessful, medications are used to control the heart rate.

> **When defibrillating a narrow complex tachycardia,** the timing of the shock should coincide with the R wave and not the T wave. This prevents the 'R on T' phenomenon, which may induce ventricular tachycardia or fibrillation (cardiac arrest)(**Figure 12.8**).

# Broad complex tachycardia

Patients with broad complex tachycardias have a heart rate > 100 beats/min and abnormally long QRS durations (> 0.12 s) (see page 226).

Broad complex tachycardias compatible with life include the following.

- Rhythms with regular complexes, such as monomorphic ventricular tachycardia (**Figure 12.9**)
- Irregular complexes, such as atrial fibrillation with bundle branch block, pre-excitation and polymorphic ventricular tachycardia (**Figure 12.10**)

They represent either a ventricular rhythm, or a supraventricular rhythm with abnormal conduction. Around 85% of regular broad complex tachycardias are secondary to ventricular tachycardia. In patients with a history of structural heart disease this rises to 95%. Broad complex tachycardia should be considered as ventricular tachycardia until proven otherwise. Ventricular tachycardias are more unstable than supraventricular tachycardias because they can quickly degrade into ventricular fibrillation,

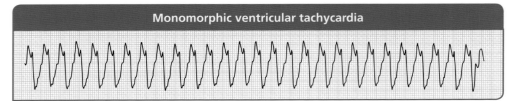

**Monomorphic ventricular tachycardia**

**Figure 12.9** Rhythm strip typical of monomorphic ventricular tachycardia.

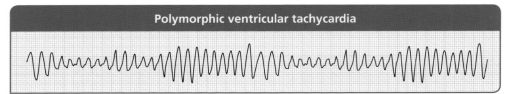

**Polymorphic ventricular tachycardia**

**Figure 12.10** Rhythm strip of polymorphic ventricular tachycardia.

cardiac arrest and death, and are considered an emergency even in the absence of overt adverse features.

Patients with broad complex tachycardia should be managed according to **Figure 12.4**.

Polymorphic ventricular tachycardia, also known as torsade de pointes (where the QRS axis appears to twist around the baseline), necessitates the immediate cessation of QT-prolonging drugs **(Table 12.4)**, defibrillation and magnesium therapy.

| QT-prolonging drugs | |
| --- | --- |
| Drug class | Examples |
| Class 1 antiarrhythmics | Flecainide and propefanone |
| Class 3 antiarrhythmics | Amiodarone and sotalol |
| Antihypertensives | Indapamide and nicardipine |
| Antihistamines | Hydroxyzine and terfenadine |
| Macrolide antibiotics | Clarithromycin and erythromycin |
| Quinolone antibiotics | Ciprofloxain and ofloxacin |
| Antifungals | Fluconazole and ketoconazole |
| Antipsychotics | Quetiapine and risperidone |
| Antidepressants | Amitriptyline and citalopram |
| Antimigraine | Sumatriptan |
| Miscellaneous | Salbutamol, opiates and domperidone |

**Table 12.4** Drugs that can cause QT prolongation increasing the risk of torsade de pointes ventricular tachycardia

# Cardiac tamponade

Cardiac tamponade occurs because fluid accumulates between the myocardium and the pericardium at a faster rate than the pericardial sac can accommodate. The exerts pressure on the heart preventing the chambers from filling during diastole, leading to reduced stroke volume, reduced cardiac output, cardiogenic shock and eventually cardiac arrest.

Causes of cardiac tamponade include chest trauma, cardiac surgery, myocardial rupture, malignancy, renal failure, pericarditis and hypothyroidism.

Patients have palpitations, anergia and breathlessness. Signs include tachycardia, quiet heart sounds, elevated jugular venous pressure, Kussmaul's sign, pulsus paradoxsus and decreased blood pressure (**Table 12.5** and **Figure 12.11**).

> **Kussmaul's sign** is a rise in the jugular venous pressure during inspiration. The jugular venous pressure normally falls during inspiration. A rise suggests impaired filling of the right ventricle, resulting from the presence of pericardial fluid in cardiac tamponade.
>
> **Pulsus paradoxus** is an abnormally large drop in blood pressure (> 10 mmHg) during inspiration. It occurs for the same reasons as Kussmaul's sign.

Electrographic findings can be helpful (**Table 12.6**). Chest X-ray may show cardiomegaly and a globular cardiac silhouette. Echocardiogram shows a pericardial effusion with collapsing chambers (**Figure 12.12**), and abnormally large respiratory swings in the mitral and tricuspid flow velocities.

### Beck's triad: signs of cardiac tamponade

| Feature | Cause |
|---|---|
| Hypotension | Reduced stroke volume |
| Quiet heart sounds | Fluid in the pericardial space |
| Raised jugular venous pressure | Impaired diastolic filling |

**Table 12.5**  Beck's triad: the signs of cardiac tamponade

### ECG features of cardiac tamponade

| Feature | Cause |
|---|---|
| Sinus tachycardia | To maintain cardiac output |
| Small complexes | Damping effect of fluid layer |
| Electrical alternans | Movement of heart in the pericardial space |

**Table 12.6**  Key electrocardiographic features of cardiac tamponade

Treatment is pericardiocentesis, which involves inserting a needle into the pericardial sac to aspirate the pericardial fluid.

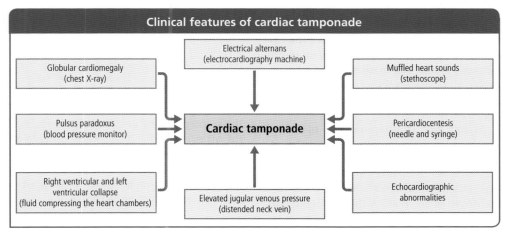

**Figure 12.11**  Key clinical features in cardiac tamponade.

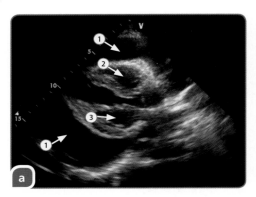
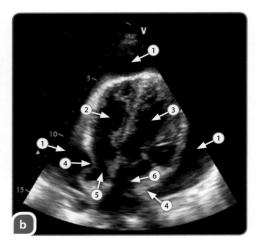

**Figure 12.12** Transthoracic echocardiogram demonstrating cardiac tamponade. (a) A parasternal long axis view showing ① a large 4–5 cm rim of pericardial fluid  surrounding the heart. The apex is to the left of the image and the base to the right. ② Right ventricle ③ left ventricle. (b) Apical view with the apex pointing upwards and the base at the bottom. ① The surrounding effusion is causing the ⑥ left and ⑤ right atria to collapse ④ secondary to the tamponade. ② Right ventricle ③ left ventricle.

# Bradycardia

Bradycardia is a pulse rate below 60bpm (see page 217). Initially, bradycardia is accompanied by an increased stroke volume which compensates for the low heart rate and maintains cardiac output. However, once the cardiovascular system cannot compensate any further cardiac output falls, blood pressure drops and patients experience syncope or pre-syncope. This can cause myocardial ischaemia and heart failure.

Mobitz type II atrioventricular block and complete heart block are bradycardic rhythms associated with increased risk of cardiac arrest, especially if there is loss of consciousness or ventricular pauses of > 3s. These rhythms constitute an emergency. The non-emergency management of bradycardia is described in Chapter 5.

## Management

Rhythms causing adverse features or with an increased risk of asystole are initially managed with intravenous bolus doses of atropine (**Figure 12.13**). Atropine is an anticholinergic drug that increases the depolarisation rate of the sinoatrial node and conduction through the atrioventricular node. After atropine an intravenous infusion of either a beta adrenergic agonist (e.g. isoprenaline, adrenaline, dopamine) or aminophylline can be used to maintain an acceptable heart rate.

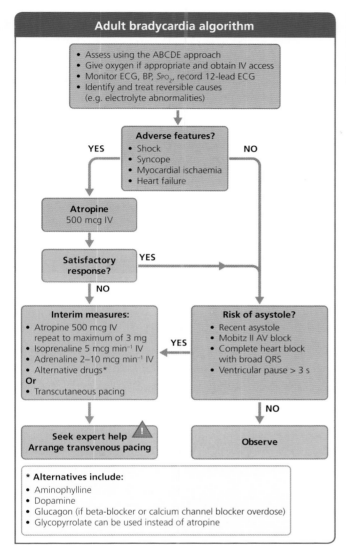

**Figure 12.13** The adult bradycardia algorithm for the initial management of bradycardia. Reproduced with the kind permission of the Resuscitation Council (UK).

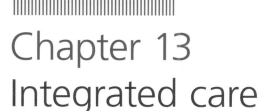

# Chapter 13
# Integrated care

## Starter questions

Answers to the following questions are on page 371.

1. Are public health campaigns effective?
2. Why is it important to check renal function when increasing the doses of spironolactone?
3. Why should patients not drive following a shock from an implantable cardiac defibrillator?
4. Why is cardiac rehabilitation such an important part of the management of myocardial infarction?
5. Why is familial hypercholesterolaemia an important condition to diagnose and treat?

## Introduction

Many cardiovascular diseases first present to primary care. Primary care is the term used to describe physicians who work in the community and not in hospitals. They are often called General Practitioners (GPs). GPs must decide which patients to refer and whether the referral is urgent. This can be challenging because cardiovascular conditions are common and patients present with varying levels and tolerance of symptoms.

GPs are also usually responsible for the day-to-day treatment of patients with cardiovascular diseases. Medications prescribed at a hospital require monitoring and possible up-titration. Furthermore, patients often need ongoing support and advice.

# Case 16 Breathlessness 2 months after a heart attack

## Presentation

Frank Smith is a 66-year-old retired firefighter. He was fit and healthy until 2 months ago, when he had an unheralded anterior myocardial infarction and was admitted to hospital. He underwent primary percutaneous coronary intervention and a stent was inserted.

Mr Smith was discharged after 5 days in hospital. Last week, he attended his first session of cardiac rehabilitation with a physiotherapist. However, he was short of breath on minimal exertion.

## Initial interpretation

Mr Smith had a large anterior myocardial infarction. Therefore the left anterior descending artery was probably occluded. Consequently, the anterior wall of the left ventricle was temporarily deprived of blood.

Breathlessness on exertion suggests the development of some left ventricular failure secondary to the myocardial infarction.

## History

The physiotherapist advised Mr Smith to see his GP which he did the next day. Mr Smith described feeling progressively breathless since his myocardial infarction. He also told the GP that he had noticed he could no longer lie flat at night, and that his ankles were swollen. Although he had had no further chest pains, he explained that he felt tired and generally unwell, and mentioned that he was bruising easily.

Mr Smith gave his GP a list of medications. These included aspirin 75 mg once daily, ticagrelor 90 mg twice daily, atorvastatin 80 mg once daily, ramipril 1.25 mg twice daily, bisoprolol 1.25 mg once daily, spironolactone 25 mg once daily and a glyceryl trinitrate spray.

## Interpretation of history

The symptoms described are those of left ventricular failure; they include orthopnoea (shortness of breath when lying flat) and peripheral oedema. Patients receive antiplatelet therapy after stent insertion, and the two antiplatelet agents (aspirin and ticagrelor) are the cause of the bruising (because of platelet inhibition caused by these two drugs).

## Examination

Mr Smith is breathless at rest. The bruising on his arms is obvious. His blood pressure is 130/70 mmHg, and his heart rate is 80 beats/min. His jugular venous pressure is elevated 4 cm above the manubriosternal angle. A pansystolic murmur is audible at the apex and radiates to the axilla, and bilateral coarse crepitations are heard at the lung bases. Pitting oedema is present to the mid shin.

## Interpretation of findings

Mr Smith has left ventricular failure, as evidenced by the raised jugular venous pressure, the bilateral crepitations at the lung bases and the peripheral oedema. The pansystolic murmur is caused by mitral regurgitation resulting from lack of coaptation of the mitral valve leaflets.

## Diagnosis

In this case, the diagnosis of left ventricular failure is made clinically using the information from the history and examination. Left ventricular impairment and consequent left ventricular failure is always considered in patients who have had a myocardial infarction.

# Up-titration of medication

Many cardiac conditions that are followed up in primary care settings require the up-titration of medications. Up-titration is when a patient's medication is gradually increased in dose, to establish them on the maximum tolerated dose or the maximum dose required to treat their symptoms while monitoring for side effects (**Figure 13.1**). This requires regular review while medications are being increased (every 2–4 weeks) and assessments for symptom and risk factor control (e.g. blood pressure measurements for hypertension) and side effects.

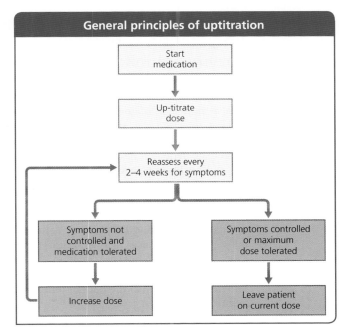

**General principles of uptitration**

**Figure 13.1** General principles of uptitration.

# Management of chronic heart failure

Patients with heart failure fall into two broad categories:

- those presenting with acute cardiac failure (e.g. after a large myocardial infarction)
- those presenting with a more chronic, indolent pattern of disease (e.g. secondary to valvular heart disease)

Patients who develop acute heart failure usually first present to the hospital, where their condition is stabilised. These patients require ongoing follow-up in the community, either with visits to their GP surgeries or during home visits; they are discharged from hospital on standard medications (see page 247) that often need to be up-titrated.

Patients with chronic heart failure usually present to primary care first. They are then referred to hospital to confirm the diagnosis. These patients also require ongoing community care. Heart failure specialist nurses are often available to provide such support, including help with the up-titration of medications.

# Treatment

Brain natriuretic peptide is measured in all patients with clinically suspected heart failure; its concentration increases with disease severity. Patients are also referred to hospital for an echocardiogram and specialist assessment to confirm the diagnosis and establish the cause.

Once the diagnosis and cause have been determined, the cause is treated, often in hospital. Diuretics, angiotensin-converting enzyme (ACE) inhibitors, beta-blockers and spironolactone are also prescribed to help stabilise the patient's condition. These medications are started at low doses and require up-titration in the community by either the GP or the heart failure specialist nurse.

> **Great care should be taken when giving a diagnosis of heart failure to a patient.** Patients somtimes cannot grasp the importance of a diagnosis or, conversely, think that they are going to die very soon. Careful explanation and reassurance should be given in easy-to-understand terms.

# Monitoring response to treatment

The clinical response to medications started in hospital is monitored by their GP after they have been discharged (either at the surgery or in the patient's home). All patients are weighed regularly, because weight gain is one of the first signs of increasing fluid overload. Ideally, the same set of scales is used for accuracy.

Patients with more severe heart failure may need to restrict their intake of fluids; the usual limit is 1.0–1.5 L per 24 h. When possible, and in the early stages, patients are advised to complete an input–output (fluid balance) chart to assess their response to therapies such as diuretics.

## Diuretics

Diuretic therapy is used to control symptoms associated with fluid retention. They are up-titrated if there is clinical evidence of raised jugular venous pressure, peripheral oedema or lung crepitations. Renal function should be closely monitored by measuring urea and electrolytes about 7 days after each dose change (because the drugs used to treat heart failure are all associated with possible adverse effects on renal function, e.g. raised urea, creatinine and/or potassium). In chronic heart failure, diuretic therapy improves symptoms but does not affect long-term prognosis.

# Angiotensin-converting enzyme inhibitors

All patients with heart failure caused by left ventricular systolic dysfunction should receive an ACE inhibitor, or if ACE inhibitors are not tolerated, an angiotensin II receptor blocker. This is because these drugs infer prognostic benefit to patients with heart failure caused by left ventricular systolic dysfunction.

It is important to be cautious when starting ACE inhibitor therapy in a patient with an estimated glomerular filtration rate < 40 mL/min. This is because ACE inhibitors may cause deterioration in renal function. When renal function is already impaired, any additional insult may push the patient into renal failure.

Urea and electrolytes are checked within 7 days of each dose increment. Particular attention is given to creatinine and potassium concentration.

- An increase in creatinine is normal with the addition or up-titration of an ACE inhibitor. However, if creatinine concentration increases to > 26 µmol/L with each dose increment, do not increase the dose further to prevent significant deteriorations in renal function.
- A few patients develop hyponatraemia. In these patients, the dose of ACE inhibitor may need to be reduced if their condition is not improved by other interventions, such as stopping proton pump inhibitor therapy and reducing the use of diuretics (thiazide or loop) and aldosterone antagonists.

Heart failure care should be coordinated by a cardiologist to ensure an appropriate plan is made. However, multiple disciplines are also involved including the family physician, specialist nurses, physiotherapists, dieticians, occupational therapists, palliative care doctors and psychologists. This multi-disciplinary team should communicate effectively to ensure optimal continuity of care.

Based on these principles, the plan for ACE inhibitor therapy in patients with heart failure caused by left ventricular systolic dysfunction is as follows:

1. Prescribe an ACE inhibitor and arrange for a blood test for urea and electrolytes 1 week later
2. In the following week, check the results of the test, review the notes, and call the patient at home to monitor their symptoms and weight and to advise a dose increment, if appropriate
3. After up-titration of the dose, check urea and electrolytes 1 week later
4. Repeat steps 2 and 3 until the maximum tolerated dose is reached and check urea and electrolytes every 3 months.

## Contraindications

Angiotensin-converting enzyme inhibitors and angiotensin II receptor blockers are contraindicated in cases of:

- known angio-oedema
- critical aortic or mitral stenosis
- advanced chronic renal disease in the absence of renal replacement therapy

## Beta-blockers

Low dose beta-blocker therapy has been shown to improve prognosis in chronic heart failure caused by left ventricular systolic dysfunction. A cardioselective beta-blockers such as bisoprolol, metoprolol or carvedilol are used.

Before starting beta-blocker therapy, an electrocardiogram (ECG) is done to ensure that there is no evidence of heart block or bradycardia. The beta-blocker is started at the lowest dose possible. The dose is then slowly increased every 2 weeks to the maximum tolerated.

Heart rate and blood pressure are rechecked before each change in dose. If heart rate is ≤ 55 beats/min and systolic blood pressure is ≤ 100 mmHg, the dose is not increased without specialist advice.

### Contraindications

Beta-blockers are contraindicated in cases of:

- advanced atrioventricular block in the absence of pacing
- asthma or chronic obstructive pulmonary disease with evidence of reversibility to inhaled bronchodilator therapy
- heart rate ≤ 55 beats/min
- systolic blood pressure < 100 mmHg

## Aldosterone antagonists (spironolactone and eplerenone)

In patients with New York Heart Association class 3 or 4 heart failure or post–myocardial infarction heart failure the use of aldosterone antagonists, such as spironolactone or eplerenone, improves prognosis (**Table 13.1**). Renal

| Pharmacological treatment for chronic HFREF | | | | |
|---|---|---|---|---|
| Drug | NYHA I | NYHA II | NYHA III | NYHA IV |
| ACE inhibitor* | ✓ | ✓ | ✓ | ✓ |
| Beta-blocker* | ✓ | ✓ | ✓ | ✓ |
| Diuretic | | ✓ | ✓ | ✓ |
| Aldosterone antagonist* | | | ✓ | ✓ |
| Digoxin | | | | ✓ |

\* These drugs improve prognosis in patients with chronic HFREF. The other medications reduce symptoms but do not effect the prognosis

**Table 13.1** Pharmacological treatment for chronic HFREF. A tick indicates that a particular agent is indicated

function is monitored by measuring urea and electrolytes at 1, 4, 8 and 12 weeks, and every 3 months thereafter to ensure potassium levels remain within the normal range.

## Contraindications

Spironolactone and eplerenone are contraindicated in conditions that predispose to hyperkalaemia:

- pre-existing hyperkalaemia
- Addison's disease
- anuria

## Palliative care

End-stage heart failure is distressing for patients and their relatives. Patients who remain severely symptomatic (NYHA stage 4 or American Hear Association American College of Cardiology stage D) with a poor prognosis are referred to the local palliative care unit for advice and guidance. Palliative care input includes increasing doses of diuretics (even at the expense of renal function) and opioids to help relieve their symptoms. Specialist palliative care teams manage end-stage symptoms and provide psychological and social support.

# Management of stable angina

Angina is the clinical manifestation of stable ischaemic heart disease. Patients usually complain of central chest tightness, with or without associated shortness of breath.

All cases of new-onset chest pain with a possible ischaemic cause are referred for further investigation at their local hospital. In the interim, the GP should start patients on aspirin 75 mg once daily. Patients also require a baseline ECG to look for evidence of ischemia; a fasting lipid profile and to have their haemoglobin A1c checked.

Secondary prevention is started as soon as possible. Many patients require a lipid-lowering agent, preferably a statin (these drugs are thought to have pleiotropic effects). If patients have angina attacks more than twice a week, regular antianginal medication is started and patients are referred to a cardiologist for further assessment.

> Sublingual glyceryl trinitrate can cause hypotension, so advise patients to take this medication when sitting down. Warn patients starting glyceryl trinitrate therapy that severe transient headaches are a common adverse effect.

## Treatment

Many different agents are used to treat angina. First-line therapy is usually with a beta-blocker or calcium channel blocker (**Figure 13.2**). Beta-blockers relieve symptoms of angina by reducing cardiac work load. Calcium channel blockers relax vascular smooth muscle cells to cause vasodilation.

If symptoms continue despite these therapies, another agent is added that has vasodilating effects. There are several to choose from, including:

- long-acting nitrates, such as isosorbide mononitrate and isosorbide dinitrate
- potassium channel activators, such as nicorandil

Acute attacks of angina are treated with sublingual glyceryl trinitrate. This drug is also used as a preventive therapy and can be taken before activities known to trigger an angina attack (e.g. climbing a hill).

## Follow-up

Response to therapy is assessed by their GP every 2–4 weeks. Drug doses are increased to the maximum tolerated or additional agents

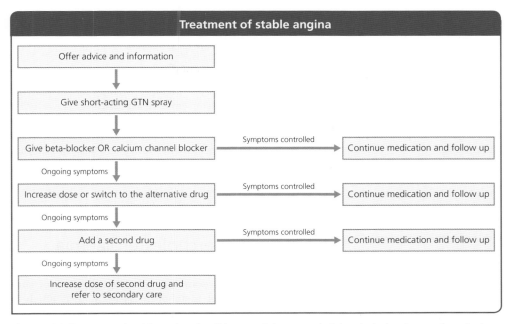

**Figure 13.2** Treatment of stable angina. Possible second drugs to administer include a long-acting nitrate, nicorandil, ivabridine or ranolazine.

are added to the patient's current therapy until symptoms are controlled. If symptoms are uncontrolled despite the use of two or more agents, patients are referred to their local hospital for further investigation.

> **Patients on antiplatelet therapy often experience bruising.** However, aspirin reduces the risk of myocardial infarction by up to 30% in patients with angina, so the benefits usually outweigh this adverse effect. If bruising is excessive, discuss with a cardiologist before stopping treatment, because of the associated risk of potentially fatal acute stent thrombosis in stented patients.

# Other interventions for primary and secondary prevention

Primary and secondary prevention are both important considerations for a GP. When patients visit the surgery it is important to use that opportunity to check blood pressure and ask about smoking habits, to try and prevent heart disease. Once patients are above 40 years old, lipid profiles can be checked with a simple blood test and may help prevent the occurrence of heart disease in the future. Once a patient has had a cardiovascular event then secondary prevention (to stop further events) must be addressed when the patient is reviewed. This will include regular blood pressure checks, monitoring of fasting lipids and continued advice for people who smoke.

## Lipid regulation

Hypercholesterolaemia is a risk factor for the development of atherosclerotic plaques. High levels of low-density lipoprotein (LDL) cholesterol cause atherosclerotic plaques to progress.

The aim of lipid-lowering therapy is to decrease LDL cholesterol (the so-called bad cholesterol) and increase high-density lipoprotein cholesterol (the so-called good cholesterol). Therefore fasting lipid profile is checked for all patients with a diagnosis of ischaemic heart disease. This is vital if the patient has a strong family history of premature coronary artery disease; in such cases, familial hypercholesterolaemia should be excluded (see page 337).

## Statins

Statins are competitive inhibitors of 3-hydroxy-3-methylglutaryl coenzyme A reductase, an enzyme involved in lipid synthesis. These drugs exert their effects in the liver and are very effective at lowering LDL cholesterol.

In some patients statins are associated with muscle pains (myalgia) and myositis. If patients complain of muscle pains, their creatine kinase is measured. If creatine kinase concentration is over twice the upper limit of normal, the dose is reduced or the drug stopped and an alternative drug used instead.

> **Statins are uniformly prescribed to patients with ischaemic heart disease, regardless of starting cholesterol level, because they reduce cardiac events and total mortality.** If lipid levels are not controlled by a single agent, combination therapy is required. In such cases, the risks of adverse effects such as myositis or even rhabdomyolysis are increased, so patients are monitored closely.

Liver function can also be affected. Therefore liver function is monitored either by primary and/or secondary care in patients receiving statin therapy. Statins are unsuitable for patients with pre-existing liver disease; other agents are used instead.

## Other agents

Statins are first-line therapy for all patients with ischaemic heart disease. However, if these drugs are contraindicated or not tolerated, then ezetimibe, a fibrate (e.g. fenofibrate) or a bile acid sequestrant (e.g. colestyramine) are used. Ezetimibe inhibits the intestinal absorption of cholesterol and is often better tolerated than fibrates and bile acid sequestrants.

# Familial hypercholesterolaemia

Familial hypercholesterolaemia is an autosomal dominant inherited disorder of cholesterol metabolism (see Chapter 10). It is under-recognised and may be undiagnosed in as many as 90% of patients. This is because cholesterol is often not checked in people unless they are over 40 years old or complain of chest pain. A family history for high cholesterol is rarely asked for.

Early identification with a simple fasting lipid blood test is important to allow prompt treatment. Treatment improves outcomes. All patients with definite, possible or suspected familial hyperlipidaemia are referred to a specialist centre for diagnosis and management.

# Atrial fibrillation

Patients with atrial fibrillation may be asymptomatic or complain of symptoms such as palpitations, shortness of breath and chest pain. The diagnosis is first made on clinical examination, when patients are found to have an irregular pulse. Atrial fibrillation is then confirmed by an ECG showing an absence of P waves.

Once diagnosed, general management requires two distinct steps (which can be made in primary or secondary care).

- A decision about whether a rate or rhythm control strategy is most appropriate
- A decision about whether anticoagulation is necessary

To determine whether anticoagulation is necessary to reduce vascular risk, predominantly the risk of stroke, the $CHA_2DS_2$-VASc and HASBLED scoring systems are used to assess an individual patient's risk (see page 231). This can be done in either primary or secondary care. The $CHA_2DS_2$-VASc is an assessment of vascular risk and gives an annual estimate of stroke risk without anticoagulation. The HASBLED score gives an annual risk of bleeding while taking anticoagulants such as warfarin. The two scores are combined to determine whether anticoagulation is indicated.

# Driving regulations

Many countries have regulations covering when patients can resume driving after a major cardiac problem, and these should be checked before advising patients. Drivers may have to inform an appropriate authority (in the UK, the Driver and Vehicle Licensing Agency, DVLA) of their condition. Their license may be suspended until they have been judged to have recovered.

Further information from the DVLA is available through the www.gov.uk website. Depending on the condition, it is often a legal requirement to report any new diagnoses (such as myocardial infarction or syncope) to the DVLA. Failure to do so can result in a patient's driving license being suspended. Different conditions require different lengths of abstinence from driving, e.g. in the UK you cannot drive for 4 weeks after a heart attack and for 6 months after insertion of a cardiac defibrillator for ventricular tachycardia. More stringent rules apply to drivers with passenger carrying or large or heavy goods vehicle licenses.

## Answers to starter questions

1. The number of people smoking has dramatically decreased over the last decade. This is partly due to the effects of a worldwide anti-smoking campaign. This had led to the prevention of advertising by tobacco companies, increasing the cost of cigarettes and a mass advertising campaign highlighting the dangers of cigarette smoking.

2. Spironolactone is a potassium-sparing diuretic and consequently hyperkalemia is a possible side-effect. Patients' renal function should be monitored for this as it can cause cardiac arrhythmias.

3. An appropriate shock from an implantable cardiac defibrillator is given for ventricular fibrillation or ventricular tachycardia. Patients with either of these rhythm abnormalities will have impaired consciousness and are not safe to drive. A shock from an ICD often incapacitates the patient for a short period of time as it can be painful and is distressing rendering them unsafe to drive.

4. There are many lifestyle modifications required post-heart attack and so it is important that patients receive the relevant information and continuing support to make these changes and optimise their recovery. Cardiac rehabilitation provides an appropriate forum for this to take place. Patients are able to meet in groups over a period of several weeks and are given a supervised exercise program. This allows them to meet other people who have been through the same experience and to regain confidence in getting back to a full and active lifestyle. There is a also a patient forum where appropriately qualified people are available to offer advice.

5. Familial hypercholesterolaemia is underdiagnosed and undertreated; as many as 90% of sufferers may not have a formal diagnosis. In part, this is because patients who have FH but have not suffered any clinical sequelae from the condition remain well and so are unlikely to present to their GP with symptoms. When patients present with a heart attack they are started on a high dose statin but baseline cholesterols are often not checked or followed up.

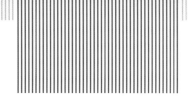

# Chapter 14
# Self-assessment

## SBA Questions

### Ischaemic heart disease

**1.** A 68-year-old woman has a 4-day history of intermittent chest pain. Her worst pain was 2 days ago. Her ECG shows anterior T-wave inversion and her high sensitivity troponin is 465 ng/ml. She is currently pain-free.
What is the single next best step?

   **A** Discharge and refer to outpatient clinic for review
   **B** Immediate coronary angiography
   **C** Immediate echocardiography
   **D** Start secondary prevention and admit to hospital for further assessment
   **E** Start secondary prevention and discharge from hospital for outpatient follow-up.

**2.** A 55-year-old man has had primary percutaneous coronary intervention with insertion of a drug-eluting stent into his proximal left anterior descending.
Which single length of time should he take dual anti-platelet therapy for?

   **A** 1 month
   **B** 3 months
   **C** 6 months
   **D** 8 months
   **E** 12 months.

**3.** A 56-year-old woman has chest pain when she walks her dog in the evenings. The pain is central and radiates to her neck. She has a family history of premature ischemic heart disease, but no other risk factors. She is referred to hospital for further investigations.
What is the single most appropriate set of investigations to perform?

   **A** 24 h blood pressure monitor, cardiac echo and coronary angiogram
   **B** 24 h blood pressure monitor, cardiac echo and myocardial perfusion scan
   **C** 24 h tape, cardiac echo and coronary angiogram

   **D** ECG, CT pulmonary angiogram and a myocardial perfusion scan
   **E** ECG, myocardial perfusion scan and CT coronary angiogram.

**4.** A 60-year-old man works as a heavy goods vehicle lorry driver. Last week he had a myocardial infarction.
According to UK law, what is the single most appropriate advice you should give him regarding his return to work?

   **A** 2 weeks if he completes an exercise tolerance test
   **B** 4 weeks if he completes an exercise tolerance test
   **C** 4 weeks, no additional requirements
   **D** 6 weeks if he completes an exercise tolerance test
   **E** 6 weeks, no additional requirements.

**5.** A 49-year-old man has acute central chest pain, which started 4 hours ago. He has no significant past medical history and takes no regular medications. His ECG shows ST segment elevation in leads V2, V3 and V4. There is ST segment depression in leads II, III and aVF.
What is the single best next management step?

   **A** Admit for troponin measurement
   **B** Admit for dual antiplatelet therapy and start secondary prevention
   **C** Emergency referral and transfer for primary percutaneous coronary intervention
   **D** Investigate for ischaemia once the pain settles
   **E** Thrombolysis.

**6.** A 75-year-old man had an anterior ST elevation myocardial infarction 6 hours ago and underwent primary percutaneous coronary intervention. He has been transferred to the coronary care unit and has experienced a sudden recurrence of chest pain. His blood pressure is 80/60 mmHg and his pulse rate is 110 bpm.

What is the single most appropriate next step in his management?

**A** Resuscitation and intravenous beta-blocker
**B** Resuscitation, ECG and echocardiogram
**C** Urgent ECG and chest X-ray
**D** Urgent referral to cardiothoracic surgery
**E** Urgent transfer to the catheter laboratory for repeat angiography.

**7.** A 60-year-old woman develops central crushing chest pain that radiates to her throat, which is associated with shortness of breath for 1 hour. An ambulance takes her immediately to the emergency department. She has an initially normal ECG, normal chest X-ray and normal troponin concentration.
What is the single most appropriate next step?

**A** Admit to hospital for observation and a repeat troponin concentration
**B** Discharge to the outpatient department for further investigations
**C** Immediate cardiac echocardiogram
**D** Immediate coronary angiogram
**E** Urgent gastroscopy.

**8.** A 66-year-old man has had acute central chest pain for < 3 hours. His ECG has ST segment elevation in leads II, III and aVF. He is urgently transferred to the catheter laboratory for primary percutaneous coronary intervention.
What is the single most likely angiographic finding?

**A** Diffuse disease affecting all three main coronary arteries
**B** Dissection of the circumflex artery
**C** Normal coronary arteries
**D** Occluded left anterior descending artery
**E** Occluded right coronary artery.

**9.** A 22-year-old man has pleuritic chest pain and global concave ST elevation on his ECG. He was previously fit and well with no past medical or family history of ischaemic heart disease.
What is the single most likely diagnosis?

**A** Acute myocardial infarction
**B** Chest infection
**C** Musculoskeletal chest pain
**D** Pericarditis
**E** Pulmonary embolus.

# Hypertension

**1.** A 54-year-old Caucasian man is diagnosed with essential hypertension after a period of home monitoring. He is otherwise fit and well and has no known drug allergies. There is no evidence of any target organ damage.
What single drug should he be treated with as first line therapy?

**A** Amlodipine
**B** Bendroflumethiazide
**C** Bisoprolol
**D** Doxazosin
**E** Ramipril.

**2.** A 78-year-old woman has a resting blood pressure of 183/112 mmHg. She is asymptomatic and has no known drug allergies. She has a family history of premature ischaemic heart disease. A urine dip is negative and fundoscopy reveals grade 2 hypertensive retinopathy. There are no other abnormal features on clinical examination.
What is the single best next step?

**A** Assess her risk of cardiovascular disease
**B** Commence antihypertensive drug therapy
**C** Perform home monitoring with a view to commencing drug therapy very soon
**D** Refer her for urgent secondary care
**E** Request investigations for a secondary cause.

**3.** A 56-year-old man has a blood pressure of 148/98 mmHg during an occupational health check. He is otherwise fit and well and there are no abnormal findings on clinical examination.
What is the single best next step?

**A** Assess his risk of cardiovascular disease
**B** Commence first line drug therapy
**C** Investigate for target organ damage
**D** Perform ambulatory blood pressure monitoring
**E** Re-check the blood pressure in five years or less.

**4.** A 44-year-old woman is admitted to hospital with headaches. Her neurological examination is normal but fundoscopy reveals silver wiring and a-v nipping.
Which single option best describes findings on fundoscopy?

**A** Benign intracranial hypertension
**B** Hypertensive emergency
**C** Stage 2 hypertensive retinopathy
**D** Normal finding
**E** Proliferative diabetic retinopathy.

**5.** A 57-year-old Afro-Caribbean man attends his annual diabetes review. His blood pressure is 155/100 mmHg. He is asymptomatic. Past medical history includes hypertension and gastro-oesophageal reflux disease. Clinical examination is unremarkable. His regular medications include metformin, amlodipine, simvastatin and omeprazole.
What is the single best next course of action?

**A** Add a beta-blocker
**B** Add a diuretic

C   Add an alpha-blocker
D   Add an angiotensin-converting-enzyme inhibitor
E   Stop his amlodipine and start an angiotensin-converting-enzyme inhibitor.

6.  A 72-year-old man has a headache and blurred vision. His blood pressure is checked in primary care and is 210/118 mmHg. He has a past medical history of ischaemic heart disease and hypertension. Fundoscopy reveals swollen optic discs. His regular medications include: ramipril 5 mg od, bisoprolol 5 mg od, aspirin 75 mg od, simvastatin 40 mg od, amlodipine 10 mg od and bendroflumethiazide 2.5 mg od.
    What is the single most appropriate next step?

    A   Emergency referral to secondary care for urgent investigation and controlled blood pressure reduction
    B   Increase antihypertensive medication dose
    C   Routine referral to hypertension specialist
    D   Urgent investigations for a potential secondary cause
    E   Urgent referral to eye clinic to treat the swollen optic discs.

7.  A 28-year-old woman has stage 2 hypertension. Because of her age and high blood pressure, the general practitioner is concerned there may be a secondary cause.
    Which is the single most appropriate combination of conditions that should be excluded?

    A   Acromegaly, Addison's disease, phaeochromocytoma and renal artery stenosis
    B   Acromegaly, Cushing's disease, phaeochromocytoma and pulmonary artery stenosis
    C   Acromegaly, Cushing's disease, phaeochromocytoma and renal artery stenosis
    D   Cardiomegaly, Addison's disease, phaeochromocytoma and renal artery stenosis
    E   Coarctation, Cushing's disease, phaeochromocytoma and pulmonary artery stenosis.

8.  A 56-year-old man is under investigation for elevated blood pressure.
    Which single answer is most consistent with a diagnosis of hypertension?

    A   Blood pressure of 200/110 mmHg during exercise
    B   Persistent blood pressure > 140/90 mmHg
    C   Persistent blood pressure of 135/80 mmHg
    D   Single recording of blood pressure at 140/90 mmHg
    E   Single recording of blood pressure at 150/80 mmHg.

9.  A 61-year-old woman has essential hypertension following a period of monitoring by her GP. Apart from being a smoker, she is fit and

well. She is completely asymptomatic.
Which single set of conditions she should be investigated for?

A   Nephropathy, neuropathy and left ventricular hypertrophy
B   Retinopathy, nephropathy and biventricular hypertrophy
C   Retinopathy, nephropathy and left atrial hypertrophy
D   Retinopathy, nephropathy and left ventricular hypertrophy
E   Retinopathy, neuropathy and left ventricular hypertrophy.

# Arrythmias

1.  A 61-year-old woman is newly diagnosed with asymptomatic atrial fibrillation. She is anticoagulated with warfarin with good international normalised ratio control and takes bisoprolol 2.5 mg od. On the Holter monitor, the daytime rate varies from 56 bpm at rest to 136 bpm during exertion. In the early hours of the morning (during sleep) her rate is 48 bpm and she has occasional pauses of up to 2.5 seconds.
    What is the single best next step?

    A   Check troponin concentration and request an echocardiogram
    B   Do nothing and reassure her
    C   Refer for pacemaker insertion
    D   Start digoxin
    E   Stop the beta-blocker.

2.  A 72-year-old woman has palpitations occasionally accompanied by feeling light-headed. Her blood tests are normal. Her 12-lead ECG shows normal sinus rhythm at a rate of 68 bpm. Her Holter monitor report states: 'eight sinus pauses of up to 3 seconds, occasional runs of atrial tachycardia, sinus bradycardia and 3 episodes of atrial fibrillation during the afternoon'.
    What is the single most likely underlying diagnosis?

    A   Heart block
    B   Normal rhythm
    C   Paroxysmal atrial fibrillation
    D   Paroxysmal atrial flutter
    E   Sinus node disease.

3.  A 24-year-old woman has palpitations at night before she goes to sleep. She is distressed by them but denies any loss of consciousness or light-headedness. She has a past medical history of fibromyalgia. Her Holter monitor report states: 'sinus rhythm throughout with very occasional premature ventricular ectopic beats not corresponding to diary events'.

What is the single most appropriate next step?

A  Prescribe digoxin
B  Reassure her
C  Repeat Holter monitor
D  Request exercise ECG
E  Request troponin concentration.

4.  A 53-year-old woman has occasional episodes of light-headedness. She is admitted to hospital because her 12-lead ECG reveals sinus bradycardia at a rate of 40 bpm. She is transferred to coronary care unit and undergoes continuous cardiac rhythm monitoring. Her blood pressure is 152/86 mmHg.
What is the single best next step?

A  Arrange temporary pacemaker insertion
B  Check thyroid function and electrolytes
C  Prescribe antihistamines
D  Request Holter monitor
E  Urgent referral for permanent pacemaker.

5.  An 87-year-old man has a pacemaker inserted for complete heart block. 90 minutes after the procedure, his condition has deteriorated. He is dyspnoeic, his jugular venous pressure is elevated to 7 cm and his blood pressure is 95/65 mmHg. Auscultation of his chest reveals good bilateral air entry and his oxygen saturation is 97% on room air. His pulse rate is 80 bpm. His wound and dressings are unremarkable.
What is the single most important complication to exclude?

A  Bleeding
B  Cardiac perforation
C  Infection
D  Lead displacement
E  Pneumothorax.

6.  A 76-year-old man presents with breathlessness. He states that he had a 'pacemaker' inserted 2 years ago. At the time his echocardiogram was normal, his QRS duration was <120 ms but his Holter monitor demonstrated atrial fibrillation with significant pauses. On examination, there is a fullness in his left subclavicular region.
What single option best describes his type of device?

A  Cardiac resynchronization therapy device
B  Implantable cardioverter defibrillator
C  Implantable loop recorder
D  Left atrial pressure monitor
E  Rate responsive single chamber pacemaker.

7.  A 68-year-old obese woman has occasional palpitations over 3 weeks. Her ECG demonstrates an absence of P waves and irregularly irregular QRS complexes. She has a past medical history of type 2 diabetes and takes

metformin. There are no bleeding risks.
What is the single most important next step?

A  Arrange direct current (electrical) cardioversion
B  Attempt chemical cardioversion with class IC antiarrhythmic agent
C  Prescribe anticoagulation
D  Prescribe Na$^+$/K$^+$ pump inhibitor
E  Reassure her.

8.  A 76-year-old woman has an 8-year history of atrial fibrillation. Her past medical history includes asthma. Her anticoagulation was recently switched from warfarin to rivaroxaban because of labile international normalised ratio measurements on warfarin. Other medications are inhaled salbutamol (prn) and beclomethasone bd. Her blood pressure is 135/95 mmHg and her pulse rate is 126 bpm.
What is the single best next step?

A  Arrange cardioversion
B  Prescribe atenolol
C  Prescribe digoxin
D  Prescribe phytomenadione
E  Re-start warfarin.

9.  A 26-year-old woman has fast regular palpitations. This is the first incidence and she has no significant past medical or family history. Her pulse is 140 bpm, blood pressure is 115/78 mmHg and oxygen saturation is 98% on room air. Her ECG shows a regular tachycardia with a QRS width of 100 ms with a ventricular rate of 138 bpm.
What is the single best next step?

A  Intravenous adenosine
B  Intravenous amiodarone
C  Intravenous flecainide
D  Urgent direct-current cardioversion
E  Vagal manoeuvers.

10. A 35-year-old male athlete has paroxysmal atrial flutter. He is treated with bisoprolol 5 mg od. He continues to experience symptomatic episodes.
Which single option offers the greatest chance of rhythm control?

A  Catheter ablation
B  Perform direct-current cardioversion next time he presents
C  Switch to pill-in-the-pocket strategy with flecanide
D  Switch to regular verapamil therapy
E  Up-titrate and optimise the beta-blocker dose.

11. An 88-year-old woman is breathless with a 2-year history of heart failure. Her blood pressure is 85/53 mmHg and pulse 128 bpm.

Her oxygen saturation is 93% on 10 L/min of inspired oxygen. Her jugular venous pressure is elevated to 7 cm and she has oedema up to her knees. Her ECG rhythm strip shows regular QRS complexes with a width of 138 ms. She is cardioverted back to sinus rhythm and her blood pressure improves to 122/78 mmHg. What is the single most appropriate management?

A Intravenous beta-blocker
B Intravenous digoxin
C Intravenous flecainide
D Intravenous fluid resuscitation
E Intravenous furosemide.

# Heart failure

1. An 80-year-old man has symptomatic left ventricular systolic dysfunction heart failure, secondary to ischaemic heart disease. He is taking ramipril 10 mg od, bisoprolol 10 mg od and furosemide 80 mg bd. He complains of ankle swelling.
What is the single most appropriate treatment?

A Amlodipine
B Bumetanide
C Metolazone
D Spironolactone
E Valsartan.

2. A 67-year-old man has a cough and breathlessness. He has a family history of diabetes and is an ex-smoker. His lung function tests are normal.
What is the single most important investigation to perform?

A Blood sugar
B Chest X-ray
C Electrocardiogram
D Transoesophageal echocardiography
E Transthoracic echocardiography.

3. A 67-year-old woman with long-standing diabetes has breathlessness walking from the kitchen to the living room next door. Her echocardiogram demonstrates an ejection fraction of 25%. She is diagnosed with left ventricular systolic dysfunction (LVSD) heart failure due to ischaemic heart disease.
What single option best describes her symptoms according to the New York Heart Association (NYHA) classification and the severity of LVSD?

A NYHA class II and moderate LVSD
B NYHA class III and moderate LVSD
C NYHA class III and preserved ejection fraction

D NYHA class III and severe LVSD
E NYHA class IV and moderate LVSD.

4. A 56-year-old man has chronic left ventricular systolic dysfunction and heart failure. He is on maximal medical therapy with New York Heart Association class III symptoms. He is suitable for cardiac resynchronisation therapy.
Which single ECG finding would support the use of this therapy?

A Atrial fibrillation
B Left atrial hypertrophy (P mitrale)
C Left axis deviation
D Left bundle branch block
E Left ventricular hypertrophy.

5. A 45-year-old man has a myocardial infarction. Several days later he becomes breathless, sweaty and hypotensive. An arterial blood gas is normal and a portable chest X-ray is requested. His ECG demonstrates anterior Q waves.
What is the single most likely finding on his chest X-ray?

A Dextrocardia
B Pericardial effusions
C Reduced cardiothoracic ratio
D Upper lobe venous diversion
E Widened mediastinum.

6. A 25-year-old woman has acute dyspnoea. Other than a recent cold, she has no significant past medical, family or drug history. A portable echocardiogram shows severe biventricular dilation and systolic dysfunction. Her coronary angiogram is normal.
Which is the single most likely cause of these symptoms?

A Apical thrombus
B Cardiac syndrome X
C Myocardial infarction
D Viral myocarditis
E Viral pericarditis.

7. A 56-year-old woman with dyspnoea has type 2 diabetes and hypertension. There is no access to an echocardiogram or chest X-ray until the following week and she refuses to be admitted to hospital.
What is the single best blood test to perform to aid diagnosis of her dyspnoea?

A Brain natriuretic peptide
B C-peptide
C C-reactive protein
D Thyroid stimulating hormone
E Troponin I.

8. A 45-year-old man with alcohol dependency has bilateral leg swelling. His GP is concerned he may have heart failure. An urgent echocardiogram demonstrates normal cardiac function.

The oedema is pitting, symmetrical and up to his knees.
What is the single best blood test to perform to aid diagnosis?

A  Clotting studies
B  Liver function
C  Protein electrophoresis
D  Renal function
E  Thyroid function.

9.  A 65-year-old man has breathlessness. He suffers from diabetes and had coronary artery bypass grafting following a myocardial infarction. He worked as an accountant and has never smoked. An echocardiogram report shows his ejection fraction is 15%.
Which single statement best describes the aetiology of these symptoms?

A  Ischaemic cardiomyopathy
B  Left ventricular non-compaction
C  Nonischaemic cardiomyopathy
D  Restrictive cardiomyopathy
E  Takotsubo cardiomyopathy.

10. A 23-year-old woman has breathlessness. On examination she has a tremor, a swollen neck and exophthalmos. An ECG demonstrates atrial fibrillation and a chest X-ray shows pulmonary oedema. She is admitted for further assessment and treatment.
Which single answer best describes the pathophysiology of her breathlessness?

A  High output heart failure due to hyperthyroidism
B  High output heart failure due to hypothyroidism
C  Low output heart failure due to hyperthyroidism
D  Low output heart failure due to hypothyroidism
E  Normal output heart failure due to euthyroidism.

11. A 49-year-old woman has breast cancer and is receiving cardiotoxic chemotherapy. A recent echocardiogram was normal. She has a sudden onset of breathlessness. She is morbidly obese, making her difficult to examine, but clinically she is unremarkable. Her ECG shows a sinus tachycardia.
What single investigation is most likely to reveal the diagnosis?

A  Chest X-ray
B  CT pulmonary angiogram
C  Serial ECGs
D  Transthoracic echocardiogram
E  Troponin I.

12. A 45-year-old man has acute chest pain and breathlessness. He is an ex-smoker. On examination he is hypotensive, has a raised jugular venous pressure but a clear chest on auscultation. His chest X-ray is clear but his ECG demonstrates inferior ST elevation myocardial infarction.
Which single answer explains why this patient is breathless?

A  Aortic root dissection
B  Left ventricular ST segment elevation myocardial infarction
C  Pericarditis
D  Pulmonary embolus
E  Right ventricular ST segment elevation myocardial infarction.

# Valvular heart disease

1.  A 70-year-old woman has exertional chest pain. She has a past medical history of hypertension and psoriasis. Her blood pressure is 115/95 mmHg and she has a slow rising pulse, a quiet second heart sound and an ejection systolic murmur.
What is the single best investigation to perform?

A  Cardiac MRI
B  Coronary angiogram
C  Exercise ECG
D  Serum troponin assay
E  Transthoracic echocardiogram.

2.  A 29-year-old man has mitral regurgitation secondary to mitral valve prolapse.
What is the single most likely finding at auscultation?

A  Loud first heart sound with low-pitched diastolic murmur
B  Mid systolic click with late systolic murmur
C  Quiet first heart sound with pansystolic murmur
D  Quiet second heart sound with an early, decrescendo, diastolic murmur
E  Quiet second heart sound with ejection systolic murmur.

3.  A 65-year-old man with mitral regurgitation is seen in the cardiology clinic for follow up. He has no other medical problems.
Which single option would most indicate that mitral valve surgery is indicated?

A  Left atrium severely dilated, mitral regurgitation moderate-severe and patient is asymptomatic
B  Left ventricle hypertrophied, mitral regurgitation moderate and patient is asymptomatic

C Left ventricle moderately dilated, mitral regurgitation moderate-severe and patient is breathless
D Left ventricle normal in dimensions, mitral regurgitation moderate-severe and patient is asymptomatic
E Left ventricle normal in dimensions, mitral regurgitation severe and patient is asymptomatic.

4. A 24-year-old man is an intravenous drug user. He has weight loss, night sweats and what sound like rigors. His temperature is 38.5°C and his pulse rate is 118 bpm. He has a rash on his legs and has a cardiac murmur.
What is the single most appropriate set of investigations to request?

A Three blood cultures, immunological screen and cardiac MRI
B Three blood cultures, troponin assay and CT head scan
C Three blood cultures, white cell count, inflammatory markers (erythrocyte sedimentation rate and C-reactive protein) and transthoracic echocardiogram
D Two blood cultures, white cell count, inflammatory markers (erythrocyte sedimentation rate and C-reactive protein) and chest X-ray and CT head scan
E Two blood cultures, white cell count, inflammatory markers (erythrocyte sedimentation rate and C-reactive protein) and transthoracic echocardiogram.

5. A 48-year-old woman with a past medical history of menorrhagia and hypertension has a cardiac murmur. She is tired and dyspnoeic on exertion. Her blood pressure is 125/84 mmHg and pulse rate is 88 bpm. She is pale. There is a mild ejection systolic murmur heard best over the right second intercostal space. The murmur does not radiate. Blood results are as follows: Hb, 8.1; WCC, 5; platelets, 128; sodium, 137; potassium, 5.2; urea, 5.2; creatinine, 82.
What is the single most likely cause of her murmur?

A Anaemia
B Aortic sclerosis
C Aortic stenosis
D Mitral regurgitation
E Thyrotoxicosis.

6. A 48-year-old man with a mechanical prosthetic heart valve feels lethargic and has lost weight. He is referred to cardiology outpatients for further investigation.
Which single option is most consistent with a diagnosis of infective endocarditis?

A Negative blood cultures, but raised inflammatory markers and signs of infection on chest X-ray
B One positive blood culture and a cardiac murmur
C One positive blood culture and evidence of prosthetic valve regurgitation on transoesophageal echocardiography
D Three negative blood cultures and a vegetation on transoesophageal echocardiography
E Three positive blood cultures and vegetation on transthoracic echocardiography.

# Congenital heart disease

1. A newborn baby initially seems well but within a few hours his lips are blue. A harsh murmur is heard.
What is the single most likely cause of his cyanosis?

A Atrial septal defect
B Coarctation of the aorta
C Ebstein's anomaly
D Fallot's tetralogy
E Ventricular septal defect.

2. A 6-year-old boy has increased breathlessness. He previously had an operation to repair a hole in his heart. He has been well until 6 weeks ago when he became short of breath and had a productive cough. A murmur can be heard.
What is the single most appropriate next step?

A CT thorax
B Chest X-ray
C Urgent cardiac echo
D Send a sputum sample to the laboratory
E Take blood to assess for anaemia.

3. A 25-year-old woman is 6 weeks pregnant. She is on warfarin for a mechanical mitral valve replacement.
What is the single most appropriate next step?

A Continue warfarin and refer routinely to the obstetric clinic
B Continue warfarin and refer urgently to the obstetric clinic
C Stop warfarin and refer urgently to the obstetric clinic
D Stop warfarin and refer routinely to the obstetric clinic
E Stop warfarin and request immediate review with the anticoagulation clinic.

4. A 47-year-old man has palpitations and an atrial arrhythmia. An echocardiogram suggests a congenital heart defect.

What is the single most likely defect?

**A** Atrial septal defect
**B** Fallot's tetralogy
**C** Pulmonary stenosis
**D** Transposition of the great vessels
**E** Ventricular septal defect.

**5.** An 8-year-old girl has undergone surgical correction of an aortic coarctation. She has been well ever since and is seen annually in clinic. When assessing her in clinic, what is the single most important investigation to perform?

**A** Blood pressure in both arms
**B** Blood pressure in her left arm
**C** Blood pressure in her right arm
**D** Chest X-ray to assess aortic size
**E** ECG to look for signs of heart block.

**6.** A 34-year-old man has a ventricular septal defect. It has been present from birth but is small. He has not had any corrective surgery and is under regular follow-up. He and his wife want to start a family.
Regarding the risk of his children having a congenital heart defect, what is the single most appropriate piece of advice to give him?

**A** The risk is 1%
**B** The risk is 3%
**C** The risk is 10%
**D** The risk is 15%
**E** There is no risk.

# Peripheral vascular disease

**1.** A 68-year-old man has been complaining of abdominal pain for several days. After his dinner, he clutched his stomach and collapsed. His blood pressure is 90/60 mmHg and his pulse rate is 90 bpm.
Which single finding best supports a diagnosis of a ruptured abdominal aortic aneurysm?

**A** Abdominal guarding
**B** Abdominal pain
**C** Pulsatile abdominal mass
**D** Shock
**E** Tachycardia.

**2.** A tall 15-year-old girl with learning difficulties has a family history of aortic dissection and the family would like her to be screened.
Which single condition puts her at the highest risk of aortic dissection?

**A** Aortic unfolding
**B** Down's syndrome
**C** Marfan's syndrome
**D** Noonan's syndrome
**E** William's syndrome.

**3.** A 77-year-old man has chest pain that radiates to his back. He has a 60-pack year history of smoking. On examination, an early diastolic murmur is heard. An aortic dissection is suspected.
What is the single best investigation to confirm this diagnosis?

**A** Chest-X ray
**B** CT chest
**C** ECG
**D** Transthoracic echocardiogram
**E** Troponin I.

**4.** A 67-year-old woman has had intermittent claudication for many years and had a previous angioplasty to her iliac artery. She is a lifelong smoker. She says her leg 'feels funny' and she is having difficulty walking.
Which single sign suggests an acutely ischaemic lower limb?

**A** Absent pulse
**B** Bounding pulse
**C** Collapsing pulse
**D** Peripheral cyanosis
**E** Pitting oedema.

**5.** A 52-year-old woman has a swollen right leg. She has recently returned from Australia. Other than a basal cell carcinoma aged 45, she has no past history. On examination there is unilateral calf swelling, 4 cm more than the left, and tenderness along the deep venous system, but no oedema, erythema or pyrexia.
What is her single score using the Well's criteria?

**A** 0
**B** 1
**C** 2
**D** 3
**E** 4

**6.** A 55-year-old diabetic man has persistent 9/10 pain in his left leg at rest. His capillary refill is 5 seconds, pulses are impalpable and he has difficulty moving his ankle with a stocking shaped sensory loss over his lower limb.
What is the single most likely diagnosis?

**A** Critical lower limb ischaemia
**B** Deep venous thrombosis
**C** Intermittent claudication
**D** Nonviable lower limb ischaemia
**E** Viable lower limb ischaemia.

**7.** A 78-year-old woman has atrial fibrillation and is prescribed warfarin. She is concerned because she already takes a lot of other medications for blood pressure, diabetes, cholesterol and angina. While on warfarin, she develops a chest infection.

Which single antibiotic is most likely to interact with warfarin?

**A** Amoxicillin
**B** Augmentin
**C** Ciprofloxacin
**D** Doxycycline
**E** Tazocin.

8. A 65-year-old man has an incidental abdominal aortic aneurysm found on ultrasound following cholecystitis. The diameter is 4.5 cm. The following year it is 4.7 cm. The patient is now anxious that it may burst.
What is the single most likely risk of this rupturing within a year?

**A** 1 %
**B** 2 %
**C** 3 %
**D** 4 %
**E** 5 %.

9. A 64-year-old man has a fractured femur which was caused by a lytic lesion from prostate cancer. He has liver metastases and stage 5 chronic renal impairment with an estimated glomerular filtration rate of 10 mL/min/m². 
What is the single most appropriate medication to reduce his risk of thromboembolism?

**A** Aspirin
**B** Graduate compression stockings
**C** Low molecular weight heparin
**D** Unfractionated heparin
**E** Warfarin.

10. A 90-year-old woman has dizziness for several months, but no loss of consciousness. A 12-lead ECG demonstrates complete heart block and she is referred for a permanent pacemaker. The procedure is successful, but the following day she has a heavy and painful left arm. Examination and blood tests are unremarkable.
What is the single most likely diagnosis?

**A** Axillary vein thrombosis
**B** Brachial artery stenosis
**C** Compartment syndrome
**D** Pacemaker syndrome
**E** Thoracic outlet syndrome.

11. A 35-year-old woman has unsightly varicose veins. They are painful and cause her legs to swell during the day. She has no family history of varicose veins. Her BMI is 23 and she is a competitive swimmer.
Which single treatment will provide the best long-term outcome?

**A** Compression stockings
**B** Exercise program

**C** Laser therapy
**D** Sclerotherapy
**E** Surgery.

12. A 60-year-old man has a swollen left leg following a total knee replacement 4 weeks ago. He is breathless and is known to have chronic obstructive pulmonary disorder. His clinical examination is unremarkable. His Well's score is 4. His ECG is unremarkable and a chest X-ray shows chronic changes only.
What is the single most appropriate investigation to perform?

**A** CT pulmonary angiogram
**B** D-dimer
**C** Leg Doppler
**D** Troponin I
**E** Ventilation/perfusion scan.

13. A 78-year-old woman with dementia has an acutely ischaemic right lower limb. She was discharged 1 week ago following an anterior ST elevation myocardial infarction which was managed conservatively. Her ECG demonstrates sinus rhythm with anterior Q waves and persisting ST elevation.
Which single location is the most likely source of the thromboembolism?

**A** Left atrial appendage
**B** Left ventricle
**C** Right atrium
**D** Right long saphenous vein
**E** Right ventricle.

14. A 36-year-old woman has intermittent left hand pain, swelling and numbness. She has no past history and is a non-smoker. Blood tests and an ultrasound are normal. She recently underwent surgery for an elbow fracture/dislocation following a horse-riding accident. On examination her hand is swollen, red and tender.
What is the single most likely diagnosis?

**A** Buerger's disease
**B** Complex regional pain syndrome
**C** Raynaud's disease
**D** Raynaud's syndrome
**E** Thoracic outlet syndrome.

15. A 56-year-old man has an upper gastrointestinal bleed. He takes warfarin for previous deep vein thrombosis. 2 weeks ago, he had gastric bypass surgery for obesity. His international normalised ratio was stable for many years (2–3), but is currently not recordable. Endoscopy is unremarkable, his international normalised ratio responds to 10 mg of vitamin K intravenously, but not orally.
What is the single most likely cause of his upper gastrointestinal bleed?

**A** Complications from gastric bypass
**B** Impaired vitamin K absorption
**C** Peptic ulcer disease
**D** Oesophageal varices
**E** Unintentional warfarin overdose.

# Inherited cardiac conditions

1.  A 37-year-old woman's identical twin sister dies suddenly in her sleep. She is referred for an assessment of her cardiac risk.
    What is the single best set of investigations to perform?

    **A** 24 h tape, echocardiogram and 24 h blood pressure monitor
    **B** ECG, 24 h blood pressure recording and echocardiogram
    **C** ECG, 24 h tape and 24 h blood pressure recording
    **D** ECG, 24 h tape and echocardiogram
    **E** ECG, echocardiogram and abdominal ultrasound.

2.  A tall, thin, 35-year-old man is breathless on exertion and has developed chest pain. His paternal uncle and grandfather both had heart conditions diagnosed when they were young. What is the single most likely cause of his chest pain?

    **A** Brugada syndrome
    **B** Down's syndrome
    **C** Hypertrophic cardiomyopathy
    **D** Long QT syndrome
    **E** William's syndrome.

3.  The parents of an 8-year-old boy are concerned because they have read about a local boy who has Marfan's syndrome and, based on his description, feel that their son may also have the condition.
    What is the single most appropriate next step?

    **A** Assessment of Beighton score
    **B** Assessment of Ghent criteria
    **C** Assessment of symptoms
    **D** Genetic testing of him and his parents for the Fibrillin-1 gene
    **E** Measurement of height relative to peers.

4.  A 35-year-old man has hypertrophic cardiomyopathy, diagnosed because his father's aunt had an out-of-hospital cardiac arrest and died. He has had chest pain and 4 unexplained episodes of syncope over the last 5 years. A 24 h tape shows several runs of non-sustained ventricular tachycardia.

    What is the single most important factor when assessing his risk?

    **A** 24 h tape showing several runs of non-sustained ventricular tachycardia
    **B** Age
    **C** Episodes of syncope
    **D** Family history of sudden cardiac death
    **E** Recurrent episodes of chest pain.

5.  A 44-year-old man has a dilated cardiomyopathy. He drinks no alcohol and has never taken drugs. His creatine kinase, thyroid function tests and ferritin concentration are normal. An echocardiogram shows a normal right heart and his angiogram is normal. There is no family history of this condition.
    What is the single most likely cause?

    **A** Cardiac amyloidosis
    **B** Haemochromatosis
    **C** Inherited cardiomyopathy
    **D** Ischaemic heart disease
    **E** Myotonic dystrophy

6.  A 24-year-old man has palpitations while cycling. A 24 h tape shows ventricular ectopics at the time of his symptoms. His ectopic burden is 25%. An echocardiogram shows a dilated right heart but normal left ventricle. What is the single next best investigation to perform?

    **A** Cardiac CT scan
    **B** Cardiac memo for 7 days
    **C** Cardiac MRI scan
    **D** Exercise tolerance test
    **E** Myocardial perfusion scan.

# Cardiac emergencies

1.  A 76-year-old man has recently had a myocardial infarction and is undergoing rehabilitation. During his exercises he develops a tachycardia with a rate of 160 bpm, and a cardiac monitor shows a QRS duration of 130 ms.
    Which single finding would indicate that immediate direct-current cardioversion is required?

    **A** Critical leg ischaemia
    **B** Digital ischaemia
    **C** Mesenteric ischaemia
    **D** Myocardial ischaemia
    **E** Transient ischaemic attack.

2.  A 46-year-old man has an ST elevation myocardial infarction. He is awaiting transfer to the cardiac catheter laboratory for primary percutaneous coronary intervention. He has

been loaded with dual antiplatelet agents and low molecular weight heparin. While waiting he develops further pain.
Which single drug is the analgesia of choice?

**A** Aspirin
**B** Codeine
**C** Morphine
**D** Paracetamol
**E** Tramadol.

**3.** A 78-year-old woman is undergoing chemotherapy for breast cancer. She complains of gradually increasing dyspnoea. A pericardial effusion is suspected because on examination she has a raised jugular venous pulse and a displaced apex beat.
Which single ECG finding would best support this diagnosis?

**A** Absent QRS complexes
**B** Broad QRS complexes
**C** High voltage QRS complexes
**D** Low voltage QRS complexes
**E** Narrow QRS complexes.

**4.** A 29-year-old man has palpitations. His examination is unremarkable other than a regular pulse of 180 bpm. His ECG shows a tachycardia with a QRS duration of 100 ms and his blood pressure is 120/60 mmHg. He is otherwise asymptomatic.
What is the single most appropriate next step?

**A** Adenosine 6 mg intravenously
**B** Amiodarone 300 mg intravenously
**C** Atropine 400 µg intravenously
**D** Synchronised direct-current cardioversion
**E** Vagal manoeuvres.

**5.** An 80-year-old woman is found on the floor by a neighbour. It is unclear how long she was there. She has no past medical history of note. She is found to be bradycardic, drowsy and confused.
What single test will reveal the cause of the bradycardia?

**A** Blood sugar
**B** Chest X-ray
**C** Echocardiogram
**D** Electrocardiogram
**E** Thermometer reading.

# Integrated care

**1.** An 88-year-old man has a past medical history of myocardial infarction 20 years ago and hypercholesterolemia. His is currently taking aspirin, ramipril, bisoprolol and simvastatin. His blood pressure is 150/80 mmHg and pulse rate 56 bpm. Examination is otherwise normal. He has muscle pains in his legs at night and these aches are preventing him from going on his usual walks.
What is the single most appropriate next step?

**A** Increase angiotensin-converting-enzyme inhibitor
**B** Increase bisoprolol
**C** Increase simvastatin
**D** Stop bisoprolol
**E** Stop simvastatin.

**2.** A 66-year-old woman has heart failure. She is intolerant of angiotensin-converting-enzyme inhibitors because of renal dysfunction. She is currently taking bisoprolol 10 mg od, spironolactone 50 mg od, hydralazine 50 mg bd and isosorbide mononitrate 60 mg od. At the last renal function check her potassium concentration is 6.4 mmol/L.
What is the single most appropriate next step?

**A** Recheck potassium concentration in 1 week
**B** Reduce hydralazine and recheck potassium concentration in 1 week
**C** Reduce spironolactone and recheck potassium concentration in 1 week
**D** Stop hydralazine and recheck potassium concentration in 1 week
**E** Stop spironolactone and recheck potassium concentration in 1 week.

**3.** A 54-year-old woman has stable angina. She has been taking aspirin and simvastatin for many years and was started on isosorbide mononitrate 1 week ago. She has used her glyceryl trinitrate spray daily for the past 4 days and is concerned. The spray takes the pain off very quickly.
What is the single most appropriate next step?

**A** Add a further antianginal medication
**B** Admit to hospital immediately
**C** Increase isosorbide mononitrate
**D** Perform an ECG
**E** Reassure and do nothing.

# SBA Answers

## Ischaemic heart disease

**1. D**

This patient's diagnosis is non-ST elevation myocardial infarction. This puts her at high risk; she should therefore be admitted to hospital. Secondary prevention should be commenced and a coronary angiogram should be performed, but this is not needed immediately. An echocardiogram should be performed during her hospital stay to assess cardiac function post infarct but again, this doesn't have to be done immediately. The last pain is over 12 hours ago and the troponin level is high and so there is no need to wait for 12 hours.

**2. E**

Dual anti-platelet therapy should be continued for 12 months following the insertion of a drug-eluting stent to reduce the risk of stent thrombosis. Dual anti-platelet therapy is required for 4–6 weeks in bare metal stent cases because the risk of stent thrombosis is present in the first few weeks only.

**3. E**

The patient has angina. There is no evidence of arrhythmia in this case, and no other risk factors; 24 h tape and 24 h blood pressure monitor are therefore not first line test. A CT pulmonary angiogram is used to assess for pulmonary embolus and does not assess the coronary arteries. An ECG is an important diagnostic tool for anyone with chest pain and both CT coronary angiography and myocardial perfusion scans are appropriate non-invasive tests of coronary artery disease and cardiac ischemia.

**4. D**

Any group 2 driver (e.g. heavy goods vehicle drivers) who has a myocardial infarction in the UK must inform the DVLA (the UK regulatory body for driving), undergo a satisfactory non-invasive test for ischemia and receive permission prior to driving again; the standard DVLA advice is that patients must not drive for at least 6 weeks. Standard car and motorcycle licence holders do not need to routinely inform the DVLA of a myocardial infarction but must refrain from driving for at least one month and only start driving again after being informed by their doctor that it is safe to do so.

**5. C**

He is having an anterior ST segment elevation myocardial infarction. He needs emergency primary percutaneous coronary intervention (PCI) to identify the occluded artery (likely left anterior descending) and to stent it open to restore blood flow, i.e. revascularisation. Thrombolysis is only appropriate if primary PCI is not possible due to logistic or geographical problems. Waiting for a troponin will only delay life-saving treatment. Dual antiplatelet therapy and secondary prevention will be appropriate after primary PCI. Investigation for ischaemia is not needed: he is ischaemic.

**6. B**

This patient is displaying signs of cardiogenic shock. Resuscitation should be the first step followed by diagnosis of the cause. The major concerns are the development of cardiac tamponade, arrhythmia or recurrent ischaemia. Therefore, an ECG and an emergency echocardiogram are essential. He may well need urgent transfer back to the catheter laboratory for repeat angiography but the cause of his deterioration must be elucidated first. A chest X-ray will not accurately exclude any of the major concerns. He is tachycardiac because he is in cardiogenic shock and given his hypotension, a beta-blocker is contraindicated.

**7. A**

This patient is describing cardiac chest pain and an acute coronary syndrome should be excluded as a matter of priority. A troponin concentration needs be taken at least 6 hours, but ideally 12 hours, post maximal chest pain before it can truly be regarded as 'negative'. No further decision on management can be made until a 12-hour troponin concentration indicates myocardial infarction or not. Neither an echo nor an angiogram is urgently indicated as her ECG is normal. If the suspicion of acute coronary syndrome is high, and there are no contraindications, it is usually safest to treat as if there is an acute coronary syndrome until the troponin result is known.

**8. E**

In the context of acute chest pain and typical, territory specific ECG changes, the diagnosis here is an inferior territory ST segment elevation myocardial infarction. ECG leads II, III and aVF correspond to the inferior myocardial territory. The inferior myocardium is usually supplied by the right coronary artery (see pages 19 and 178). In the context of acute chest pain, ST segment elevation is usually caused by acute, complete occlusion of a coronary artery.

**9. D**

Pericarditis presents with pleuritic chest pain (see page 343) and global (i.e. not territory specific) concave ST changes on the ECG. The other diagnoses may all cause chest pain but are not associated with these ECG changes. The ST elevation of an acute myocardial infarction is usually convex.

# Hypertension

**1. E**

In this case essential hypertension should be treated with an angiotensin-converting-enzyme inhibitor as first line therapy. Angiotensin-converting-enzyme inhibitors are appropriate in those who are 55 years of age or under and Caucasian. If the patient was Afro-Caribbean and/or over 55 years of age, first-line treatment would be a calcium channel blocker (see page 205).

**2. B**

This woman has stage 3 hypertension. Drug therapy should be commenced straight away. Home or ambulatory monitoring may be useful in the future to assess her response to treatment. She does not require urgent referral to secondary care because there are no features of accelerated hypertension. A secondary cause would be unlikely in a woman of this age unless her hypertension is resistant to drug therapy. She will benefit from an assessment of cardiovascular risk but commencing drug therapy is the most important in terms of her prognosis.

**3. D**

In this case it is important to establish whether he has hypertension or not. Only then can drug therapy be commenced. The best way to do this is with ambulatory monitoring. If this is not available, a period of home monitoring should be performed. An assessment of cardiovascular risk is useful but the next step should be to establish whether he has hypertension or not.

**4. C**

Silver wiring and a-v nipping are features of stage 2 hypertensive retinopathy (see pages 196–197). The absence of papilloedema rules out any cause of intracranial hypertension, such as benign intracranial hypertension or hypertensive emergency. This is not a normal finding and is not proliferative diabetic retinopathy as there are no new blood vessels on the retina.

**5. D**

This man is not optimally controlled on appropriate fist line therapy. He therefore needs to be escalated to second line therapy. This means adding in a second drug as opposed to converting therapies. The best choice is an angiotensin-converting-enzyme inhibitor (see page 205). If this does not control his blood pressure, he may require a diuretic as well but this would be third line treatment. There is no evidence supporting the commencement of insulin.

**6. A**

A blood pressure of 210/118 mmHg is severely high. The combination of this severely high blood pressure, his headache and the blurred vision (secondary to optic disc oedema) indicate that the diagnosis is accelerated hypertension. This is a hypertensive emergency and requires urgent referral to secondary care for assessment and controlled blood pressure reduction. In the long term he may require an increase in his antihypertensive drug doses. However, the next step is urgent referral (page 202).

**7. C**

Acromegaly, Cushing's disease, phaeochromocytoma and renal artery stenosis are all secondary causes of hypertension. Addison's, pulmonary artery stenosis and cardiomegaly are not.

**8. B**

To diagnose hypertension the blood pressure must be persistently > 140/90 mmHg, e.g. 3 or more recordings, or persistently elevated measurements on home monitoring or on a 24 h blood pressure monitor. Measurements of blood pressure should be taken at rest. It is normal for blood pressure to rise with exercise.

**9. D**

Signs of hypertensive end organ damage include retinopathy, nephropathy and left ventricular hypertrophy. Neuropathy and right/biventricular hypertrophy are complications of many conditions but not hypertension per se.

# Arrythmias

**1. B**

This woman has asymptomatic atrial fibrillation and is appropriately anticoagulated. The key fact in this question is that she is asymptomatic. The daytime range is normal and occasional nocturnal pauses are a normal phenomenon in atrial fibrillation. Therefore, there is no reason to change any of her medications and there is no indication for pacemaker insertion (see page 220), a troponin concentration, or an echocardiogram in this situation.

**2. E**

The combination of bradycardia with atrial tachycardias in the same patient, on different occasions, is known as tachy-brady syndrome and is suggestive of sinus node disease, also known as sinus node dysfunction and sick sinus syndrome. Sinus node disease character-istically causes a mixture of atrial arrhythmias, as in this case. Sinus pauses are not a feature of heart block and the rhythm is certainly not normal. Although she does have paroxysms of atrial fibrillation, the question asks for the most likely underlying diagnosis.

3. **B**
Premature ventricular ectopics are a nor-mal phenomenon. They do not require any intervention unless they are very frequent. This woman has normal sinus rhythm, i.e. she is normal. Reassurance is vital here; it is not unusual for patients to become distressed and anxious when they think they might have 'heart disease'. Patients are asked to complete a symptom diary during the recording period. The fact that her symptoms do not match the premature ventricular ectopics indicates that her palpitations are occurring during times of normal sinus rhythm. This should be explained to her.

4. **B**
All patients with arrhythmia should have their electrolytes and thyroid function checked. Profound hypothyroidism is a cause of sinus bradycardia and, with replacement therapy, is a reversible cause. There is no need for a Holter when she is undergoing constant rhythm monitoring already. A permanent pacemaker may be indicated, but only if reversible causes are excluded. A temporary pacemaker is reserved for unstable and/or high risk patients until they are stable or a permanent system can be implanted. There is no indication for antihistamines as this is not Ménière's disease (vestibular neuronitis).

5. **B**
All of these options are complications of pace-maker insertion. Cardiac perforation resulting in tamponade (see page 358) is consistent with all of these clinical findings and the timing of his deterioration. Lead dislodgement is unlikely given he has a pulse rate of 80 bpm. Pneumo-thorax is also a major concern and should be excluded. However, this is less likely given that he has good bilateral air entry with normal oxy-gen saturation on room air. His deterioration is too early for infection. Bleeding is possible but is unlikely to account for such a profound decline, especially since his wound is okay.

6. **E**
The patient has a rate responsive single cham-ber pacemaker in situ for sick-sinus syndrome.

He has atrial fibrillation and so there is no point pacing the atria. He was diagnosed 2 years ago, so there is no indication for a loop recorder as the pacemaker already records the activity of the heart. Left atrial pressure moni-tors are used for patients with heart failure, but are not yet in routine use. His QRS duration and left ventricular function were normal 2 years ago, so there is no indication for a resyn-chronisation or defibrillator device.

7. **C**
The description of this patient's ECG indicates she has atrial fibrillation. The primary concern with atrial fibrillation is thromboembolic com-plications such as stroke. The question gives enough information to indicate an elevated stroke risk (age, female, diabetes) without any additional bleeding risks beyond her age (see page 231). Anticoagulation is therefore the first priority. Rate control is not appropri-ate because we do not know her pulse rate. In those with symptoms over longer than 48 hours, cardioversion should only be performed after a 6-week period of anticoagulation. Flei-cainide is a class IC agent and digoxin is a Na+/K+ pump inhibitor.

8. **C**
This woman has a problem with elevated heart rate secondary to atrial fibrillation. She is already appropriately anticoagulated. She needs rate control. Two options would help reduce her rate (B and C). Digoxin would be preferable to atenolol because of her asthma. Cardioversion is highly unlikely to be success-ful after an 8-year history of atrial fibrillation. Phytomenadione is vitamin K, but there is no indication to reverse warfarin in this case.

9. **E**
This patient has a narrow complex tachycardia, i.e. a supraventricular tachycardia. Based on the information provided in the question, it is impossible to know the precise underlying diagnosis (see page 223). However, the first line treatment for any undifferentiated regular and narrow complex tachycardia is vagal manouvres to see if the arrhythmia can be terminated. If this fails, then adenosine is considered.

10. **A**
The best course of action should be discussed between him and his cardiologist. However, the best chance of rhythm control for any patient is offered by catheter ablation (see page 226). Options B and C, aim to cardio-vert the flutter back to sinus rhythm once it has begun. Options D and E, may reduce the frequency of flutter but not nearly as much as catheter ablation.

**11. E**

The description of the ECG is consistent with ventricular tachycardia and this is likely to have been caused by her decompensated heart failure. After successful cardioversion, treatment should be aimed at reducing the risk of recurrence and in this case, that means controlling her heart failure. It is dangerous to treat patients who are acutely unwell and unstable with heart failure with beta-blockers or intravenous fluids. Digoxin may improve her symptoms but will not affect her prognosis or the chance of ventricular tachycardia recurrence. Flecanide is contraindicated in heart failure.

# Heart failure

**1. C**

The management of refractory oedema in heart failure involves the use of thiazide diuretics such as metolazone which works synergistically with loop diuretics such as furosemide. Bumetanide is another loop diuretic; amlodipine is contraindicated in heart failure. Mineralocorticoid antagonists such as spironolactone augment cardiac function but do little in the way of diuresis and finally angiotensin receptor blockers are only indicated if patients are intolerant of angiotensin-converting-enzyme inhibitors, but are not diuretics.

**2. E**

All cases of suspected heart failure need blood tests to rule out other causes, an electrocardiogram for myocardial ischaemia and a chest X-ray for pulmonary oedema. The most sensitive and specific test for heart failure, however, is an echocardiogram, which assesses ventricular function and possible causes. A trans-oesophageal echocardiogram is performed if standard trans-thoracic images are poor. This patient has not complained of any pain, making myocardial ischaemia unlikely and a family history of diabetes is not relevant at this stage.

**3. D**

Breathlessness on minimal exertion, e.g. walking a short distance on the flat equates to New York Heart Association class III and an ejection fraction of 25% represents severe left ventricular systolic dysfunction. A preserved ejection fraction is normal, e.g. > 50%.

**4. D**

Cardiac resynchronisation therapy is used for patients with New York Heart Association II-III heart failure secondary to left ventricular systolic dysfunction who are on maximal medical therapy. Patients with prolonged QRS duration, typically left bundle branch block morphology, have a higher probability of success with this therapy. Findings like left anterior descending, atrial fibrillation, P mitral and left ventricular hypertrophy are not indicative of dyssynchrony and are not pre-implant criteria for cardiac resynchronisation therapy.

**5. D**

This man has most likely developed left ventricular systolic dysfunction and pulmonary oedema following his myocardial infarction. In pulmonary oedema there is upper lobe venous diversion, increased cardiothoracic ratio, pleural effusions, batwing shadows and Kerley B lines. Dextrocardia (heart on the right) is of no consequence, pericardial effusions cannot be seen on chest X-ray (other than cardiomegaly), finally reduced cardiothoracic ratio is not a pathological entity. A widened mediastinum is seen in aortic dissection.

**6. D**

In the absence of any other causes and with a recent cold, fulminant myocarditis following a viral infection is the most likely cause. A normal angiogram rules out a myocardial infarction, apical thrombus is a consequence but not a cause of heart failure, pericarditis does not affect the heart muscle and finally cardiac syndrome X is not a cause of heart failure.

**7. A**

Brain natriuretic peptide has high sensitivity and specificity for the diagnosis of heart failure and is a first line investigation, particularly when echocardiography is not available. C-reactive protein is a marker of infection and inflammation, C-peptide a marker of insulinoma causing hypoglycaemia, thyroid stimulating hormone is a marker of thyroid function and troponin I a marker of myocardial ischaemia and not diagnostic of heart failure.

**8. B**

The patient is an alcoholic, with bilateral pitting oedema and this is likely to be due to impairment of synthetic liver function, leading to reduced albumin and therefore plasma oncotic pressure, with resultant leaking of fluid into tissues. Clotting studies, renal function, protein electrophoresis and thyroid function won't answer this question. His echocardiogram is normal so he doesn't have heart failure, but liver failure.

**9. A**

This man has developed heart failure as a consequence of macro and microvascular ischaemia leading to left ventricular systolic dysfunction and so ischaemic, not non-ischaemic, cardiomyopathy is the answer. Left ventricular non-compaction is a rare and inherited form of heart failure, restrictive cardiomyopathy is due to conditions such as amyloid or sarcoid and finally Takotsubo cardiomyopathy occurs following a significant life stress, e.g. bereavement.

**10. A**

The patient is clinically hyperthyroid and most likely has Graves' disease and co-existing eye involvement. Hyperthyroidism can cause a high output state, with reduced vascular resistance, increased metabolic rate and tachycardiomyopathy which can lead to heart failure. Hypothyroidism can cause low output heart failure, but the patient is neither eu- nor hypothyroid.

**11. B**

The patient is likely to be suffering from a pulmonary embolism; malignancy and chemotherapy are risk factors. As a result, a CT pulmonary angiogram is the best modality to demonstrate this pathology. The patient has no chest pain and so further ECG's or troponin is not indicated. The most recent echocardiogram was normal and so a further one is unlikely to be helpful. A chest X-ray is non-diagnostic in the presence of a pulmonary embolism.

**12. E**

The ST changes affecting the inferior surface of the heart are due to a right ventricular myocardial infarction causing chest pain. This is leading to right ventricular systolic function, impaired pulmonary artery perfusion and dyspnoea. The chest is clear and there is no pulmonary congestion because the left ventricle is not affected. The ECG changes do not fit with pericarditis, pulmonary embolus or aortic dissection.

# Valvular heart disease

**1. E**

Aortic stenosis is the only diagnosis which explains all of these clinical findings and is best diagnosed, and assessed, with a transthoracic echocardiogram (see page 260). Coronary artery disease is possible, but this would not cause the other clinical examination findings. A serum troponin would indicate whether there was any acute myocardial damage, but would not reveal the underlying diagnosis. An angiogram might be appropriate if the echo is normal (this is unlikely) or if she is listed for valve surgery (more likely). There is no indication for a cardiac MRI.

**2. B**

In mitral valve prolapse, the mitral valve prolapses back into the left atrium during systole (often causing a 'click') after which blood leaks from the ventricle into the atrium causing the murmur which occurs mid-late systole. The other options describe mitral stenosis, mitral regurgitation, aortic regurgitation and aortic stenosis respectively.

**3. C**

The severity of the mitral regurgitation is only one consideration. Indications for mitral valve surgery include a dilating left ventricle in a symptomatic patient (usually dyspnea) with at least moderately severe mitral regurgitation. The key is to try and intervene before severe left ventricular dilatation, heart failure and pulmonary hypertension ensue. The left atrium often dilates in mitral regurgitation but this is not an indication for surgery.

**4. C**

The concern here is that this patient has infective endocarditis (see page 277). Diagnosis of infective endocarditis is by the modified Duke's criteria. Three good volume aerobic and anaerobic blood cultures should be acquired. Inflammatory markers are raised in infective endocarditis. An echocardiogram is the best test to evaluate valve function and diagnose a vegetation. A CT head scan is only indicated if there is focal neurological deficit. A chest X-ray is a useful adjunct but is not involved in the diagnosis of endocarditis. A serum troponin would indicate whether there was any acute myocardial damage but would not reveal the underlying diagnosis. An immunological screen may be useful but a cardiac MRI is not indicated.

**5. A**

A murmur does not always indicate a valvular abnormality. The presence of a murmur indicates either an abnormal valve or abnormally high flow across a normal valve. The latter are known as flow (or functional) murmurs. Causes of flow murmurs include anaemia, thyrotoxicosis, pregnancy, exercise and sepsis. The clinical history and blood test results are most consistent with anaemia.

**6. E**

Infective endocarditis is diagnosed according to the modified Dukes' criteria (see page 280). Infective endocarditis can definitely be diagnosed if: two major criteria are met, one major and three minor, or five minor. Infective endocarditis is possible if: one major and one minor criteria are met, or three minor. Only option E satisfies the criteria for a definite diagnosis. Inflammatory markers can be raised for a variety of reasons. A cardiac murmur is important. However, we do not know from this scenario if the murmur is new has changed in nature which is important.

# Congenital heart disease

1. **C**
   The causes of cyanotic congenital heart disease are shown on page 286. These include: Ebstein's anomaly; Fallot's tetralogy (cyanosis is not present in neonates); hypoplastic left heart and transposition of the great vessels. Once cyanosis is seen and diagnosed, an urgent cardiac echo should be performed to establish the nature of the cardiac lesion so best treatment (which may be surgical) can be initiated.

2. **B**
   Breathlessness is a common symptom in young children and despite the fact that the GP can hear a murmur, the most likely cause of this child's symptoms is still an upper respiratory tract chest infection. Other investigations are secondary to the chest X-ray which will also give important clues as to the heart size and presence of any chest infection or indeed heart failure.

3. **E**
   Warfarin is teratogenic and must be discontinued in pregnancy as soon as the patient realizes she is pregnant. All patients on long term warfarin and of child bearing age should receive counseling about the teratogenicity of warfarin. Low molecular weight heparin is safe and can be substituted and this should take place either when the patient is trying to conceive or as soon as the pregnancy is confirmed. In this case, the patient should be immediately started on heparin, pending referral to anticoagulation clinic.

4. **A**
   Atrial septal defects may be asymptomatic for many years and then often present with signs of right heart failure and atrial arrhythmias. Other congenital abnormalities are diagnosed in childhood and patients rarely become adults without symptoms. On examination, a split second heart sound may be heard and the ECG may show an underlying right bundle branch block.

5. **A**
   Blood pressure should be checked in both arms to see if there is a difference between the two arms as a drop in blood pressure may indicate

a recurrence of the coarctation. Heart block is not a recognised feature of coarctation and an MRI scan is required to assess the aorta rather than a chest X-ray which will not show the aorta in enough detail.

6. **B**
   Any patient with a congenital heart condition has an increased risk of passing the condition onto their children. This risk is between 2–5%. The risk of anybody having a child with a congenital heart defect is 1%.

# Peripheral heart disease

1. **C**
   The triad of a ruptured AAA includes abdominal pain, shock (hypotension and tachycardia) and a pulsatile abdominal mass. This man is hypotensive but not tachycardic and so is not in shock. Abdominal pain has many causes and abdominal guarding is typically due to a ruptured hollow viscus with resulting peritonitis.

2. **C**
   All the answers given are inherited apart from aortic unfolding which is commonly seen in the elderly and caused by hypertension. Of the conditions given, only Marfan's syndrome is a risk factor for aortic dissection. William's, Down's and Noonan's syndromes are associated with other cardiac abnormalities. Simply being tall, however, does not mean a patient has Marfan's syndrome.

3. **B**
   A chest X-ray may show mediastina widening in aortic dissection as the aorta increases in diameter, a raised troponin can occur from proximal extension of the dissection that disrupts the coronary ostia, which can lead to ST changes on the ECG. However, these can also occur due to other pathology. An echocardiogram may demonstrate aortic regurgitation but may not visualise the aorta and for this reason, a chest CT is required.

4. **A**
   A patient with an acutely ischaemic limb may present with a painless, pulseless limb that has absent capillary refill and paralysis. The limb will be painless (as it is dead), pulseless with no capillary refill (as the blood supply has stopped) and there may be paralysis because the muscles and nerves have started to die. A bounding pulse occurs with $CO_2$ retention, a collapsing pulse with aortic regurgitation and finally pitting oedema and peripheral cyanosis have many causes but not acute ischaemia.

**5. C**

According to the Well's criteria, the patient scores 2, due to unilateral calf swelling > 3 cm more than the left and tenderness along the deep venous system. The patient does not have active cancer, oedema, swollen veins, previous deep vein thrombosis, entire leg swelling or recent surgery/immobility. The lack of erythema or pyrexia makes cellulitis or a ruptured Baker's cyst, e.g. an alternative diagnosis unlikely.

**6. A**

The patient has an ischaemic lower limb, the presence of a delayed capillary refill, severe pain and the presence of motor and sensory deficit means that the ischaemia is critical and the limb may be at risk unless it is urgently revascularised. This is not a deep venous thrombosis as that does not cause ischaemia and claudication refers to pain on exertion only with normal clinical findings at rest.

**7. C**

Many drugs interact with warfarin and caution should always be used when writing prescriptions for these patients. Most drugs enhance the effects of warfarin causing the international normalised ratio to go out of range. Whilst most antibiotics can interact with warfarin, of those listed, ciprofloxacin is the most likely to do so. If in doubt, always look up any possible drug interactions in the British National Formulary.

**8. C**

The risk of a 4.7 cm AAA rupturing (regardless of age or gender) is 3% per annum. This is important to recognise, as patients need to be informed of the importance of attending for screening and regular follow up. Rapidly expanding aneurysms also cause concern and may indicate that early intervention is necessary. Patients are told to be wary of developing symptoms, such as abdominal pain.

**9. D**

Aspirin does not provide thromboembolic protection and warfarin takes at least 3 days to reach therapeutic range. Low molecular weight heparin is used in prophylaxis and treatment of venous thromboembolism but with such deranged renal function, unfractionated heparin is preferable and safest. Due to the malignancy, fracture and consequent immobility, graduated stockings would be insufficient.

**10. A**

The patient has a pacemaker implanted and subsequent to this develops a heavy arm, ipsilateral to the pacemaker, which are always implanted on the left. This is a recognised cause of axillary vein thrombosis. Compartment syndrome, brachial artery stenosis and thoracic outlet syndrome would not be normal on examination. Pacemaker syndrome is a physiological consequence of atrio-ventricular dysynchrony following pacemaker implantation and doesn't cause arm symptoms.

**11. E**

All of the options listed are recognised treatments for varicose veins; however, surgery is the most likely to provide long lasting effects as the veins are stripped out and tied off. All the other options leave the veins in situ and therefore recurrence is always a possibility.

**12. C**

The patient has developed a deep vein thrombosis (DVT) following a total knee replacement, which occurs in 25% of patients follow major joint replacement. A d-dimer is inappropriate to rule out DVT, as the Well's score is so high. A ventilation/perfusion scan would be contraindicated as the chronic changes on the chest X-ray and the chronic obstructive pulmonary disease means that there will be abnormal ventilation at baseline. A troponin is of no use when investigating DVT. The breathlessness is chronic and isn't necessarily due to a pulmonary embolism. The simplest, quickest and most cost effective investigation would be a leg Doppler.

**13. B**

This patient suffered a recent anterior ST segment elevation myocardial infarction and the resulting Q waves and persisting ST elevation suggests there may be a left ventricular aneurysm. Conservative management suggests the left ventricle may have been severely impaired, resulting in a left ventricular thrombus, making the left ventricle the likely source. Venous disease cannot cause ischaemia nor can right-sided thrombus lead to systemic arterial emboli due to the pulmonary vascular bed. The ECG does not demonstrate atrial fibrillation and this makes the left atrial appendage as a source unlikely.

**14. B**

Complex regional pain syndrome is a condition that occurs following trauma or surgery, previously known as algodystrophy or reflex sympathetic dystrophy. It leads to pain, swelling and skin changes but it is not bilateral, unlike Raynaud's disease, occurs in non-smokers and women unlike Buerger's and is unrelated to activity like thoracic outlet syndrome. Raynaud's syndrome is the presence of Raynaud's disease with an associated auto-immune condition, which this patient doesn't have.

**15. B**

The patient has a normal endoscopy and so varices, peptic ulcer disease and complications are excluded. There is no mention of the patient taking more warfarin than normal and the international normalised ratio responds only to intravenous not oral vitamin K. This suggests there is a problem with absorption of fat-soluble vitamins, which can occur following gastric bypass due to reduced gastric acid. This can lead to derangement of both coagulation pathways, which when combined with regular warfarin, can lead to catastrophic bleeding.

# Inherited cardiac condition

**1. D**

An ECG is important and will help to diagnose conditions such as hypertrophic cardiomyopathy, Brugada and long QT syndrome. An echocardiogram will diagnose either dilated or hypertrophic cardiomyopathy and will allow for aortic assessment. A 24 h blood pressure is not required as hypertension does not have a clear familial inheritance and does not usually cause sudden cardiac death. An ultrasound of the abdomen is not a first line investigation. A 24 h tape may identify arrhythmias.

**2. C**

There is a clear history of an inherited cardiac condition on his father's side which affects every generation. This makes an autosomal dominant condition the most likely. Patients with Brugada syndrome are often asymptomatic as are patients with long QT syndrome. Down's syndrome and William's syndrome are not inherited conditions, they are congenital abnormalities.

**3. B**

Ghent criteria should be used to diagnose Marfan's syndrome. There are many clinical features associated with Marfan's syndrome and the Ghent criteria assess all of these and ascertain the likelihood of Marfan's syndrome. Many tall people may appear to have Marfan's syndrome, but it is far more common to just be tall.

**4. A**

The features of hypertrophic cardiomyopathy that infer increased risk are shown on page 329. His dad's auntie is not a first degree relative and also we do not know what she died of. The chest pain is a symptom and does not infer increased risk. The syncope is too infrequent to infer increased risk.

**5. C**

The patient is male and cannot have a peripartum cardiomyopathy. His ferritin is normal ruling out haemochromatosis. He has a normal coronary angiogram excluding ischemic heart disease. Myotonic dystrophy is excluded by a normal creatine kinase. This leaves the most likely cause of his dilated cardiomyopathy as being inherited.

**6. C**

The high ectopic burden with a dilated right heart in a young person suggests a diagnosis of arrhythmogenic right ventricular cardiomyopathy. The changes in the right ventricle are often not picked up on echocardiography and therefore a cardiac MRI scan must be performed.

# Cardiac emergencies

**1. D**

Hypotension, syncope, heart failure and myocardial ischaemia all suggest significant hypoperfusion of critical organs, which requires urgent treatment of a tachycardia (regardless of QRS width) by direct-current cardioversion. Critical leg ischaemia, digital ischaemia, mesenteric ischaemia and a transient ischaemic attack do not.

**2. C**

During an acute myocardial infarction all patients should be offered morphine for pain relief, together with an anti-emetic. Aspirin, codeine, paracetamol and tramadol are all also effective analgesic agents but not first line during a myocardial infarction.

**3. D**

Pericardial effusions may be seen in patients with cancer. The ECG changes that suggest this are: small complexes due to electrical dampening by the fluid between the ECG electrodes and myocardium. Broad complexes are found in in bundle branch block, narrow QRS complexes are normal, absent QRS complexes suggests ventricular standstill and high voltage QRS complexes suggest left ventricular hypertrophy.

**4. E**

This patient has a narrow complex tachycardia with no adverse features and so the next step would be to try some vagal manoeuvres to see if the tachycardia can be terminated. If this is unsuccessful then adenosine would be the next step. Amiodarone and direct-current cardioversion are reserved for either unstable patients or those with broad complex tachycardias. Finally, atropine is used for patients with bradycardias.

**5.  E**

The patient is suffering from a bradycardia as a result of hypothermia from a long lie. This carries a poor prognosis but it is important to recognise as it will significantly alter the management. We already know the patient is bradycardic and so an ECG will only confirm this. There is no indication for an echocardiogram, chest X-ray or blood sugar.

# Integrated care

**1.  E**

Although he has a past medical history of myocardial infarction, at 88 years old there is little evidence that continuing with simvastatin will make a difference to his length of life. His muscle aches are clearly interfering with his quality of life and it would, therefore, be appropriate to stop his simvastatin.

**2.  E**

Spironolactone is a potassium sparing diuretic and causes retention of potassium. A potassium concentration of 6.4 mmol/L cannot be ignored and action must be taken. Hydralazine does not affect potassium the concentration. The spironolactone should be stopped and the concentration rechecked a week later; if the concentration has fallen it can then be restarted at a lower dose.

**3.  D**

This woman has known angina and her symptoms have worsened. Before making any alterations to her medication, an ECG should be performed to check there are no new changes or signs of myocardial ischemia. If her ECG is unremarkable then her anti-anginal medication can be increased but she must be told that if her pain does not ease with her glyceryl trinitrate spray that she needs to seek urgent medical attention.

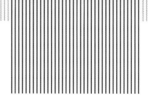

# Index

Note: Page numbers in **bold** or *italic* refer to tables or figures, respectively.